The International Libra

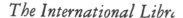

THE PSYCHOLOGY OF
RELIGIOUS MYSTICISM

Founded by C. K. Ogden

The International Library of Psychology

PSYCHOLOGY AND RELIGION
In 6 Volumes

THE PSYCHOLOGY OF
RELIGIOUS MYSTICISM

JAMES H LEUBA

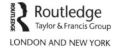

Routledge
Taylor & Francis Group

LONDON AND NEW YORK

First published in 1925 by
Routledge, Trench, Trubner & Co., Ltd.

Reprinted in 1999 by
Routledge
2 Park Square, Milton Park, Abingdon, Oxon, OX14 4RN

Simultaneously published in the USA and Canada by Routledge
711 Third Avenue, New York, NY 10017

Transferred to Digital Printing 2007

Routledge is an imprint of the Taylor & Francis Group, an informa business

First issued in paperback 2013

© 1925 James H Leuba

The publishers have made every effort to contact authors/copyright holders
of the works reprinted in the *International Library of Psychology*.
This has not been possible in every case, however, and we would
welcome correspondence from those individuals/companies
we have been unable to trace.

These reprints are taken from original copies of each book. In many cases
the condition of these originals is not perfect. The publisher has gone to
great lengths to ensure the quality of these reprints, but wishes to point
out that certain characteristics of the original copies will, of necessity, be
apparent in reprints thereof.

British Library Cataloguing in Publication Data
A CIP catalogue record for this book
is available from the British Library

The Psychology of Religious Mysticism

ISBN 978-0415-21112-3 (hbk)
ISBN 978-0-415-86448-0 (pbk)

CONTENTS

CHAPTER VIII

CHAPTER IX

CHAPTER X

CHAPTER XI

CHAPTER XII

CONTENTS

CHAPTER XIII

PREFACE

EXPERIENCES named " mystical " have played a conspicuous rôle at almost every level of culture; and yet, despite the vast literature devoted to them, the subject has remained until recently as dark as it is fascinating. Little could be expected of writers who, neglecting a close and dispassionate study of the facts, devoted themselves to religious edification or to the defence of the traditional theories. The hortatory, apologetic, and romantic character of most of the literature on religious mysticism accounts for its scientific insignificance.

Mysticism has suffered as much at the hands of its admirers as at the hands of its materialistic enemies. If the latter have been unable to see in mysticism anything else than aberrations and abnormalities, the former have gone to the other and equally fatal extreme ; no descriptive adjective short of " sublime," " infinite," " divine " has seemed to them at all sufficient.

The best among the prominent mystics are persons of pure heart and stout will from whom it is not possible to withhold admiration. Their beliefs and practices—whatever we may have to say in condemnation of them—have been to these mystics a refuge against the conflicts and the loneliness of life, and a source of strength and courage in the pursuit of worthy purposes.

*　　　　　*　　　　　*

This book is a psychological study of human nature. It includes, it is true, a philosophical chapter and also one in which are set forth the practical consequences to religion of some of its conclusions. But, whatever may be the importance of these two chapters, the book is to be judged primarily as a psychological study of aspects of human nature conspicuous in mystical religion. It represents an effort to remove that part of " inner life " from the domain of the occult, in which it has too long been permitted to remain, in order to incorporate it in that body of facts of which psychology takes cognizance. If we may not expect to have succeeded in producing a satisfactory answer to all the scientific problems raised by the mystical life, we may at least hope to have convinced the reader that there is in principle no satisfactory reason for leaving any of them outside the range of scientific research, and that, on the contrary, they are all explicable *in the same sense, to the same extent,* and *by the same general scientific principles* as any other fact of consciousness.

In this book, as in the preceding ones, we have proceeded according to the genetic method, i.e., we have begun with mystical experiences in early societies where they are simpler and, therefore, more easily understood, and we have followed them up in their main modifications and complications. We have, moreover, made use of the comparative method, for it is quite impossible to come to adequate conclusions in this field by remaining within the pale of religious life. Such phenomena, for instance, as ecstatic trance and the impression of illumination become comprehensible only when they are considered under the diverse conditions in which they appear, i.e., out of, as well as in, religious life.

The terms, " tendency," " impulse," " instinct," " motive," and the like, recur with great frequency in the following pages. This fact may serve to indicate the point of view from which the book is written. It proceeds from a dynamic conception of human nature ; it is interested in behaviour and its springs, and it gives a large place to the non-rational, and to the not-conscious.

In these directions this work falls in line with the recent trends of psychological science. The author does not, however, accept the Freudian conceptions in the form in which they are found in the books of the Viennese physician. The terms of his vocabulary, libido, introversion, extraversion, complex, psychical compensation, subconscious activity, conflict, repression, substitution, etc., are rarely used in these pages, and yet the discerning reader will not fail to realize that the facts they designate are among the conspicuous facts discussed here.

* * *

This book has been long in the making. My first studies in religious mysticism were embodied in an essay published in two parts under the titles, *Les Tendances Fondamentales des Mystiques Chrétiens* and *Les Tendances Religieuses chez les Mystiques Chrétiens* (*Rev. Philos.*, vol. LIV., 1902, pp. 1-36, 441-87).

Since that time our knowledge has been enriched by a number of contributions of which I shall mention only those which have been of particular value to me. First in date and brilliance came the *Varieties of Religious Experience*, by William James, 1902 ; then H. Delacroix's penetrating *Etudes d'Histoire et de Psychologie du Mysticisme*, 1908 ; Friedrich von Hügel's conscientious and sympathetic *Mystical Element of Religion as studied in Saint Catherine of Genoa*, 2 vols, 1909. A little later appeared *The Meaning of God in Human Experience*, by William E. Hocking, 1912, a remarkable expression of spiritual discernment served by a rare literary talent ; and, quite recently, five excellent chapters in James B. Pratt's *The Religious Consciousness*, 1920. Little of value on Christian mysticism from the point of view of psychology has been published in Germany. The book of Joseph Zahn, *Einführung in die Christliche Mystik* (*Wissenschaftliche Handbibliothek*, 1908) may be mentioned as of general interest.

Among authors in fields other than the psychology of religion, I owe most to Pierre Janet, of the Collège de France, who from the *Automatisme Psychologique*, 1894, to the *Médications Psychologiques*, 1919, has not ceased to make valuable contributions to our understanding of human nature.

*   *   *

The present volume completes the execution of a plan for a somewhat systematic study of religious life, sketched out after the publication of my Doctor's Dissertation on Conversion (*Studies in the Psychology of Religious Phenomena—Conversion, Amer. Journal of Psychol.*, vol. VII, 1896)—a plan which, unfortunately, I was unable to follow closely either with regard to content or with regard to order.

In two earlier books (*A Psychological Study of Religion : its Origin, Function, and Future*, New York, Macmillan, 1912 ; and *The Belief in God and Immortality : a Psychological, Anthropological, and Statistical Study*, 1st ed., 1916 ; 2nd. ed., Chicago, The Open Court, 1921) and in the present volume I have considered the origin, the nature, and the function of the god-ideas, of the belief in personal immortality, and of the mystical beliefs and practices. The discussion of the origin and nature of the god-ideas and of religion involved a discussion of the origin and nature of the primitive philosophy of man and of magic, and the separation of magic from religion (Parts I and II of *A Psychological Study*).

Interest in the present status of the cardinal beliefs of Christianity led me to carry out a statistical investigation of contemporary belief in personal immortality and in the kind of god implied in the worship of the existing religions (Part II, pp. 172-287 of *Belief in God and Immortality*). This investigation provides the first definite and exact information regarding the number of believers, doubters, and disbelievers in a number of classes of intellectual leaders, namely, physicists, biologists, historians, sociologists, and psychologists, and also among college students of non-technical departments. Among the important facts brought out by these statistics are regular correlations between disbelief and distinction attained in the branches of science named above.

On the basis of these studies of origin and function, I was, moreover, led to write on the *Latest Forms and the Future of Religion* (Part IV of *A Psychological Study*), on the *Present Utility of the Beliefs in God and Immortality* (Part III of *Belief in God and Immortality*) and finally, on the *Disappearance of the Belief in a Personal Superhuman Cause and the Welfare of Humanity* (last chapter of the present book).

The relation of Theology to Psychology is considered in Chapter XI of *A Psychological Study*. The conclusion is reached that in so far as the present form of the belief in God among the Christian people is maintained by facts of the "inner life," i.e., psychical experiences regarded as requiring a personal God as causal Agent, it is a belief dependent not upon metaphysics but upon psychological science. This problem reappears in Chapter XII of the present volume.

*   *   *

Any one interested in the relation of my work to that of other writers, notably Wm. James and H. Delacroix, should bear in mind that my study of Christian conversion appeared in 1896 (E. Starbuck's *Psychology of Religion* was published in 1899. It was preceded by an article, *A Study of Conversion*, Amer. Jr. of Psychol., vol. VIII, 1897) and the essay on the Christian mystics in 1902, the year in which *Varieties of Religious Experience* was published. In so far as that book is a psychological work it is based upon a study of Christian conversion and of mysticism. In my two early essays just referred to on Conversion and on Christian Mystics, numerous facts are set forth, analyzed, compared, and classified. The method followed was, therefore, as in my later work, the inductive method of the descriptive sciences.

My conception of magic and of its relation to religion appeared first in print in *The Psychological Origin and the Nature of Religion* (1909), a volume of the series of little books published by Messrs. Constable, under the name, "Religions Ancient and Modern." The substance of that booklet was incorporated, with some elaboration, in *A Psychological Study of Religion*.

*   *   *

The substance of several chapters of this book was used in a series of lectures delivered in the winter 1921-2 at Cambridge University, St. John's College (London), the Sorbonne, and at the University of Neuchâtel (Switzerland).

*   *   *   *   *   *

I wish to express my indebtedness and appreciation to E. H., L. D., and M. G. for their valuable assistance in preparing this book for the press.

CHAPTER I

MYSTICISM AND RELIGION—AN INTRODUCTION

THE term " mysticism " comes from a Greek word which designated those who had been initiated into the esoteric rites of the Greek religion. At present, however, it has at least two meanings. The wider and less definite of them signifies anything marvellous or weird, anything which seems to reach beyond human reason. We shall take the term " mystical " in a narrower sense ; it will mean for us any experience taken by the experiencer to be a contact (not through the senses, but " immediate," " intuitive ") or union of the self with a larger-than-self, be it called the World-Spirit, God, the Absolute, or otherwise[1].

The following definitions, selected from a large number of the same tenor, indicate that this use of the term is in substantial agreement with the generally accepted understanding of it in Protestantism : " Mysticism is a deification of man," it is " a merging of the individual will with the universal Will," " a consciousness of immediate relation with the Divine," " an intuitive certainty of contact with the supersensual world," etc. In this view, whatever tends to sharpen the demarcation between the self and the not-self, whatever leads to an isolation of the subject from the Principle of Life, is anti-mystical.

Among Roman Catholics, however, the emphasis is not placed upon the union of the soul with the divine Principle, but upon a superhuman knowledge. They say for instance : " We give the name of mystic to supernatural states containing a knowledge of a kind that our own efforts and our own exertions could never succeed in producing[2]." Mysticism is " the final outcome of a congenital desire for knowledge," in particular of a knowledge " which lies beyond the sphere of things and of the senses by which things are

---

[1] In the German language the word *Mystik* has the meaning in which we use the term in this book, while *Mysticismus* possesses the wider and vaguer meaning.

In an appendix to *Christian Mysticism*, William R. Inge has published twenty-six definitions of mysticism.

[2] A. Poulain, S.J., *The Graces of Interior Prayer*, 2nd ed., 1912, p.3.

perceived[1]." This emphasis upon superhuman knowledge is probably in agreement with the early Greek meaning of the term, but the experience regarded both by Roman Catholics and Protestants as mystical is, as we shall see, far too complex to be satisfactorily defined in terms of acquired knowledge. It includes, it is true, an impression of illumination or revelation, but that does not constitute the only significant part of the experience.

*   *   *

No one doubts that mysticism as defined in both these classes of definitions is included in the meaning of the term religion. But disagreement exists as to whether religion is always mystical; whether, as some put it, mysticism is at the root of every religion, so that in its absence no religion could have come into existence, and with its withdrawal all religions would die[2]. It seems to us that a reference to the facts establishes the existence of two types of religious relation : in the one, it consists in objective, business-like transactions with God ; in the other, it consists in communion or union with God or even in an absorption in the divine Substance. These two different attitudes, and the different methods of worship they involve, are observable throughout the history of religion, both in private and in public worship. We find them among uncivilized races as clearly as among ourselves. Miss Kingsley gives us an instance of objective religion in the uncivilized when she relates how the chief of a West African tribe, Anyambie, met his god. "The great man," she writes, "stood alone, conscious of the weight of responsibility on him of the lives and happiness of his people. He talked calmly, proudly, respectfully to the great god who, he knew, rules the spirit world. It was like a great diplomat talking to another great diplomat[3]."

---

[1] A. B. Sharpe, S.J., *Mysticism ; its True Nature and Value*, London, Sands & Co., 1910, pp. 1-3.

[2] William James, for instance, affirms, that " personal religious experience has its root and centre in mystical consciousness," *The Varieties of Religious Experience*, p. 379. Similarly, William Hocking writes of the mystics, " their technique which is the refinement of worship, often the exaggeration of worship, is at the same time the essence of all worship," *Mind*, vol. XXI, N. S., p. 39. Delacroix, who in the preface to *Etudes d'Historie et de Psychologie du Mysticisme* says that mysticism, understood as the immediate apprehension of the divine, is " at the origin of all religion," recognizes nevertheless, on p. 306, that " The Christianity of Bossuet excludes the Christian mysticism of Mme. Guyon. One cannot deny that there are here two different forms of Christianity." He opens a more recent article on *Le Mysticisme et la Religion* with the words, "There exist religions without mysticism." *Scientia*, vol. XXI, 1917.

[3] Mary H. Kingsley, *The Forms of Apparitions in West Africa*, Proc. Soc. for Psychical Research, vol. XIV, 1898, pp. 334-5.

Under other circumstances this same Anyambie might have behaved in a totally different way toward a less clearly defined superhuman Power, if not this same god. He might, in a sacred ceremony, have imbibed some narcotic beverage in company with men of his tribe, and have regarded the wonderful feelings, the hallucinations, the sense of enlargement and power he would have enjoyed, as participation in divine nature. For the uncivilised maintain not only the objective, business-like religious relation, they are usually familiar also with the mystical type of worship. "The negroes of the Niger had their 'fetish water,' the Creek Indians of Florida, their 'Black Drink.' In many parts of the United States the natives smoked stramonium, the Mexican tribes swallowed the *peyotl* and the snake plant, the tribes of California and the Samoyeds of Siberia had found a poisonous toadstool—all to bring about communication with the Divine and to induce ecstatic visions[1]." Mescal is one of the plants venerated by the Indians in certain parts of Mexico and in neighbouring regions. The Kiowa Indians use it at night, usually in front of a camp-fire, to the constant beating of drums. The men swallow at intervals from ten to twelve buttons of mescal between sundown and 3 a.m. They sit quietly until noon of the following day, when the effect of the drug has worn off. It is regarded as the food of the soul. It has tutelary deities and a special goddess. "Its psychic manifestations are considered as supernatural grace bringing men into relation with the gods[2]."

The ancient worship of the Hebrew was altogether of the objective type. Yahweh did not even maintain a relation with individuals, his dealings were with the nation as a whole. When, later, personal relations appeared, they remained for a long time external. Certain Psalms and the later Prophets contain the earliest expressions of mysticism in the religion of Yahweh[3]. Among the Greeks the worship of the Olympian divinities was altogether non-mystical, and it is still an open question how much mysticism is to be found in the mysteries.

Perhaps no semi-civilized people was ever more free from mysticism, in our sense of the term, than the old Romans. "These

---

[1] Daniel Brinton, *The Religion of Primitive Peoples*, p. 67.

[2] Havelock Ellis, "Mescal, a Study of a Divine Plant," *Popular Science Monthly*, vol. LXI, 1902, pp. 52-71.

[3] The mystical practices and theories before that time did not belong to the religion of Yahweh. They were remnants of other and older cults. We refer, for instance, to the excitement, reaching a contagious frenzy, generated among bands of "prophets" and regarded as a mark of divine possession. See 1 Sam. x, 5,ff ; xix, 20,ff.

people," says J. B. Carter, "could know nothing of their gods, beyond the activity which the gods manifested in their behalf; nor did they desire to know anything. The essence of religion was the establishment of a definite legal status between these powers and man, and the scrupulous observance of those things involved in the contractual relation, into which man entered with the gods. As in any legal matter, it was essential that this contract should be drawn up with a careful guarding of definition, and an especial regard to the proper address. Hence the great importance of the name of the god, and failing that, the address to the ' Unknown God.' A prayer was therefore a vow (votum), in which man, the party of the first part, agreed to perform certain acts to the god, the party of the second part, in return for certain specified services to be rendered. Were these services rendered, man, the party of the first part, was compos voti, bound to perform what he had promised. Were these services not rendered, the contract was void. In the great majority of cases the gods did not receive their payment until their work had been accomplished, for their worshippers were guided in this by the natural shrewdness of primitive man, and experience showed that in many cases the gods did not fulfil their portion of the contract which was thrust upon them by the worshippers. There were, however, other occasions, when a slightly different set of considerations entered in. In a moment of battle it might not seem sufficient to propose the ordinary contract, and an attempt was sometimes made to compel the god's action by performing the promised return in advance, and thus placing the deity in the delicate position of having received something for which he ought properly to make return[1]." That is the objective religious relation in all its nakedness.

Among Christian nations both the objective and the msytical type of religion are usually found side by side. In the controversy about Quietism, in which Bossuet and Félénon were the great protagonists and Mme. Guyon the victim, Bossuet represents rational Christianity, a Christianity in which man and God—the creature and the Creator, the sinner and the Judge—remain face to face with each other. While Mme. Guyon represents Christian mysticism in a form with which common sense could have nothing to do. It is a relation in which the self dissolves in God.

The Christian mystics themselves realize clearly enough this dualism. They say that these two attitudes are " diametrically contrary to one another." "There are," they tell us, "two sorts of spiritual persons, internal and external : these seek God without, by discourse, by imagination, and consideration : they endeavour mainly to get virtues by many abstinences, maceration of body, and mortification of the senses ; bear the presence of God, forming Him present to themselves in their idea of Him, or their imagination, sometimes as a Pastor, sometimes as a Physician, and sometimes as a Father and Lord.

" But none of these ever arrives by that only to the mystical, way, or to the excellence of union, as he doth who is brought by the Divine grace, by the mystical way of contemplation. These men of learning, who are merely scholastical, don't know what the spirit is, nor what it is to be lost in God[1]."

Christianity as expressed in its official creeds and books of worship is clearly an objective religion. According to the ritual the worshipper comes into the presence of his God to acknowledge his sins and to be cleansed from them, to receive protection from bodily and moral harm, to return thanks for God's goodness, to praise him, and to rejoice in the assurance of his favour. But, just as intercourse between sympathetic persons constantly tends .to pass from externality to the intimacy of united feeling and will, so, in the Christian religion, the objective worship of a loving God tends ever to glide into the trustful, self-surrendering attitude which constitutes the first step towards complete mystical union.

Mysticism, in its incipient stages at least, is encouraged in the Christian Church[2], but when it assumes the amazing aspects with which the famous mystics have made us familiar, the Church becomes uneasy and watchful. For, in his search for God, the mystic goes his own way. He is ready to brush aside rites and formulae—even the priest who would serve him as mediator—and

---

[1] Molinos, *The Spiritual Guide*, John Thomson, Glasgow, 1885, Part I, chap. I, 54, 65 ; Part II. chap. XVIII, pp. 126-7.

[2] In recent times, Ritschl has altogether rejected mysticism. He " will hear nothing of direct spiritual communion of the soul with God. Pietism in all its forms is an abomination to him. The one way of communion of the soul with God is through His historical manifestation in Jesus Christ, and experience due to a supposed immediate action of the Spirit in the soul can be regarded as an illusion. This is the side of Ritschl's teaching that has been specially taken up and developed by his disciple, Hermann." Professor Orr, as quoted by Garvie in the *Ritschlian Theology*, p. 143.
Of Ritschl's main disciples, Garvie writes : " Kaftan, with Ritschl and Hermann, condemns mysticism in the two types which they describe, both as an attempt to secure union with God conceived as the Absolute, and as an endeavour to be joined through the imagination and the affections to Christ in His glorified state. But in his antagonism to mysticism he is not led, as Ritschl is, to deny there is in Christian experience a mystical element, a real communion of the soul with Christ." *Ibid.*, p. 157. See also Hermann's work, *Verkehr des Christen mit Gott.*

he issues from the divine union with a sense of superior, of divine, knowledge. Persons of this kind may obviously be dangerous to the stability of old institutions which have come to regard their truths as the only truths. But these god-intoxicated persons may also perform the invaluable function of innovators, revelators, and inspirers.

*   *   *

Types of behaviour so general and so persistent as those expressed in the objective and the subjective types of worship must, it seems, have their bases in different and fundamental traits of human nature. These traits are not very difficult to discover. Most of the specific tendencies and instincts with which man is endowed are roughly classifiable in two groups. In the one there is fear and the various expressions of aggression and aversion. In the other there is curiosity and the expressions of liking and affection. The former finds satisfaction by the disregard, or at the expense, of other selves ; it leads to methods of life which would separate the individual from the rest of the world and sharpen self-consciousness. The latter seeks co-operation with other selves ; its method is that of association, co-operation, and union.

Animal life began, it seems, with an endowment of conflict-instincts. The appearance of the parental instincts marked probably the introduction of the other type of endowment : the animal family became the cradle of the co-operative method of life. In humanity, the aggressive, self-sharpening attitude was for a long initial period the conspicuous one ; the other attitude was called forth mainly, or only, in the narrower circles of family and tribe. Even there, its expression was easily inhibited by the dividing, destructive instincts. Only very slowly did men discover the objective value of good-will and the subjective delight of spiritual union.

The powerful instinctive tendencies which incline man to seek union of will and feeling with other selves receive assistance from another quarter : striving with resisting other selves and inanimate objects brings recurrent moments of weariness when the zest for the strife disappears. How delightful it is then to close one's eyes to the multiplicity of things, to ignore the challenge of other wills, to renounce effort, and to lose oneself in the silent, peaceful current of undifferentiated life ! Both physical and moral causes bring on this inclination to self-surrender. The pace has been too fast and the jaded nerves demand rest, or dispiriting queries have arisen : " What matter gains and conquests ; what boot fortune, knowledge, human loves ? Nothing is perfect and nothing endures. Would that I could overcome my spiritual isolation, destroy the barriers which separate me from my fellow men, be one with them, instead of struggling against them[1]." In this mood the will-to-union is given full career.

---

[1] The roots out of which the two types of relation with the Invisible World have developed penetrate so deep into human nature that their growth may be traced in other directions, in particular in the processes of thought. Thinking includes a double movement. Consider the man of science or the philosopher; they do their work by alternating analyses and syntheses; they cannot do it by one of these alone. There must be observation and discrimination; but when objects have multiplied under the analysing activity of the mind, the severed things must somehow be united again; they must be seen in their connections. And, at least for some men, a unification of all things must be reached; a universe must be built out of the discreet objects. Completed thinking implies these two movements: sundering and uniting.

CHAPTER II

MYSTICAL ECSTASY AS PRODUCED BY PHYSICAL MEANS

Only by looking low, ere looking high,
Comes penetration of the mystery.
BROWNING.

AMONG most uncivilized populations, as among civilized peoples, certain ecstatic conditions are regarded as divine possession or as union with the Divine. These states are induced by means of drugs, by physical excitement, or by psychical means. But, however produced and at whatever level of culture they may be found, they possess certain common features which suggest even to the superficial observer some profound connection. Always described as delightful beyond expression, these ecstatic experiences end commonly in mental quiescence or even in total unconsciousness. Common features should not, however, lead to a disregard of dissemblances. The presence, for instance, of an ethical purpose places some of these states in a separate and higher class.

In this chapter we shall confine ourselves to mystical experiences induced by physical means, and chiefly by drugs. Our main task is to discover their forms, their motives, and the gratification they yield. Why their fascination and why the religious significance ascribed to them? These questions once answered, we shall be prepared to undertake the study of higher forms of mysticism and to recognize a continuity of impulse, of purpose, of form, and of result between the ecstatic intoxication of the savage and the absorption in God of the Christian mystic.

* * *

I. The Use of Drugs and Other Physical Means.

We have already had occasion to remark that in nearly every savage tribe is found a knowledge of narcotic plants employed to induce strange and vivid dreams or hallucinations. And we have quoted Brinton who writes that " in many parts of the United States the natives smoked stramonium, the Mexican tribes swallowed the *peyotl* and the snake plant, the tribes of California and the Samoyeds of Siberia had found a poisonous toad-stool ;—all to bring about communication with the Divine and to induce ecstatic visions[1]."

[1] Daniel Brinton, *The Religion of Primitive Peoples*, p. 67.

8

The priest among certain Indian tribes had apparently learned to snuff a " certain powder called *cohoba* [perhaps tobacco] up his nose which makes him drunk, so that he knows not what he does[1]." The Indians of New Mexico are " unacquainted with intoxicating liquors, . . . yet find drunkenness in the fumes of a certain herb smoked through a stone tube and used chiefly during their festivals[2]."

Of the New Mexicans, Bancroft says, " drunkenness prevails to a great extent among most of the tribes ; their liquors are prepared from the fruit of the ptahaya, mezquite-beans, agave, honey, and wheat. In common with all savages, they are immoderately fond of dancing, and have numerous feasts, where, with obscene carousals and unseemly masks, the revels continue until the dancers, from sheer exhaustion or intoxication, are forced to rest[3]." These feasts have nearly always a religious character.

Taken in moderation, mescal enables a man to face the greatest fatigues and to bear hunger and thirst for several days. A sort of pilgrimage is organized to gather the plant for festivals and for private consumption. As the Indians approach the plants, they uncover their heads and display every sign of veneration. Before gathering them they sprinkle themselves with copal incense. In some tribes mescal is consumed only by medicine men and certain selected Indians who sing invocations to it to grant a " beautiful intoxication[4]." A rasping noise is made with sticks while men and women dance before those who are under the influence of the god. The remarkably beautiful coloured hallucinations produced by mescal have been described by several experimenters.

In the Indic and Iranian cult there was a direct worship of deified liquor analogous to Dionysiac rites. It has even been maintained that the whole Rig Veda is but a collection of hymns for Soma worship. It contains, in any case, a large number of such hymns. Soma, an intoxicating liquor, was prepared from a plant unknown to us. It became identified with the moon, and hence was called moon plant. The brahmanic priest crushed in a small mortar the stalk of the plant and poured into the fire a libation, usually to

---

[1] Quoted by G. M. Stratton, *The Psychology of Religious Life*, p. 111, from Wilson, *Prehistoric Man*, 1865, p. 323, *ff*.

[2] H. H. Bancroft, *Native Races*, vol. I, pp. 566-7. Among the old Mexicans, the most powerful of the ingredients used to make their festival drinks intoxicating " was the *teonanacatl*, ' flesh of god,' a kind of mushroom which excited the passions and caused the partaker to see snakes and diverse visions." *Loc. cit.*, vol. II, pp. 360, 601.

[3] *Loc. cit.*, vol. I, v. 586. For intoxication among many different peoples, see Edward B. Tylor, *Primitive Culture*, vol. II, pp. 377-9, and G. M. Stratton, *The Psychology of Religious Life*, pp. 108-14.

[4] *Ibid.*

Indra; but he himself drank the greater part of what he had prepared, until he became inebriated, or at least until he felt the stimulating effect of the beverage. The drinking ceremony was accompanied by magical incantations and invocations. The officiating priest offered the liquor with these words: "O, Indra, accept [our offering] . . . drink of the soma, thou the friend of prayer and of the liquor, well disposed God, drink in order to intoxicate thyself." Here is one of the numerous invocations made during the sacrifice: "Come to us who have pressed out the soma, come; to our good praises drink, O helmeted hero, of the juice of the plant, I pour it out, into the double cavity of thy belly; may it spread through thy members; may it be sweet to thy taste; may it steal upon thee, veiled, as women seeking a *rendez-vous*. Hero with the strong neck, full-bellied, strong of arms, . . . O Indra, hurl thyself forward upon them triumphing by thy strength. . . . O Indra, praised by many, accept the pressed out soma, father of divine energy: drink, make the assuaging sap rain in upon thee. . . . Let those who desire the inexhaustible celestial glories attach themselves to Indra[1]." The desire for sexual vigour is one of the dominant notes of the soma hymns.

[1] W. Caland and V. Henri, *L'Agnistoma*, vol. I, pp. 162, 155, 249 ; vol. II, p. 311. According to these authors, soma was a usual beverage or was perhaps reserved for totemic sacrifices, and later on came into use as a sacrificial offering. They do not agree with Oldenberg in his opinion that soma never had any importance in the Vedic cult. See vol. II, pp. 471-3. It is not to be supposed that the use of intoxicating drugs in connection with religion has vanished from India, according to the findings of the Indian Hemp Commission, the use of narcotics in religion was on the increase in 1893, the date of their report. The commissioners wrote :

" It is chiefly in connection with the worship of Siva, the Mahades or great god of the Hindu trinity, that the hemp plant, and more especially perhaps ganja [one of the preparations from hemp] is associated. The hemp plant is popularly believed to have been a great favourite of Siva, and there is a great deal of evidence before the Commission to show that the drug in some form or other is now extensively used in the exercise of the religious practices connected with this form of worship. Reference to the almost universal use of hemp drugs by fakirs, yogis, sanyasis, and ascetics of all classes, and more particularly of those devoted to the worship of Siva, will be found in the paragraphs of this report dealing with the classes of the people who consume the drugs. These religious ascetics, who are regarded with great veneration by the people at large, believe that the hemp plant is a special attribute of the god Siva, and this belief is largely shared by the people. Hence the origin of many fond epithets ascribing to ganja the significance of a divine property, and the common practice of invoking the deity in terms of adoration before placing the *chillum* or pipe of ganja to the lips. There is evidence to show that on almost all occasions of the worship of this god, the hemp drugs in some form or other are used by certain classes of the people. In a specialized recent form of worship of Siva, called Trinath, the use of ganja is considered to be essential."

" The custom of worshipping the hemp plant, although not so prevalent as that of offering hemp to Siva and other deities of the Hindus, would nevertheless appear from the statements of the witnesses to exist to some extent in some provinces of India." *Report of the Indian Hemp Commission*, vol. I, 1893-4, pp. 160, 161, 165.

In Greece also, intoxication was customary in connection with established cults. The Pythia at Delphi after a fast of three days, chewed laurel leaves, and in a state of intoxication stood upon a tripod placed over an opening from which issued noxious vapours. Her body shook, her hair stood on end, and out of her convulsed and frothing mouth came the answers to the questions addressed to her. Wine drunkenness was prominent in the worship of Dionysus. To the effect of the wine was added that of dancing, music, shouting, and the expectation of divine ecstasy. Rhode makes a vivid picture of the worship of the Thracian Dionysus : " The celebration took place in the dead of night on the mountain tops by ,the flickering light of torches. Noisy music resounded ; the pealing tones of cymbals, the hollow thunder of kettle-drums, mingled with the ' frenzy-summoning harmony ' of the deep-voiced flutes. Stirred by this wild music, the crowd of worshippers danced and shouted in exultation. We have no mention of songs ; for these, the vigorous dancing left no breath. This was not the rhythmic dance with which, perhaps, the Greeks of Homer's age accompanied their pæans, but a frenzied, whirling, plunging sort of round in which the crowd of inspired devotees rushed about over the mountain slopes. For the most part it was women, oddly clad, who whirled about to the point of exhaustion. They wore ' Bassaren,' long flowing garments, apparently made of fox-skins ; over these they wore besides, deer-skins with the horns sometimes remaining on the head. . . . Thus they raved, until they reached the utmost excitement. In this ' holy madness ' they rushed upon the animals chosen for the sacrifice, and tore off with their teeth the bloody flesh, which they devoured raw[1]."

* * *

But drugs are not the only physical means of producing the ecstacy dear to men of every degree of culture. Deprivations of food and sleep, isolation, even active tortures are well-known and frequent means of religious ecstasy. Rhythmic bodily movements and shouting or singing, when long continued, yield results similar in several respects to that of alcohol, stramonium, mescal, and other drugs.

The American Indians made much use of fasting. In certain ceremonies " they fasted sometimes six or seven days, till both their bodies and minds became free and light, which prepared them to dream. The object of the ancient seers was to dream of the sun ; as it was believed that such a dream would enable them to see

[1] Erwin Rhode, *Psyche, Seelencult und Unterblichkeitsglaube*, 4th ed., Tübingen, 1907, vol. II, pp. 9-10.

everything on the earth. And by fasting long and thinking much on the subject, they generally succeeded. Fasts and dreams were at first attempted at an early age. What a young man sees and experiences during these dreams and fasts, is adopted by him as truth and it becomes a principle to regulate his future life. He relies for success on these revelations. If he has been much favoured in his fasts, and the people believe he has the art of looking into futurity, the path is open to the highest honours[1]."

" We may judge of the mental and bodily condition of the priest and sorcerer in Guyana, by his preparation for his sacred office. This consisted in the first place in fasting and flagellation of extreme severity; at the end of his fast he had to dance till he fell senseless, and was revived by a potion of tobacco-juice, causing violent nausea and vomiting of blood; day after day this treatment was continued till the candidate, brought into or confirmed in the condition of a ' convulsionary,' was ready to pass from patient into doctor[2]."

From *The Beginnings of Art*, by Grosse, I take the following description of native dances known throughout the Australian continent. They leave the participants in a condition in many respects similar to that produced by intoxicating drugs.

" The corroborries are always performed at night, and generally by moonlight. The largest and most noteworthy festivals apparently take place on the conclusion of a peace; moreover, all the more important events of Australian life are celebrated by dances—the ripening of a fruit, the beginning of the oyster dredging, the initiation of the youth, a meeting with a friendly tribe, the march to battle, a successful hunt.

" It is astonishing how accurately the time is kept; the tunes and the movements are all in unison. The dancers move as smoothly as the best-trained ballet-troupe. The dancers gradually become more excited; the time-sticks are struck faster; the motions become more rapid and vigorous; the dancers shake themselves, spring into the air to an incredible height, and finally utter a shrill cry, as if from one mouth. The excitement is at its height; the dancers cry out, stamp, and jump; the women beat time as if they were crazy, and sing with all the strength of their lungs; the fire, which is blazing up high, scatters a shower of red sparks over the wild scene; and then the director raises his arms high over his head; a loud clapping breaks through the tumult, and the next instant the dancers are gone. No protracted research is needed to estimate the pleasure these gymnastic and mimetic performances afford to the performers

[1] Edward B. Tylor, *Primitive Culture*, vol. II, p. 373.
[2] *Loc. cit.*, pp. 379-80, quoted from Meiners, vol. II, p. 162.

and spectators. There is no other artistic act which moves and excites all men like the dance. In it primitive men doubtless find the most intense aesthetic enjoyment of which they are generally capable[1]."

But aesthetic pleasure is certainly not the only thing we are to take into account in connexion with the frequent wildly exciting ceremonies of the native Australians. There is, above all, in these performances as in drug-intoxication, a delightful surrender of self-restraint, a sense of power, an enjoyment of the sensuous pleasures arising from unrestrained, intense movement, and, in addition, the fascination of belief in the superhumanness of the experience. Spencer and Gillen report several ceremonies characteristic of a mental condition in several respects comparable with that of intoxication by drugs. The fire ceremony of the Warramunga tribe is one of these. It takes place at night. The preparations completed, the performance opens with one of the men " charging full tilt, holding his *wanmanmirri* like a bayonet, and driving the blazing end into the midst of a group of natives, in the centre of which stood a man with whom, a year before, he had had a serious quarrel. Warded off with clubs and spear-throwers, the torch glanced upwards. This was the signal for the commencement of a general *mêlée*. Every *wanmanmirri* was blazing brilliantly, the men were leaping and prancing about, yelling wildly all the time ; the burning torches continually came crashing down upon the heads and bodies of the men, scattering lighted embers all around, until the air was full of falling sparks, and the weird, whitened bodies of the combatants were alight with burning twigs and leaves. The smoke, the blazing torches, the showers of sparks and the mass of dancing, yelling men with their bodies grotesquely bedaubed, formed altogether a genuinely wild and savage scene of which it is impossible to convey any adequate idea in words[2]."

The Mohammedans, whose religion forbids wine, contrive nevertheless to secure a condition similar to liquor intoxication. An order of Sufis, founded probably in the twelfth century, distinguish themselves from their co-religionists by strange and extravagant dancing, continued until partial anæsthesia and even unconsciousness resulted. These Sufis were divided, according to the nature of the dancing, into shouting, gyrating, and dancing dervishes. The following is part of a detailed description by an eye-witness.

[1] E. Grosse, *The Beginnings of Art*, chap. VIII, much abbreviated.

[2] *Northern Tribes of Central Australia*, pp. 389-91. The use of narcotics among Australians is very rare. I find, however, in *Native Tribes of Central Australia*, p. 528 mention of " native tobacco " as being given to the young men to chew when they are made medicine men.

" The exercises which are followed in these halls are of various kinds, according to the rules of each institution ; but in nearly all they commence by the recital, by the sheikh, of the seven mysterious words of which we have spoken.   He next chants various passages of the Koran, and, at each pause, the Dervishes placed in a circle round the hall, respond in chorus by the word ' Ahhah ! ' or ' Hoo ! '   In some of the societies they sit on their heels, their elbows close to each other, and all making simultaneously light movements of the head and body.   In others, the movement consists in balancing themselves slowly, from the right to the left, and from the left to the right, or inclining the body methodically fore and aft."

The ceremony is completed in five scenes ; we may omit the description of the first three.   " After a pause commences the fourth scene.   Now all the Dervishes take off their turbans, form a circle, bear their arms and shoulders against each other, and thus make the circuit of the hall at a measured pace, striking their feet at intervals against the floor, and all springing up at once.   This dance continues during the Ilahees chanted alternately by the two elders to the left of the sheikh.   In the midst of this chant the cries of ' Ya Allah ! ' are redoubled, as also those of ' Ya Hoo ! ' with frightful howlings, shrieked by the Dervishes together in the dance. At the moment that they would seem to stop from sheer exhaustion the sheikh makes a point of exerting them to new efforts by walking through their midst, making also himself most violent movements.

" The fourth scene leads to the last, which is the most frightful of all, the wholly prostrated condition of the actors becoming converted into a species of ecstasy which they call Halet.   It is in the midst of this abandonment of self, or rather of religious delirium, that they make use of red-hot irons.   Several cutlasses and other instruments of sharp-pointed iron are suspended in the niches of the hall, and upon a part of the wall to the right of the sheikh.   Near the close of the fourth scene two Dervishes take down eight or nine of these instruments, heat them red-hot, and present them to the sheikh. He, after reciting some prayers over them, and invoking the founder of the order, Ahmad or Rufâee, breathes over them, and raising them slightly to the mouth, gives them to the Dervishes, who ask for them with the greatest eagerness.   Then it is that these fanatics, transported by frenzy, seize upon these irons, gloat upon them tenderly lick them, bite them, hold them between their teeth, and end by cooling them in their mouths.   Those who are unable to procure any, seize upon the cutlasses hanging on the wall, with fury, and stick them into their sides, arms, and legs.

" Thanks to the fury of their frenzy, and to the amazing boldness which they deem a merit in the eyes of the Divinity, all stoically bear up against the pain which they experience with apparent gaiety. If, however, some of them fall under their sufferings, they throw themselves into the arms of their *confrères*, but without complaint or the least sign of pain. Some minutes after this, the sheikh walks around the hall, visits each one of the performers in turn, breathes upon their wounds, rubs them with saliva, recites prayers over them, and promises them speedy cures. It is said that twenty-four hours afterward nothing is to be seen of their wounds[1]."

Very recently a " new " religion, called the Ghost-Dance religion, has arisen among the semi-civilized Indians of the United States[2]. In this instance, more conspicuously than in those before mentioned—except, perhaps, in the dervish dancing—psychic means are added to the physical : auto-suggestion in the form of a definite intention and expectation of transcending the limitations of ordinary life and entering into relation with the gods is a very influential factor in producing ecstasy.

Dancing in order to arouse a divine furore is not of course confined to the religions of the savages and of the Mohammedans. Civilized Europe has had its dancing sects, and new ones continue to appear now and again. As late as 1907, New York City received the missionary visit of the " Holy Jumpers," a Christian dancing sect moved to compassion by the wickedness of the great city[3].

[1] From Brown's *Dervishes,* pp. 218-22, as quoted by J. W. Powell, in *Fourteenth Annual Report of the Bureau of Ethnology,* Part II, 1896, pp. 948-52. What is said above of the Dervishes is, of course, not to be taken as adequately representing Sufism which really belongs with the ethical religions.

[2] For a description of the Ghost-Dance religion, see the *Fourteenth Report of the Bureau of Ethnology,* (U.S.), 1892-3, pp. 915-28.

[3] The " Holy Jumpers " are now preparing to move from their idyllic country home in western New Jersey to the wickedest quarters here. Between their dances, which include every manner of step, from the Dervish's whirl to the sailor's horn-pipe, they will warn New Yorkers of the destruction that is bound to come in the shape of a pillar of fire. The Jumpers will make extraordinary efforts to interest the city in the weird gyrations which give them their name, and if they are successful they will establish a colony and missionary school such as they have in Denver, their parent city. At any stage of the " Holy Jumpers' " meetings the inspiration to dance is likely to seize on members, with a shout of joy one begins. Perhaps he starts by waltzing alone around the ring. Another joins him. They grasp shoulders, and the waltz livens into a movement like a very rapid two-step. Then they stop, face each other, and whirl like Dervishes, ending their performance by jumping high in the air, and sometimes half turning before reaching the ground. Excited by the dance and singing and the shouts, others join, women skip about like school-girls, and seize and drag one another into the circle. By and by the whole assemblage is whirling and jumping and shouting, but the women never dance with the men.—From a newspaper report.

* * *

But with the dawn of a spiritual conception of the Divine, the use of drugs and of mechanical means could hardly continue in favour. These grossly material methods are incongruous with a spiritual conception of the gods. Furthermore, they produce after-effects which, because disagreeable or debasing, or both, cannot easily be reconciled with the theory of god-possession. Yet, ecstatic states are too delightful, too wonderful; they gratify too many deep needs, to be given up. Therefore it was that, groping in the dark, men gradually evolved a method of ecstasy apparently consistent with a higher conception of divine nature: the *psychical* method. That method is to occupy our attention in subsequent chapters.

The displacement of physical by psychical means was, of course, gradual and never complete. As a matter of fact, in the ceremonies of savages psychical influences are present; while, in the production of even the highest forms of religious ecstasy, assistance is obtained from a diversity of physical means. As far as actual causation is concerned, the difference is rather one of the degree in which these two classes of factors contribute to the result.

Both physical and psychical means are clearly in evidence in the worship of Dionysus and of Soma. In Moslem mysticism and in Yoga practices, to which a special chapter will be devoted, physical means vie in importance with the psychical. In Christian mysticism, the latter only are officially recognized, although physical influences have not ceased to lend their aid. The inclination to employ even some of the coarser physical means still lingers among us. In the so-called "revival meeting," the monotonous repetition of rhythmical songs, accentuated by shouts and bodily movements, helps to produce a condition similar to that through which the dervish attains partial anæsthesia and visions of Allah.

*   *   *

We have set forth a fact as surprising as undeniable: both among savage and civilized peoples, states of ecstatic intoxication are regarded as the culmination of man's commerce with a superhuman world. Why this association? The usual answer, that ecstasy brings superhuman powers such as healing, making rain, destroying enemies, forcasting the future, controlling spirits, and the like, leaves unmentioned the deeper and most influential causes of the fascination.

That superhuman powers are supposed to be acquired by the ecstatic is well attested and perhaps already sufficiently illustrated. It is in a state of inebriation that the Hottentot conjurer is thought to act most successfully upon spirits[1]. The *Ololiuhqui* of the old Mexicans was used by priests to produce visions of hidden and future things[2]. " In Peru the priests whose special office it was to converse with the gods of towns or provinces were accustomed to produce in themselves ecstasy by a narcotic drink called ' tonca ' ; and while in this ecstatic state it was believed that they were inspired[3]." The present-day dervish obtains peculiar " spiritual " powers, called *Kuvveh i roohe*, through long performances ending in a hallucinatory condition. Thus he gains " the faculty of foreseeing coming events ; of predicting their occurrence ; of preserving individuals from harm and evil which would otherwise certainly result for them, . . . of restoring harmony of sentiment between those who would otherwise be relentless enemies[4]." The opinion that frenzy had in it something of the divine was still widespread among the Greeks in Plato's time. In the *Phaedrus*, Socrates is made to say : " For the prophetess at Delphi, you are well aware, and the priestesses of Dodona, have in their moments of madness done great and glorious service to the men and the cities of Greece, but little or none in their sober mood. As much then as divination is a more perfect and a more precious thing than augury, both in name and efficiency, so much more glorious, by the testimony of the ancients, is madness than sober sense, the inspiration of Heaven than the creation of men[5]."

That superhuman knowledge and marvellous powers do not account completely for the fascination of ecstatic states appears clearly enough when it is recalled that, even when these powers are known to be illusory, intoxicating drugs continue to inspire the pen of the poet and to allure the ordinary mortal beyond all power of resistance. To the reality of these other attractions, the numberless lovers of wine, opium, hasheesh, and other drugs, who, uninfluenced by thoughts of a superhuman world have gone to their ruin with eyes

---

[1] H. H. Bancroft, *Native Races*, vol. II, p. 601.

[2] *Ibid.*

[3] Rivero and Tschudi, *Peruvian Antiquities*, English translation by Hawks, 1853, p. 184, quoted by Stratton, *loc. cit.*, p. 108.

[4] Brown's *Dervishes*, p. 129, ff. It might be said that the condition produced by, let us say, mescal, is regarded as divine because mescal is a sacred plant, i.e., it contains a sacred, god-like principle. But this would be an invertion of the true causal relation. It is *because* of real and imaginary effects that mescal is supposed to possess divine power.

[5] " There is a possession and a madness inspired by the Muses, which seizes upon a tender and a virgin soul, and, stirring it up to rapturous frenzy, adorns in ode and other verse the countless deeds of elder time for the instruction of after ages. But whosoever without the madness of the Muses comes to knock at the doors of poesy, from the conceit that haply by force of art he will become an efficient poet, departs with blasted hopes, and his poetry, the poetry of sense, fades into obscurity before the poetry of madness."— Plato's *Phaedrus*.

wide open, offer a tragic testimony.   We are here in the presence of a fact of the widest and deepest social significance[1].

There are those who are satisfied when they have described these states as divine possession or union.   But nothing is thereby explained, unless first the meaning of these expressions be set forth in concrete detail ; for, the term " divine " in itself throws no light upon these facts.   It is the reverse ; *" divine " gets whatever significance it may possess from the experiences to which it is applied.* In undertaking a psychological analysis of these so-called divine experiences, we shall, therefore, enter upon an investigation of the meaning ascribed to the term " divine " in so far as it is applied to them.   According to the measure in which we shall succeed in fulfilling that task shall we escape the barrenness and confusion of those who think they have explained this or any other phenomenon when they have referred it to a " divine " agent.

*   *   *

II.   Description of the Effects produced by Certain Drugs.

Alcohol.—We may preface the following description with a few words on the similarity of the effects produced by different drugs. Some years ago the Roman Catholic Church undertook in Ireland a crusade against whisky.   It met with considerable success but, to the surprise of all, ether took the place of whisky.   In a few years, ether drunkenness became so common among the Romanists in a district

[1] Statistics of the amount of alcohol and opium consumed, in the face of strenuous opposition due to a definite knowledge of the serious material and spiritual harm they produce, help us to realize their fascination.

The amount of alcohol consumed in the civilized world is one of the staggering facts of modern history.   In the United States the *per capita* consumption of alcohol in its several forms has steadily increased up to 1914. The total consumption of malted liquors,. beers, wine, and spirits in the U.S. rose in 1914 to 2,252,272,000 gallons.   Of this 52,417,000 gallons were wines, about 150,000,000 spirits, and 2,050,000,000 malt liquors.   The total expenditure involved in this consumption reaches almost 600,000,000 dollars—the value of our entire wheat crop at that time.

The *per capita* consumption of alcoholic beverages was in 1914 considerably higher in Germany than among us.   For wine, it was twice as large.   In England at the same date, the use of distilled liquor and wine was less than in this country, but that of malted liquors much more considerable.

In China the consumption of opium had reached in 1906, 22,588 tons. The significance of this figure is evident when it is recalled that about seven grains make a dose.   The Government, realizing the seriousness of the danger, entered at that time upon a compaign destined to bring to an end after ten years, both the manufacture and the use of opium.   This purpose is still far from having been attained.

Anyone with enough imagination to estimate the moral degradation and the physical decay produced by these drugs, and the financial waste their use entails, will stand aghast at the prodigious sway they possess over mankind.

on the borders of Tyrone and Derry that a writer in the *Medical Times* declared : " The odor of the breath is enough to learn to what religion a man belongs ; alcohol characterizes the Protestant, ether the Roman Catholic[1]."

Not only can certain drugs be successfully substituted one for another, but methods of ecstasy as dissimilar as the mechanical and the psychical may, as we have seen, replace drugs, *in so far as the " divine " significance of their effects is concerned*. The extent of these similarities cannot be discussed before we have made ourselves familiar with the whole range of ecstatic, mystical phenomena. At this time we shall remark only that successful substitution is a token of the presence not merely of common effects but of *essential* common effects.

If literary descriptions are neither complete nor exact, they bring out at least dominant features, and so we may begin with this eloquent panegyric of whisky by one who saw in its effects no religious significance : " I send you," writes Ingersoll to a friend, " some of the most wonderful whisky that ever drove the skeleton from the feast, or painted landscapes in the brain of man. It is the mingled souls of wheat and corn. In it, you will find the sunshine and the shadow that chased each other over the billowy fields, the breath of June, the carol of the lark, the dew of night, the wealth of summer, and autumn's rich content, all golden with imprisoned light. Drink it and you will hear the voices of men and maidens singing the ' Harvest Home,' mingled with the laughter of children. Drink it and you will feel within your blood the star-led dawns, the dreamy, tawny dusks of many perfect days. For forty years this liquid joy has been within the happy staves of oak longing to touch the lips of men[2]."

Alcohol is forbidden by the Koran. Yet, wine is extensively used among the Persian Mohammedan sects known as Sufi. No poets have sung with more conviction the delights that are in wine than Persian poets. In the following passage Dr. Lehman points to some of the attractions of alcohol that are independent of a transcendental interpretation. " A state of exquisite exhaustion in which every limb is in complete repose, in which thinking becomes brooding absorption, while the soul revels in melancholy sensuality or senselessness, is the Oriental's most cherished experience, his paradise on earth." " The more he is weakened by the oppressiveness

---

[1] *Lancet*, 1879, Tome I, p. 870.

[2] Quoted by William James in *Principles of Psychology*, vol. II, p. 469. Comp. Oliver Wendell Holmes, *The Autocrat of the Breakfast Table*, Boston, 1892, VIII, p. 189.

of the climate, or languishes under arbitrary administration, poverty, national disorder, or individual disadvantages, the more comfort he finds in roaming those nameless distances which are untouched by earthly change, or in losing himself in ecstatic self-abandonment. And therefore he drinks; drinks, regardless of Koran and bastinado, drinks to-day like the Persian poets of the Middle Ages drank before him. ' Drunkenness,' says Gobineau, ' is the hereditary sin of the central Asiatic.' This vice, which Mohammed fought against so zealously, all the people succumb to[1]."

" Hear what Hafiz says : ' The rose has unfolded its petals, and the nightingale is in a transport of delight. Now up and rejoice, ye Sufis, if ye love wine ! *See how the crystal goblet breaks the stony wall of remorse! Bring wine, for in the royal abode of contentment there is no difference between king and serf, between wise and foolish*[2] '."

If we are to believe these and similar descriptions, alcohol is valued because it introduces us into a world throbbing with delightful, sensuous life, or produces a peaceful inactivity equally desirable. In the former case, it peoples the mind with pleasant imagery, promotes gaiety, and obliterates painful memories and distracting apprehensions.

Recent observations under controlled conditions have added precision to the literary descriptions of the effects of alcohol. As we proceed with a brief summary of some of these, we remind the reader that our primary purpose is the discovery of the meaning of " divine," as used by those who see in the effects of various drugs a divine transfiguration. We may expect to learn much that will be useful in the subsequent investigation of the nature and meaning of Christian mystical ecstasy.

To four observers, mature University students and total abstainers, Partridge[3] gave, at intervals of from half an hour to an

---

[1] Dr. E. Lehmann, *Mysticism in Heathendom and Christendom*, London, 1910, pp. 61-3, The inner quotations are from Gobineau, *Les religions èt les philosophies dans l'Asie centrale*, 2nd. ed., p. 68,ff.

[2] *Loc. cit.*, pp. 70-1. The italics are mine.
The following impressionistic description of a phase of opium consciousness may perhaps find place here : " The dream commenced with a music of preparation and awakening suspense, a music which gave the feeling of vast march, of infinite cavalcades filing off, and the tread of innumerable armies. The morning was come of a mighty day ; a day of crisis and of final hope for human nature, then suffering some mysterious eclipse, and labouring in some dread extremity. Somewhere, I knew not where,—somehow, I knew not how, by some being, I knew not whom,—a battle, a strife, an agony, was conducting, was evolving like a great drama or piece of music."—*De Quincey's Confessions*.

[3] G. E. Partridge, *Studies in the Psychology of Intemperance*, New York, Sturgis and Walton, 1912, chap. VII.

hour, six doses of alcohol, each of 100 grams of 16 per cent. alcohol. Soon after the first dose he noted in everyone of them the appearance of an increased feeling of self-confidence " which gradually deepened into recklessness and bravado." At the same time, although no noticeable decrease of sensibility had as yet taken place, there was a considerable decrease of alertness to external stimuli and of precision in following the instructions received. After several doses it became very difficult to induce the subject to conform to them.

At a definite stage of the experiments, the observers desired " to throw off all restraint," and realized that they were losing their self-control. Dunbar's subject under the influence of ether expressed in picturesque language the same desire ; and Robinson, after taking hasheesh, exclaimed, throwing off his blankets, " throw off the bonds of all existence[1]."

There was also a period during which every one of Partridge's subjects was inclined to be humorous. Their attempts frequently betrayed a sense of superiority which, in a normal state, is either not felt or carefully concealed. This is apparent in the results of " free association " tests. These tests bring out also the presence in one phase of intoxication of a conviction of power, of efficiency, of freedom. Whereas, when the subject was in a normal condition, the words " muscle," " blue," " free " and " disappointed," brought out respectively the following associations, " strength," " blazes," " generous," " regretful " ; after alcohol they called up the following ideas : (muscle) " when a man is on his muscles, folks have to look out for him " ; (blue) " I am never blue " ; (free) " makes a man independent of any restriction " ; (disappointed) " something I never was." A man who can say sincerely that he never was disappointed, has forgotten a large part of his past. The exaltation of the self indicated in these responses is not constant throughout the increasing intoxication ; there may be moments of depression. But it is sufficient for us to point out those features that bear upon our special problem.

The foregoing description does not fit in every respect each and every case. There are, for instance, persons *qui ont le vin triste*, as the French say. We are not concerned with them. Those whom alone we must take into consideration are the ones who have made the reputation of alcohol as a " divine " beverage. Neither are we to regard its undesirable later effects, temporary or permanent. Men drink and sing the glory of intoxicating drugs in spite of these after-effects.

[1] Victor Robinson, *An Essay on Hasheesh, Medical Review of Reviews*, New York, 1912, p. 59.

The observations of Partridge indicate wide disturbances, the whole body seems more or less involved. There is, in particular, incoordination of the limbs and well marked tendencies to illusion or hallucination due to functional disturbances of the external and internal sense-organs. In one instance, the sensory disturbances were considerable enough to produce a feeling of the unreality of the body or of a changed body, and to invest the outside world with extraordinary aspects. In several, if not in all the subjects, there appeared at a certain stage of intoxication, a sense of well-being, of power, and of freedom, expressed with an abnormal degree of conceit.

Result of the more exact, quantitative, study of the effects of alcohol. An important outcome of the quantitative study of alcohol is the demonstration of the incorrectness of the current opinion that alcohol increases the capacity for work, physical or mental. At a certain stage of its action it may increase muscular activity and produce exuberance of spirit, but although the number of movements and the mental vivacity may increase, muscular energy and mental efficiency, as measured by the amount of work performed, never do ; on the contrary, they decrease.

Kraepelin, Partridge, and others have found that taken in small doses alcohol stimulates motor activity for a relatively short time, but from the first it decreases sensory acuity and discrimination[1]. In the more exact research of Rivers[2], made with doses varying from five to twenty cubic centimetres, little or no effect was produced upon the work done by the hand muscles. Several experimenters, notably Kraepelin, announced a slight shortening of the reaction-time after alcohol.

In a very careful research, Dodge found clear evidence that moderate doses of alcohol (30cc.) produce a depressing effect, even on the simplest motor mechanisms such as the knee-jerk and the eyelid reflex[3]. If this conclusion of Dodge had to be rejected—and I see no reason why it should be—in favour of that of his predecessors, the most that could be claimed for the action of ethyl alcohol upon muscle activity would be that moderate doses produce a very slight improvement, of short duration, in certain motor functions. That

---

[1] Emil Kraepelin, *Ueber die Beeinflüssung einfacher psychischer Vorgänge durch einige Arzneimittel*, Jena, Gustav Fischer, 1892, p. 258 ; G. E. Partridge, *Studies in the Psychology of Intemperance*, p. 95.

[2] W. H. R. Rivers, *The Influence of Alcohol and other Drugs on Fatigue*, London, Edward Arnold, 1908. Rivers used the Mosso ergograph in the improved form given it by Kraepelin. In his experiments, the hand lifted a weight of 4.5 kilograms. By means of a " control " beverage he succeeded usually in hiding the alcohol from the subject. Thus the error (auto-suggestion) that may arise from the knowledge that one has taken alcohol was eliminated. With a dose of 40cc. he found variable results. " Sometimes a dose of 40cc. of pure alcohol may produce a decided increase in the amount of work (muscular), . . . at other times, this increase may be wholly absent, and may possibly be replaced by a decrease." p. 87. In any case, and in this he agrees with nearly all previous investigations, when there is an improvement, it is not in the extent of the contractions but in their number.

[3] Raymond Dodge and Francis G. Benedict, *The Psychological Effects of Alcohol*, Washington, Carnegie Institute, 1915, pp. 243-4 ; see also the more complete results obtained by Walter R. Miles, *Effect of Alcohol on Psychophysiological Functions*, Carnegie Institution, 1918, pp. 1-144. Upon one of the subjects of Dodge and Benedict, Miles' findings are in substantial agreement with theirs. " In twenty-seven out of thirty measurements (of physiological and psychical functions) inferior functioning was discovered after the ingestion of doses containing 30 cc. of absolute alcohol." P. 134.

improvement, if it takes place is, according to all observers, soon followed by a reduction in the normal activity. As to large doses, it is unanimously agreed that from the first they decrease the amount of muscular work done.

Regarding the action of alcohol upon sensory acuity and discrimination, there is now complete agreement : the experimental evidence indicates a loss. Several experimenters found that even very moderate doses affected unfavourably accuracy in shooting. This may be due either to decreased exactness of the accommodation and convergence reflexes of the eye, or to unsteadiness of the arm and body or to both. Lange and Sprecht have found that even small doses of alcohol lower the threshold of auditory sensation, while the difference-threshold is raised. Those two effects they found also in the case of vision.[1]

Upon higher mental processes (recall, reasoning, judgment, volition), moderate doses of alcohol either have no effect or act detrimentally. That is the conclusion reached by Kraepelin in the pioneer work already mentioned, and that conclusion has been confirmed by the investigators who followed him. Aschaffenburg, for instance, studying the effect of 200 grammes of Greek wine containing 18 per cent. of alcohol (36 to 40 grams.), upon typesetters who were habitual users of the beverage, found a marked decrease in the amount of work done on the days the wine was taken[2]. It is to be noted that the dose was a relatively small one. The work of Dodge upon the higher mental processes was not extensive enough to have much significance. The only dose he used in an experiment on memory (30cc.) produced no observable effects[3].

Lange and Sprecht found that small doses of alcohol lower the stimulus threshold and raise the difference-threshold for both hearing and vision. They think that these effects of alcohol are common to all the senses.—*Ztschr. f. Pathopsych.*, 1915, III, 155-256.

J. B. Jorger, in an investigation upon the sequence of thought in inebriates, observed modifications, all of which made for decreased mental efficiency—*Monat. f. Pschiat. u. Neur.*, 1915, XXXVII, 246-66, 323-32.

A relatively large dose of alcohol produces, as everybody knows, muscular inco-ordination, particularly obvious in the gait and speech ; it also plays havoc with the intellectual life. Very large doses result in total motor inefficiency, loss of consciousness, and even death.

*   *   *

The Action of Mescal and of Hasheesh.—Mescal, known until recently to Mexican and American Indians only, is found in the brittle little discs that form at the end of the branches of a cactus belonging to the Melocacteæ group (Anhalonium Lewinii). Careful studies of its action have been made by Dr. Weir Mitchell[4] and Havelock Ellis[5]. Four hours after taking the drug, Dr. Mitchell recorded the following observations : " Yawning at times, sleepy, deliciously at languid ease." "At this stage of the mescal

---

[1] J. Lange and W. Sprecht, *Neue Untersuchungen uber die Beeinflüssung der Sinnesfunktionen durch geringe Alcoholmengen*, *Ztschr. f. Patopsych.*, 1915, vol. III, pp. 155-256.

[2] *Psychol. Arbeiten*, 1896, vol. I, pp. 608-26. See the conclusions, p. 626 ; see also Ernst Kürz and Emil Kraepelin, *Ueber die Beeinflüssung psychischer Vorgänge durch Regelmässigen Alkoholgenuss*, *Psychol. Arbeit*, 1901, vol. III, pp. 417-57.

[3] *Loc. cit.*, pp. 126-33.

[4] Weir Mitchell, *The Effect of Anhalonium Lewinii*, *Brit. Med. Jour.*, 1896, vol. II, pp. 1625-8.

[5] Havelock Ellis, *Popular Science Monthly*, 1902, vol. LXI, pp. 52-71.

intoxication, I had a certain sense of the things about me as having a more positive existence than usual. It is not easy to define what I mean." He had also a " decisive impression " that he was more competent in mind than in his every-day moods. " I seemed to be sure of victoriously dealing with problems." Testing this, he found that he could understand a certain paper on psychology no better than when in his normal condition. He tried other mental tasks, and did as well as usual or less well. Much effort was required to write a few lines of poetry. The making of complicated sums found him as usual. Ellis confirms in this, as in all other important particulars, the observations of Dr. Mitchell. The former writes, mescal " leaves the intellect almost unimpaired[1]." This is, of course, to be understood as referring to moderate doses. The same author noted that, whereas the effect of alcohol on the emotions is marked, mescal hardly affects them ; " even in large doses . . . there is no stage of maudlin sentimentality[2]."

Dr. Mitchell had taken mescal chiefly for the sake of colour hallucinations. His expectations were not disappointed : " The display which for an enchanted two hours followed was such as I find it hopeless to describe in language which shall convey to others the beauty and splendour of what I saw." Havelock Ellis speaks of the visions with the same enthusiasm. Of their general character, he says, " If I had to describe the visions in one word, I should say that they were living arabesques." But, brilliant as these visions are, Dr. Mitchell finds them no more so than those which may appear in some ophthalmic megrims.

Mescal, like cocaine, makes possible without fatigue unusual muscular performances. Dr. Mitchell records, for instance, that he went rather quickly, taking two stairs at a time and without pause, to the fourth story of an hotel, and did not feel oppressed or short of breath. But, if mescal decreases the sense of fatigue, it also probably decreases the capacity for muscular work ; in any case, it disinclines to exertion.

From the notes of one of his subjects, Ellis quoted this interesting observation. " The connexion between the normal condition of my body and my intelligence had broken—my body had become, in a measure, a stranger to my reason." A deadening of certain classes of sensations, particularly the touch sensations and those arising from movement (kinæsthetic sensations), might account for this impression. It is probably, as we shall see, in that direction that one must look to find a justification for certain theories in which in ecstasy the " soul " is said to become separated from the body.

[1] *Ibid.* p. 65.   [2] *Loc. cit.*

A phenomenon, well-known to the psychologist, the reinforcement of sensations of one kind by the stimulation of another sense organ, is apparently present with unusual intensity. "Casual stimulation of the skin at once heightened the brilliance of the vision or produced an impression of sound," and music added beauty to light and colour. This accounts probably for the practice of the Indians of remaining while under the influence of mescal, in front of a glowing camp fire and of beating drums.

The after-effects of mescal are often, perhaps usually, neither painful nor serious. For two days afterwards Dr. Mitchell had headaches, and for one day a smart attack of gastric distress. Ellis suffered some nausea and headache during the experiment, but the next day he arose at the usual time, not tired and with an excellent appetite. "The only after-effect was a slightly hyperæsthetic vision for coloured objects[1]."

No other drug approaches mescal so nearly as hasheesh. I take from Ellis the following comparison. Both slow the heart and both affect the respiration, exaggerate the knee-jerk, and dilate the pupil; both produce visions. These two drugs differ, however, in a number of particulars. Mescal has a more restricted action. It does not produce motor exhilaration, nor loss of self-control. Hasheesh may do so. Mescal depresses action of the muscular system, creates a tendency to tremulousness. The space relations may be affected. "The positive and active manifestations of mescal are always mainly, if not entirely, on the sensory side, and the motor weakness and sense of lassitude which is often present only throw the subject of mescal intoxication more absolutely at the mercy of the waves of unfamiliar sensory impetus which strike him from every side. Every sense is affected . . . the simplest food seems to possess an added relish, . . . and to the sense of touch, the body seems as unfamiliar as everything else has become." "The 'trailing clouds of glory,' the tendency to invest the very simplest things with an atmosphere of beauty, a 'light that never was on sea

---

[1] As my manuscript goes to press I receive a paper reprinted from the *Amer. Jour. of Psychol.*, vol. XXXIV, 1923, 267-70 : *Observations on Taking Peyote* [Mescal], by Samuel W. Fernberger. To the facts noted in the above pages, he adds certain information, especially with regard to the clearness of kinæsthetic and other sensations. He accounts for the illusion of distance as we have done in chapter X, and, like the subjects of Partridge quoted above, who had taken alcohol, he notes that despite the distortion of visual space (" I extended my arm and fixated the finger-tips, and then stretched the arm away from me. The hand seemed to move to a distance of at least ten feet "), he was able to express correctly distances by means of words.

As the impression of increased ability was very notable he attempted to read a paper which a week before he had laid down in despair, but " it was less to be comprehended than ever."

or land,' the new vision of even ' the simplest flower that blows,' all the special traits of Wordsworth's peculiar poetic vision correspond as exactly as possible to the actual and effortless experience of the subject of mescal[1]." Similar sensory phenomena will be noted in connexion with Christian religious experiences. We shall see in particular that a glorious freshness and brightness of visual sensation may be observed after intense moral crises, as Christian conversion, or after certain nervous disorders, as on recovering from a fever

Of experiments with hasheesh, Dunbar wrote : " It seemed as if the moment that had gone with its myriad impressions was forgotten[2]." A person who had taken thirty minims of hasheesh is asked to let his pulse be felt. He stretches forth his hand, saying : " In the interest of science, I am willing." But after a few seconds he pulls his hand impatiently away and exclaims angrily, " You have been holding it half an hour[3]." Ether produces a similar effect : " Time seemed to have no existence. I was continually taking out my watch, thinking that hours must have passed, whereas only a few minutes had elapsed. This, I believe, was due to a complete loss of memory for recent events[4]." Amnesia accounts, in part at least, for the freedom from the past enjoyed by the experimenter. " I was free," says the same author, " from all sense of care and worry, and consequently felt very happy[5]." Partridge found that moderate doses of alcohol also caused time to pass more slowly. This however may not be true of each emotional phase through which the drinker usually passes[6].

A hilarious mood is often a symptom in hasheesh, as it is in alcohol intoxication. " The flood of laughter was loosed, the deluge of mirth poured forth," writes Robinson of the beginning of the action of hasheesh[7]. One of the persons with whom he was experimenting exclaimed : " Cast aside all irrelevant hypotheses, and get to the laughing. I proclaim the supremacy of the laugh, laughter inextinguishable, laughter eternal, the divine laughter of the gods[8]."

[1] Ellis, *loc. cit.*, p. 65.

[2] Ernest Dunbar, *Proc. Soc. Psychical Research*, 1905, vol. XIX, p. 71.

[3] Victor Robinson, *An Essay on Hasheesh, Medical Review of Reviews*, New York, 1912, p. 62.

[4] Dunbar, *Ibid.*, p. 68.

[5] *Loc. cit.*, p. 68.

[6] G. E. Partridge, *Studies in the Psychology of Intemperance*, New York, Sturgis and Walton, 1912, p. 122.

[7] *Loc. cit.*, p. 52.

[8] *Ibid.*, p. 61.

Ether and nitrous oxide gas also transport the mind into a wonderful world of freedom, efficiency, and ineffable feelings. Sir Humphrey Davy, under the influence of nitrous oxide, speaks of his emotions as "enthusiastic and sublime." Frequently the conviction becomes established that something great is happening; at times it is some momentous problem that seems to have received a solution. As we shall have to return to the effects of these two last-mentioned drugs in connexion with the several roots of the conviction of revelation, nothing more will be said in this place[1].

* * *

III. Summary of the Effects of Narcotics and Interpretation of their Religious Significance.

We are now prepared to formulate with some precision the main effects to which narcotic drugs owe a favoured place in the religious life of the non-civilized. These effects vary widely as to kind, frequency, and intensity, not only according to the drug but also with the same drug, according to the person; and different doses of a drug may induce not only different but antagonistic effects. These facts are, however, immaterial here; it is enough for us to know that these drugs produce at some stage or other of the intoxication process, in most if not in all persons, effects regarded as divine; for it is these persons who have established the sacredness of narcotic drugs.

(a) *Alteration of sensation and feeling; illusion and hallucination.* The mind does not perform its perceptual functions with improved accuracy; on the contrary, it exhibits an activity which is to an abnormal degree independent of external stimuli. The type of these perturbations vary with the drug. We have seen, for instance, that mescal induces delightful, coloured hallucinations of a somewhat definite pattern. Hallucinations of other types may convince the ecstatic that he sees and hears, unhampered by opaque obstacles and distances, or that he travels bodily through space, now here, now there, according to his good pleasure.

[1] Macht and Isaacs measured the reaction time to light, sound, and touch, and tested the ability to add and multiply after taking morphine doses varying from $\frac{1}{12}$ to $\frac{1}{4}$ of a grain,—this last dose is an ordinary therapeutic dose. With every dose there was a period of shortened reaction, a decrease in mean variation, and a reduction in the number of errors. But this period became increasingly brief with the increase of the dose; with the largest, it was extremely brief. This period was followed by a lowering of these functions.—*Action of some Opium Alkaloids on the Psychology of Reaction Time, Psychobiology,* 1917, 1, 19-31.

It is obviously not because of the very brief stimulation of sensory functions and of mental activities such as those involved in arithmetic that men become opium fiends. One must look elsewhere in order to understand its power of attraction.

The sensations and feelings arising from the moving limbs and from the internal organs are also modified. Some of these are dulled or even disappear altogether. Frequently, particularly in the more interesting period of intoxication, the dominant result seems to be a multiplication, intensification and qualitative alteration of these feelings.

Now these kinæsthetic and visceral feelings, obscure though they are ordinarily, constitute nevertheless a substantial background of the consciousness of self. Let them be changed or removed, and the feeling of self is altered. This may give rise to remarkable delusions. One of the subjects we have quoted felt separated from his own body. In more ordinary instances, a sense of the unreality of the body and of the outside world is reported or the outside world and body seem altered in particulars difficult to formulate.

Psychiatry provides numerous and striking instances of delusions arising on the basis of a disordered visceral sensitivity. Patients feel that they have lost part of their body, that their stomach is of glass, of lead, etc. Delusions such as these fit in very well with the theory of supernatural possessions—they are often ascribed, according to their nature, to evil or to good spirits.

The intensification and perhaps also the qualitative alteration of certain organic feelings account for one of the most enticing characteristics of ecstatic consciousness. It is as if usually dormant parts of the organism had awakened ; feelings well up from unknown depths and raise their multitudinous voices in a pæon of life. Horizons open up as warm and unlimited as the work-a-day world is cold and circumscribed.

We shall have occasion to illustrate from observations on neurasthenic patients how dullness, motor inertia, may impel one to seek relief in drugs or in illicit love. The apparent paradox of people seeking and enjoying pain becomes intelligible when one takes into account the passion for vivid consciousness. The self-wounding of the Dervish, the painful ascetic practices of the Yogi, the frenetic dances and shouting of the " Maenads" all may yield a sense of new or of increased life. Yejo Hirn, in his excellent work on *The Origins of Art*, remarks that " in pain as in pleasure, in suffering as in voluptuousness, we attain a heightened and enriched sensation of life," and he quotes this passage of a letter of Lessing to Mendelsohn : " We are agreed in this, my dear friend, that all passions are either vehement cravings or vehement loathings, and also that in every vehement craving or loathing we acquire an *increased consciousness of our reality, and that this consciousness cannot but be pleasurable.* Consequently, all our passions, even the most painful, are, as passions, pleasurable." Not the pain nor the wound does the martyr enjoy, but the exaltation that comes with the quivering of the flesh. "The suffering of insensibility is," as Hirn well says, "the highest form possible of tedium." Entrancing relief from normal fatigue, as well as from the insensibility of exhaustion is found at times in the early stages of drug intoxication.

(b) *Alterations of intellectual functions and of emotional attitude.* The intellectual functions—retentiveness, recall, observation, classification, judgment, etc.—stand, as everyone knows, in a relation of close dependence upon each other and upon the activity of the senses. In narcotic intoxication an impairment of these functions goes hand in hand with that of the senses.[1] It is one of the main causes of the impression of self-exaltation, of power, and of freedom.

But drugs seem to act otherwise than as inhibitors of mental activity, some of them appear to exercise a direct stimulating effect upon certain tendencies and emotions. Alcohol increases self-confidence, optimism, and courage. A man never appears or thinks himself braver than after a bottle of wine, and never is his mouth so full of arrogant self-praise. Opium, on the other hand, exaggerates diffidence, apprehension and fear. It makes of its victim a shrinking and self-deprecating object. It may, however, be maintained that the change in the emotional tone following upon the use of alcohol is due entirely to the general reduction of the activity of higher nervous organizations, and not to a stimulation of those parts of the nervous system that are correlated with instinct and emotion. We must remember in this connexion that even when motor activity is temporarily enhanced, the action of alcohol is regarded by the most competent students as a paralysing one. Dodge, for instance, accounts both for the initial increase in motor ability and for the reduction of mental efficiency by a depressing action of alcohol: "Whenever apparent excitation occurs as a result of alcohol, it is either demonstrably or probably due to a relatively overbalancing depression of the controlling and inhibitory processes[2]."

We have seen that in the case of alcohol, scientific measurements demonstrate a deficiency in acuity of perception, in recall, discrimination, and, therefore, in every mental function dependent upon these. But this fact is not realized by the intoxicated ; on the contrary, he delights in a directly opposite conviction ; never is he so sure of himself, and so ready to undertake the impossible. A

---

[1] The initial slight improvement resulting from the taking of certain narcotic drugs when the dose is very small may be disregarded here. The doses used in the production of mystical ecstasy surpass that minimum.

[2] *Ibid.*, p. 253.

limitation of mental activity would suffice to account for this delusion. If, in any particular situation, I do not recall all the essentials that bear upon it ; or if I do not discriminate correctly and analyse completely, I shall necessarily conclude wrongly. Dreams provide abundant illustrations of this kind of defective thinking. A dreamer will, for instance, soar over wide spaces without the use of any machinery ; or he will pass from one country to another in an impossibly short time ; and yet he wonders not at these marvels. He does not wonder, for mental dissociation has gone so far that it does not occur to him that the quickest available method of displacement is far too slow to make the dream possible. Why should the intoxicated hesitate if he is not aware of the presence of conditions of success impossible for him to realize ? Unaware of the difficulties or of his deficiencies, why should he doubt his ability to cope with any task ?

The self-confidence, boastfulness, and raw pugnacity characteristic of inebriation may also arise from a weakening of the control usually exercized upon instinct by the higher mental life. If the well-bred person checks manifestations of pugnacity, it is because he recognizes objections to their instinctive expression ; *i.e.*, other and antagonistic tendencies are brought to bear upon pugnacity. Fear of making himself ridiculous, because of the superficiality of his acquaintance with the topic under discussion might make a man hesitate to speak in a meeting, although he be urged to do so by an impulse to seek social recognition. Let the knowledge of his deficiency fail to appear in his mind and he will behave with the egotism characteristic of the callow youth, the untutored, and the partially intoxicated.

Excessive motor activity is one of the obvious characteristics of a phase of alcohol intoxication. This might be due altogether to decreased self-control, itself the result of the inhibition of the higher nervous centres. For, the quietness of the well-mannered person, his moderation in gesture and in facial expression are not signs of inertness, but the result of a self-control established under social tuition. Remove this control and the organism will behave like a machine without a fly-wheel. When, as in the case of hasheesh intoxication, motor activity is not increased, and there is less inclination to physical arrogance, the higher mental functions are found not to be so unfavourably affected as in the case of alcohol ; i.e., self-control is not so markedly decreased. The action of hasheesh is exerted first of all upon the external senses and the organic feelings.

To the intoxicated, the way seems clear ; the required virtues, the knowledge, and the ability seem present. What there is to be done can be done; done with ease, with exuberance, with joyous laughter or crushing scorn. Imagination is no longer restricted to rational channels or checked by the sense of the irrelevant, the improper, or the grotesque. Its quality, judged objectively, may not be high, but what matters so long as the subject thinks differently and is proudly happy? The mind seems to have broken its earthly shackles, taken wings, and soared, unrestricted. in a world of infinite possibility. If to be human means to be hemmed in at every turn by physical and moral infirmity, then intoxication must in truth seem divine[1].

Here and there, a poet is said to have found "inspiration" in wine, opium, or other drug. But when those of his works that have been written with the assistance of narcotics are examined, they turn out to be inferior *in point of intellectual and ethical* content to his other productions. It is only in the rhythmic and phonetic expression of a peculiarly amorphous mood that they may possess distinction and superiority. But superior word-music should probably be regarded as a consequence of an abnormally complete surrender to the enjoyment of feeling at the expense of purposive, rational thinking. Helmholtz is reported to have declared that when trying to give form and being to some dimly apprehended conception, the smallest quantity of alcohol sufficed to dispel from his mind every idea of the creative order.

*   *   *

The impression of free and unlimited life, the great boon conferred upon man by intoxicants, owes much to the disappearance of the social restraints. The importance of this fact is so considerable that we must dwell upon it. Life in society, at every level whatsoever, implies control and guidance of the individual's instincts and desires for the sake of the group to which he belongs. Even the lowest societies are compelled to make war on the disruptive manifestations of self-affirmation, of anger, of lust, etc. To this constraint, placed upon each individual, is added also at every level of social organization, but more especially among highly civilized peoples, the strain of continuous and systematic work. Manual workers, business and professional men alike, remain at work day after day, and year after year, with only brief intermissions, in the face of vigorous natural promptings to give up and relax, to play and enjoy.

[1] A condition strikingly similar is observed in certain types of nervous disintegration. In the disease known as progressive paralysis, entailing a gradual lessening of the mental life, there appears, parallel with the decrease of motor control, sensory acuity, discrimination, association, etc., a conviction of power and efficiency strangely at variance with reality. Here delusions of grandeur and power are definitely correlated with a progressive deterioration of the nervous system.

This moral restraint imposed by law and custom, and this sustained effort of work required under conditions of competitive existence, produce a state of tension and restlessness that cry out for relief. The need for easing the strain of voluntary effort is everywhere in evidence ; it is the " call of the wild." Savages and civilized, slaves and masters, must at times free themselves from the great social fly-wheel that regulates the individual's behaviour. The moment comes to every man, though not with equal frequency or intensity, when the sustained effort required in living up to established standards, in conforming to social usage and moral laws, passes endurance, and he lapses to a more easily maintained level. An escape to the country; a dinner with song and wine ; or, perchance, a less respectable diversion, disposes him again to take up the straight-jacket we are all wearing[1].

The more stringent the control, the greater the probability of a violent reaction. Hence the riotous festivities following periods of moral strain. When the Faculty of Paris threatened to abolish the Feast of Fools, they were petitioned in these terms : " Wine casks would burst if we failed sometimes to remove the bung and let in air. Now we are all ill-bound casks and barrels which would let out the wine of wisdom if by constant devotion and the fear of God we allowed it to ferment. . . . Thus on some days we give ourselves up to sport, so that with the greater zeal we may afterwards return to the worship of God[2]." The forward swing of the pendulum is followed by a backward swing—a temporary victory of the " natural man." Thus we understand in part the well known tendency of sober ceremonies, religious or otherwise, to pass into extravagant and indecent conduct. A burial ceremony, a marriage feast, a birth celebration, readily drift into a carousal. " The religious gladness of the Semites," writes Robertson Smith, " tended to assume an orgiastic character and become a sort of intoxication of the senses, in which anxiety and sorrow were drowned for the moment. This is apparent in the old Canaanite festivals, such as the vintage feasts at Shechem described in Judges ix. 27, and not less in the service of the Hebrew high places, as it is characterized by the prophets. Even at Jerusalem the worship must have been boisterous indeed, when Lament. ii. 7, compares the shout of the

---

[1] George T. W. Patrick in *The Psychology of Relaxation*, p. 208, points out very effectively the relaxation value of alcohol. He ascribes " the desire for alcohol to the inherent need of mind and body for relaxation, a need normally supplied by all the varied forms of play and sport. Psychologically it is the expression of the desire for release from the tension of the strenuous life."

[2] Quoted in a foot-note to Havelock Ellis, *Studies in the Psychology of Sex*, " Sex in relation to Society," Philadelphia, 1911, p. 219.

storming party of the Chaldeans in the courts of the temple with the noise of the solemn feast. . . . In evil times, when men's thoughts were habitually sombre, they betook themselves to the physical excitement of religion as men now take refuge in wine. That this is not a fancy picture is clear from Isaiah's description of the conduct of his contemporaries during the approach of the Assyrians to Jerusalem (Isaiah xxii. 12, 13. Compare with i. 11, seq.) when the multiplied sacrifices offered to avert the disaster degenerated into a drunken carnival[1]."

The cult of Dionysus was noteworthy for the licence that went along with it[2].

The demand for relaxation is so uncompromising that everywhere, even among savages, some official provision is made for it. Stated times are set apart and occasions provided when one may with impunity " kick over the traces." Thus the danger threatened to the state by outbreaks of the " natural man " are minimized. We of a highly cultured age have not found it possible to dispense

[1] W. R. Smith, *Religion of the Semites*, pp. 243-4.

[2] " In Etruria," we are told, " the cult of Dionysus developed rapidly and lost its original dignity to become a pretext for debauchery and a school of open immorality. But it was at Rome that the cult of Dionysus assumed the foulest cast. At Rome the founder of the cult soon changed its ritual and its character. Livy says : 'All crimes, all excesses find place there . . . Those who rebel against the shame and are unwilling to take part in it are sacrificed as victims. The great religious principle consists in regarding nothing as prohibited by morality. Men, as if inspired, prophesy, with violent gestures of drunkenness, of fanaticism. . . The membership is very great, a whole people ; it includes men and women of noble birth. Two years ago they decided not to initiate any one more than twenty years old.' A great trial followed which included seven thousand accused and resulted in numerous capital condemnations. This happened in 186 B.C." *Bacchanalia*, by F. Lenormant, in *Dictionnaire des Antiquités Grecques et Romaines*, vol. I, p. 590. Numerous other illustrations of the connexion of Satturnalia with religious celebrations will be found in Stratton, *Psychology of the Religious Life*, London, 1911, pp. 97-100. See for the customs of many tribes, otherwise more or less chaste, of meeting occasionally for the purpose of holding indiscriminate intercourse, H. H. Bancroft, *Native Races*, vol. I, pp. 565-6.

The following is from J. G. Frazer, *The Belief in Immortality*, London, 1913, vol. I, pp. 427-8. In the Fiji Islands certain solemn ceremonies were followed by a great feast, which ushered in a period of indescribable revelry and licence. All distinction of property was for the time being suspended. Men and women arrayed themselves in all manner of fantastic garbs, addressed one another in the foulest language, and practised unmentionable abominations openly in the public square of the town. The nearest relationships, even that of brother and sister, seemed to be no bar to the general licence, the extent of which was indicated by the expressive phrase of an old Nandi chief, who said, ' While it lasts, we are just like the pigs.' This feasting and orgy might be kept up for several days, after which the ordinary restraint of society and the common decencies of life were observed once more. The rights of private property were again respected ; the abandoned revellers and debauchees settled down into staid married couples ; and brothers and sisters, in accordance with the regular Fijian etiquette, might not so much as speak to one another."

entirely with these safety valves. We continue to tolerate carnivals, mardi gras fairs, mummeries, and their equivalents.

Among the many ways in which a moral and intellectual vacation can be secured, few are as effective—we do not say desirable—as the use of certain drugs. It may have, it is true, detrimental after effects, and it may lead to disastrous habits; but its immediate result is a relief from the intolerable strain of organized life and a readiness to take up again the social constraints. In this way it becomes an instrument of stabilization.

It might seem that the mere cessation of ordinary activities, together with sleep, should be adequate and satisfactory restoratives. The superiority of the drug-consciousness over these more normal ways of relief, lies in the fact that in intoxication the attention is not only released from the daily tasks and obligations, it becomes engrossed in pleasant and effortless activities; and there is added the already described delight of new and abundant life,—a delight none the less effective for being deceptive. Mere cessation of work does not in itself quickly give the mind all the refreshment it needs; it leaves one, for a time at least, afflicted by a sense of staleness and of the tormenting moral claims of society. Whereas the strain of effort; the disappointments of unsatisfied cravings and thwarted ambitions; the humiliating limitations of intelligence, health, and wealth; the doubts, scruples, and remorse—all these worrying, painful constituents of daily existence vanish under the spell of intoxicants.

The dreams of simple men can soar no further than the sensuous delights, the relief from painful moral efforts imposed by society, and the impression of complete freedom and unlimited power bestowed upon them by narcotic drugs and other physical means of ecstacy. Therefore, they regard drug-intoxication as divine possession or union.

It is interesting to bring the foregoing remarks in connexion with the behaviour of persons suffering from an abnormally insufficient sense of power. These sufferers, called *psychasthéniques*, by the distinguished French psychiatrist, Pierre Janet, seek energy wherever they may hope to find it. Sometimes the new influx of life seems to proceed from the personality of the physician himself; the patient comes to him more or less regularly to be " wound up." Sometimes the undervitalized has recourse to drugs and sometimes to religion.

From the age of fifteen, D. has been subject to attacks of depression. At that age his never strong will became weaker than ever; he ceased to be " good for anything."

" For a long period and until the age of twenty-two, he endured these painful attacks with resignation; sometimes he remained thus prostrated for a couple of hours, at other times for several days. He had a vague feeling that he needed some sort of excitement to set him up again; he ' would have liked to do some out-of-the-way thing ' to force himself out of this condition. As a matter of fact, he never did actually give way to any foolish impulse and, on each recurrence, the state gradually wore itself out,

" Towards the age of twenty-two, while at a German University, he was led by his comrades into excessive drinking. These repeated intoxications produced the remarkable result of dissipating the attacks of depression and freeing him from the horrible feeling of being plunged into the depths; hence a vague idea took root in his mind that intoxication was the sovereign remedy for his torments.

" From this time on, the character of his attacks has changed; when he feels cast down he is obsessed by the idea of drink; he struggles, hesitates, does not deliberately resolve to drink to the point of intoxication but wishes to give himself merely a little solace and decrease the horrible feeling of depression that he experiences. He drinks unwillingly, alone, without pleasure, without conviction; but he drinks, nevertheless, and soon he can no longer resist the impulse. He spends all the money he has about him, pawns his watch, borrows in a most absurd fashion, and winds up in a state of stupor which usually brings the attack to an end[1]."

Essentially similar in her psycho-physiological insufficiency, however different the remedy, is Sim, a woman thirty-one years old. She also is unable to live upon her own store of energy. She must be vivified, " emotionalized," as Janet says. Her husband, an energetic fellow, full of common sense, does not satisfy her. He does not give her any food for thought. Of him, she says, " he does not know anything, he does not teach me anything, he does not astonish me. I know myself. I have exhausted my own resources. I need to be given new ideas, new impressions, new emotions; my husband is merely a man of ordinary common sense, and that is deadly." The lover upon whom she comes to rely for the infusion of the life she lacks, is described by her as witty, vivacious, intellectual, self-controlled, heartless, aggressive. He keeps her constantly alert and expectant. He is the tonic she needs. At an earlier time, this woman had passed through a period of religious exaltation during which she had found in divine communion the stimulant later furnished by her lover.

Sim and her sort need stimulants in order to rise above the dead level of inactivity and inefficiency, with its accompanying intolerable *ennui*. " If they find this excitement in alcohol or in morphine, they become drunkards or morphine *habitués*; if they find it in divine love, they become delirious religious mystics; but if they find what they need in a human being, they become lovers. If the lover abandons them, they suffer from mental and physical disorders similar to those of the morphine victim when deprived of his hypodermic syringes[2]."

The reader is not to suppose that we regard these several methods of cure as complete equivalents. We would maintain merely that they include a common kernal roughly describable as enhancement of the life-powers, either temporary or permanent, illusory or substantial.

As we bring this chapter to a close, let us pause a moment to recall that religion and the enhancement of life are inseparably associated. The substance of religious life is frequently described as communion or union with the Source of Life. Christ came that men might have eternal life. A professor of Christian theology describes the action of God as " creating within the soul a new centre of activity and of force, introducing peace, joy, freedom, love, and light[3]." Digamma, probably a Fellow in a College of Oxford University, discovered that after earnest prayer, a state of depression from which he suffered severely was greatly relieved and at times

[1] Pierre Janet, *Les Obsessions et la Psychasthénie*, vol. II, p. 424.

[2] *Loc. cit.*, pp. 402-7.

[3] Henri Bois, *La Valeur de l'Expérience Religieuse*, Paris, 1908.

completely vanished[1]. Because of this life-enhancing experience, Digamma believed that in prayer God actually communicated himself to man. Every religion makes similar claims ; religious worship is essentially a method of securing more and better life.

It is because of similar effects, in part real and in part illusory, that the intoxication ceremonies we have passed in review are regarded by the non-civilized as uniting man to the Divine. The analysis of the effects of narcotics has revealed the meaning they attach to that term.

In later chapters we shall find that in some of its phases the mystical ecstatic trance brings to the Christian worshipper also hallucinations, incomparable sensuous delights, an impression of limitless power and freedom ; and, in other phases, of complete relaxation and perfect peace. And the Christian mystic also thinks of these ecstatic experiences as divine union.

As we turn to higher forms of mysticism, our main concern will be to trace the continuity of impulses and purposes from the ecstasies of the lower to the ecstasies of the higher religions, to note the appearance of new motives and new methods, and to record the results of these new efforts towards the establishment of relations with a transcendant Source of Life.

[1] Digamma, *An Aspect of Prayer*, Oxford, B. H. Blackwell.

CHAPTER III

THE YOGA SYSTEM OF MENTAL CONCENTRATION AND RELIGIOUS MYSTICISM

NOWHERE perhaps does mysticism fill so large a place as in India. Nevertheless, since we are not writing a history of mysticism, we may content ourselves with the consideration of the most influential of the Yoga[1] systems, that of Patanjali, accessible in the English language since 1914.[2]

To the historians of metaphysics this text is of great importance inasmuch as it forms, in the words of the translator, " a bridge between the philosophies of ancient India and the fully developed Indian Buddhism and the religious thought of to-day in Eastern Asia." Psychologists also will find much to interest them in this book besides that which it is our special task to bring out, for its conceptions of the mind and its workings are surprisingly different from those of the Western world. India's thinking has gone in different directions and dug different ruts from those in which the western mind has imbedded itself. Interesting instances of first attempts at psychological analyses and classifications may be found on pages 8, 31, 34, 60, 235, and 327.

The philosophical foundation of this Yoga is the Vedanta metaphysics. Its main articles may be briefly formulated in three propositions :

1. Individuals possess merely illusory existence. There is really no distinction between Brahman and souls or selves. The self is Brahman. Is is false perception, false knowledge, that leads to the opposition of selves to Brahman or ultimate reality.

2. The supreme aim of man is emancipation from individual existence ; i.e., absorption into Brahman.

3. This absorption is achieved when the illusion of the soul's separate existence vanishes—when the identity of the individual self with the universal self is realized. Thus, emancipation from rebirth does not come by good works but by understanding : " from knowledge comes emancipation." That knowledge consists in the immediate perception of the identity of the soul with Brahman.

This Vedanta doctrine is too abstruse and stands in too obvious antagonism with one of the most tenacious instinctive tendencies of human nature (self-preservation and enhancement) to recommend itself to the average person. The illusoriness of individual existence, the identity of the self with Brahman, the absorption in the All as the goal of man, are too remote from the conceptions and desires of the average man to become part of his common-sense philosophy Are, then, the rank and file shut off from the religion of Brahman ? Not at all. In India as elsewhere religious philosophy comes down to those who cannot ascend to it. Alongside of the esoteric doctrine sketched above, there grew

---

[1] The word " Yoga " comes from the same root as the Latin *jungo*, to unite. The aim of the Yogin is to become one with the All.

[2] *The Yoga-System of Patanjali, or the Ancient Hindoo Doctrine of Concentration of Mind.* Tr. by James Haughton Woods, Harvard University Press, 1914, Cambridge, Mass, pp. XII + 384.

up in India a popular Brahman in the form of a personal God occupying a position quite similar to that of God in the mind of the Christian worshipper. This Brahman saves from rebirth and vouchsaves to his faithful worshipper an indescribable blessedness. Strictly taken, this popular religion involves the negation of the fundamental propositions of the Vedanta. But this is conveniently concealed by the use of the same terms in both forms of the Brahmanic religion. (For a fuller account, see the excellent *Outline of the Vedanta System* by Paul Deussen, New York, 1906.)

It may be remarked in this connexion that a similar double conception of God exists in present Christianity. On the one hand, the familiar faith of the many regard him as a personal, benevolent Providence without whose will not even a sparrow falls to the ground. On the other, a lofty doctrine of God, entertained by the philosophically trained, makes of him an impassible Absolute. The latter doctrine is in radical disagreement with the phraseology of the Christian books of worship.

Our purpose remains, as heretofore, the description of mystical beliefs and practices and the discovery of their motives, intended goal, and actual results. Yoga appears as a connecting link between the religious intoxication of the savage and the mysticism of the higher religions.

The Yoga of Patanjali consists of 195 rules written between 650 and 850 A.D. Without comments they could be printed in the space of a dozen pages. They are, however, far from clear to the European reader, and presumably little more so to the Hindoo, for they are accompanied by the Yoga-Bhasya, a commentary much longer than the text, and by still more extensive explanations due to Vacaspatimicra. The treatise is divided into four books: Concentration, Means of Attainment, Supernormal Powers, and Isolation. The first two treat in the main of the means or methods of attaining the perfect state, and the last two describe chiefly that which is to be attained. But one should not look for a strict logical arrangement of parts.

To characterize Yoga as a system of philosophy or of ethics would be misleading. Its more direct analogy is with our manuals of religion, for its central purpose, like that of our own books of worship, is to teach the way to salvation. But its practical directions are imbedded in more or less fanciful psychology and unnecessary metaphysics.

The main propositions.—Life is evil and death is merely the beginning of another painful existence,—such is the double proposition upon which Yoga and, of course, Buddhistic philosophy in general, is grounded. The goal is escape from the round of rebirths.

So far nothing could be clearer. When we pass to the means of deliverance from this inacceptable situation, the text becomes more difficult. We must first note carefully the distinction Yoga makes between the " Self " and the " mind-substance " or " thinking-substance," and the respective functions it ascribes to them. The whole scheme of deliverance is dependent upon that distinction.

The Self is " the power of seeing," and the mind-substance is " the power by means of which one sees " (ii. 6, 20). It would probably agree better with our ways of speaking to describe the first as a " power " and the second as an " instrument." Without this mind-substance the Self would be " isolated " ; i.e., it would not be conscious of the world, for it is through the activity of the thinking-substance that the Self becomes aware of objects, acquires knowledge (i. 2 ; ii. 6, 20 ; ii. 17), and thus enters into relation with the world. This entering into relation with the world by means of the thinking-substance generates desires and passions and with them the sense of personality. Rebirth is a consequence of desire and passion. Deliverance can therefore be attained by disconnecting the Self from the mind-substance : " Isolate " the Self, make it " not conscious of any object " (i. 20), passionless and purposeless, and personality will have dwindled away—thus speaks Yoga.

In certain parts of the book the mere realization of the difference that exists between the Self and the mind-substance and of the rôle played by the latter, is said to be enough to bring about the deliverance of the Self. We read for instance that the fateful error of man is the confusion " of the power of perceiving " with " the power by which one perceives " (ii. 6). It is this confusion which gives rise to the sense of personality and, with it, to all human misery. Deliverance is therefore said to be obtained when one has become conscious of the distinction between Self and thinking-substance ; then the Self has " passed out of relation with the aspects or attributes of things ; and, enlightened by himself and nothing more, is stainless and isolated " (ii. 27). But this theory is contradicted by Yoga itself since it places the main emphasis upon other means of achieving the liberation of the Self.

The task before the Yogin is, then, the suppression of the activity of the mind, the " fluctuations of the mind-stuff are to be restricted." The classification of these fluctuations or activities offers one of the many instances of the naiveté of Hindoo psychology. Five kinds of fluctuations are enumerated : source-of-valid ideas, i.e., perceptions and verbal communications ; misconceptions ; predicate relations ; sleep ; memory (i. 2, 5-11). We need not try to puzzle out this analysis of the mind's activities. That which matters most is fortunately clear enough : the mind-stuff is to become quiescent, it is to be permanently in the " restricted state "

" Concentration " is the name of the condition of him who has entered upon the way to deliverance. In its lower degree it assumes the form either of deliberation or of reflection upon any object of thought (i. 17-18). At first the mind remains conscious of objects ; but in the higher stages of concentration, it loses that consciousness ; objects merge, and there remains only " subliminal impressions " (i. 17, 18). Finally the Yogin " ceases to be conscious of any object."

Hindrances to concentration ; how to overcome them.—There are many hindrances to concentration. Yoga divides them in two groups. The reason for the separation in two groups is as obscure as the reason for the composition of each group. In the first, we find " sickness, languor, doubt, heedlessness, worldliness, erroneous perception, failure to attain any stage of concentration, and instability in the state when attained " (i. 30). In the second group are put together undifferentiated consciousness (mistaking the impermanent, impure, etc., for the pure, permanent, etc.), the feeling of personality, passion, aversion, and the will-to-live (ii. 3).

In order to overcome these hindrances and attain his goal, the Yogin needs every available help, The sutras indicate eight methods and devices (ii. 29-55 ; iii. 1-3). Five are called indirect (abstentions, observances, postures, regulations-of-the-breath, and withdrawal-of-the-senses), and three are called direct aids (fixed attention, contemplation, and concentration).

Some of these aids indicate a concern for ethical perfection—the " abstensions," for instance, which are defined as " abstinence from injury and from falsehood and from theft and from incontinence and from acceptance of gifts." Abstinence from injury in which " all the other abstentions and observances are rooted," is to be understood as " abstinence from malice towards all living creatures in every way and at all times " (ii. 30). This is good-will expressed negatively. The " observances " also are in part of a genuine ethical character. Cleanliness is defined both as external, and then produced " by earth or water or the like ; and as inner cleanliness of the mind-stuff " (i. 32). The Yogin is enjoined furthermore " to cultivate friendliness towards all living beings that have reached the experience of happiness ; compassion towards those in pain ; joy towards those whose character is meritorious." The mind-stuff of him who conforms to these prescriptions " becomes calm ; and when calm it becomes single-in-intent and reaches the stable state " (i. 33). An ethical purpose and practice is, nevertheless, not logically demanded by the goal of Yoga ; for, honesty, friendliness, etc., are irrelevant to one who seeks utter detachment and isolation. Cultivating friendliness and rejoicing with those who rejoice are demands hardly in agreement with a desire for the suppression of personality. This is one of the incongruities that betray the confusion of thought from which this system suffers.

The most striking of the physical aids to concentration are the "postures." A sutra on postures enumerates them thus, "the lotus-posture and the hero-posture and the decent-posture and the mystic-diagram and the staff-posture and the posture with the rest and the bedstead, the seated curlew and the seated elephant and the seated camel, the even arrangement, the stable-and-easy and others of the same kind" (ii. 46)[1]. These postures are to be accompanied "by relaxation of effort or by a mental state-of-balance with reference to Ananta" (ii. 47). In this connexion we may remark that relaxation of effort as well as "concentration" of attention play a capital rôle in the production of various automatisms and of trance states. Relaxation is demanded of the subject in psychoanalysis ; and, in the Christian religion, it is when the sinner despairs of reforming himself by his own endeavours and surrenders to the will of God that salvation comes. In the production of hypnosis one or the other of these expressions, or both, are used to describe the attitude to be assumed by the subject. When discussing the ecstatic trance of the Christian mystics we shall have occasion to come back to this significant fact.

The physical helps to concentration include mortifications, fasts and other ascetic practises, but the one most insisted upon after the postures is perhaps the control of the breath. It is secured together with the attainment of "stable" postures (ii. 49). There are no

---

[1] Pictures of these postures are given in Richard Schmidt's *Fakire und Fakirthum*. I draw the following passage from the Bhagavadgita.
"A devotee should constantly devote his Self to abstraction, remaining in a secret place . . . fixing his seat firmly in a clean place, not too high nor too low, and covered over with a sheet of cloth, a deer-skin and blades of Kusa grass,—and there seated on that seat, fixing his mind exclusively on one point, with the workings of the mind and senses restrained, he should practice devotion for purity of self. Holding his body, head and neck even and unmoved, remaining steady, looking at the tip of his own nose, and not looking about in all directions, with a tranquil self, devoid of fear, and adhering to the rules of Brahmakârins, he should restrain his mind and concentrate it on me [the Deity], as his final goal. Thus constantly devoting his Self to abstraction a devotee whose mind is restrained, attains that tranquility which culminates in final emancipation and assimilation with me." Elsewhere the devotee is directed to exclude from his mind "external objects, concentrate the visual power between the brows, and making the upward and downward life-breaths even, confining their movements ' within the nose.'" In another place, he is directed to repeat the single syllable "om," a mystical formula for Brahma. Max Müller, *Sacred Books of the East*, vol. VIII, chaps. V and VI, pp. 68-9, 66-7.

less than four kinds of breath control : " it is external in case there is no flow of breath after expiration ; it is internal in case there is no flow of breath after inspiration ; it is the third or suppressed in case there is no flow of either kind " (ii. 50). The pueril subtleties into which sutras and commentaries enter in this connexion cannot interest us. We need note merely that the fourth and perfect control of the breath involves the total suppression of the passage of air to and from the lungs. Since death would speedily supervene should this be realized, we must suppose that the Yogin is deceived into the belief that breathing is totally suspended. That he suffers many illusions and hallucinations there cannot be any doubt. But why this unnatural behaviour ? Because, in restraint of breath, " the central organ " becomes fit for fixed attention, and complete mastery of the organs is attained (ii. 53, 55) ; *i.e.*, the sense organs are " restricted " their activity ceases, and that, as we know, is a step towards disinterestedness and passionlessness.

" Restriction " of the organs of sense is secured in drug-mysticism by the action of the drug. In Christian mysticism, absorption in the adorable personality of God or Christ or of one of the saints, is a recognized method of ascending the " ladder " that leads to ecstasy. A corresponding practice is found in the Yoga system ; it is the " devotion of the Içvara " (i. 23). That being is not easy to describe. He is a " special kind of Self," never in the bondage of time, space, and matter, " at all times whatsoever liberated " (i. 24) ; in him " the germ of the omniscient is at its utmost excellence " (i. 25) ; he is the Teacher of the Primal Sages (i. 26). This exalted Being is represented by the mystic syllable which, when reflected upon and many times repeated brings the mind-stuff to rest in the One Exalted (i. 28)[1].

The use of drugs is not recommended in the Yoga of Patanjali ; it is, however, mentioned and acknowledged as available and legitimate. Book IV opens with this sutra, " Perfections proceed from birth or from drugs or from spells or from self-castigation or from concentration " (iv. 1). The commentary says that " ageless-ness and deathlessness and the other perfections " may be had by the use of an elixir-of-life. This recognition of similarity between the condition secured by the Yoga-practices and that produced by drugs is too significant to be overlooked by the student of mystical ecstasy.

[1] It is to be noted that in the explanation of this sutra, " reflection " is defined as " an *absorption* in the mind again and again " (i. 28). We are therefore to understand by " reflection " in this connexion, not that which is ordinarily meant by it, but rather the opposite.

Results.—The *ultimate* end is, as we already know, the separation of the Self from every object of sense or thought, the suppression of all desire and passion, and the consequent elimination of personality. But just as Christian worship offers secondary attractions of an æsthetic, social, or even grossly utilitarian nature ; so among the Hindoo, the desire to pursue the goal is greatly assisted by many real or imaginary advantages that accrue to the faithful Yogin. Each practice has its reward. Postures render the Yogin unassailable " by cold and heat and other extremes " (ii. 48). Self-castigation brings perfection of the body, such as hearing and seeing at a distance " (ii. 43). As a result of concentration upon muscular powers, there arises strength like that of the elephant ; as the result of concentration upon the sun, there arises an intuitive knowledge of the cosmic spaces. Concentration upon the " wheel of the navel " brings " intuitive knowledge of the arrangement of the body " (iii. 29) ; upon the " well of the throat," " cessation of hunger and thirst " ; etc., etc. It would be futile to attempt a full enumeration of the marvellous powers promised to the faithful Yogin, and still more to try to fathom the reason for the connexion affirmed between each practice and its alleged result. If the connexion is, at times, natural or logical, it is more frequently obviously fanciful in the extreme.

One of the most alluring of the imaginary claims of Yoga is the possession of " all truth." When the Yogin has " ceased to be conscious of any object," he is said nevertheless to have gained the insight by which things are perceived " as they really are " (i. 20). This omniscience is, of course, not acquired by the ordinary way of protracted and systematic intellectual effort. It comes to him in the measure in which he discards critical reason and surrenders to the " unconscious " : it is when the Yogin has gained " the vision by the flash of insight which *does not pass successively through the serial order of the usual process of experience* " (i. 47), that he possesses the " truth-bearing " insight (i. 48). That insight reveals " all that he (the Yogin) desires to know in other places and in other bodies and in other times. Thereafter his insight sees into things as they are " (ii. 45. Compare iii. 54).

This is obviously nonsense. The Yogin cannot substantiate his claim to a knowledge of the thoughts of other persons, of the time of his death, or of his present and future incarnations ; concentration upon the moon does not give him an intuitive knowledge of " the arrangement of the stars " (iii. 27). A careful reading of Yoga discloses, however, that magical omniscience and omnipotence are not taken too seriously. After all, the Yogin keeps his eyes first of all on deliverance from pain. Consider for instance this elucidation of the nature of " insight " : " And in this sense it has been said, ' as the man who has climbed the crag sees those upon the plain below, so the man of insight who has risen to the undisturbed calm of insight, himself escaped from pain, beholds all creatures in their pain.' " (i. 47). Here the function of " insight " is deliverance from pain. That, in truth, is the gross purpose of Yoga.

The omniscience and omnipotence claimed for the Yogin should be placed in parallel with the similar claims made by the users of drugs in religious ceremonies. In both instances the claim is an expression of yearning for unlimited physical and intellectual powers and of an illusory realization of those yearnings. In the one case it is due chiefly to persistent fixation of the attention, and, in the other, mainly to the action of a drug.

If omniscience and omnipotence are, with the Yogin as with the drug-intoxicated, illusory, real advantages are nevertheless secured by both. During the early stages of the emptying process the Yogin enjoys an impression of unlimited power and the delights of an imagination freed from the control of critical reason. Physical pain is allayed or altogether removed. Moral pain also vanishes, the dread of sickness and age, the wearisome struggle to keep up with the demands of society and of one's ideal ; the wickedness of duplicity, pride, and hatred, disappear when the mind has become concentrated upon an " objectless content." Sensuous raptures, conspicuous in drug ecstasy, seem also in some measure at least to add their delights to the Yogin's experience. They are probably mainly responsible for utterances like this, " What constitutes the pleasure of love in this world and what the supreme pleasure of heaven are both not to be compared with the sixteenth part of the pleasure of dwindled craving (ii. 42.) In a similar way do Christian mystics speak about the unutterable delight of " union with God."

But does not this contradict the Yogin's conception of the final state ? Is unconsciousness, consonant with enjoyment ? Obviously not ; it is merely consonant with painlessness. This contradiction in the idea of Nirvana runs through all or most Hindoo religious litera- ture. Its existence is not difficult to account for : the delights found on the way to unconsciousness, are mistakenly ascribed to that final state. Similarly, the sufferer who contemplates ultimate deliverance from pain, can hardly refrain from speaking of that condition as one of bliss, although, in fact, it is no more than absence of suffering.

The illogical craving for moral perfection manifested in Yoga.— Attention has already been drawn to the very specific directions by which the Yoga of Patanjali encourages the practice of social virtues. Yet the removal of all ethical considerations would leave its essential structure unaffected ; for, after all, ethical considerations have no logical place in a system that aims at the breaking of all bonds connecting the individual to the physical and social world. If Yoga sets down principles and prescribes rules of intercourse with one's fellows that are not much inferior to the best in Christianity, it is probably because those who elaborated this scheme of deliverance were after all keenly conscious not only of the presence of the evils of existence and of a general desire to escape these evils but also of an ideal of social perfection, the worth of which they tacitly acknowledged.

In the western world, dissatisfaction with this life, because of physical and moral evils, did not lead to a condemnation of personal existence.   It resulted instead in a belief in an eternal life in an ideal social order beyond the grave.

Is the Hindoo so different from the rest of mankind as to seek that which others abhor ?   There is no sufficient reason to think so. He, no more than the westerner, gives up the struggle for self-realization.   To neither is the mere cessation of effort and extinction a really satisfactory solution of the problem of destiny.   The Hindoo also seeks a victorious end.   There must be no ignoble surrender ; *evil has to be overcome before he will consent to enter eternal rest.*   Is not rebirth a scheme to secure by gradual purification ultimate triumph over   evil   and   the   realization   of   individual   perfection ?   How senseless would be the prolonged torture of rebirth were it not regarded as an instrument of self-realization !

In this, then, Christianity and Buddhism substantially agree : both seek a self-realization that involves moral perfection.   But beyond this a bifurcation takes place.   The Hindoo considers that victory over his imperfections entitles him to an honorable dismissal from conscience existence, while the western mind regards the attainment of perfection as a warrant for a blessed and endless consciousness of self.

It is easy to speculate as to the source of this divergence.   A difference in the strength of certain primary instincts, as that of pugnacity, may account for it.   But here again the Hindoo does not really stand so far apart from the western world as it seems.   Nirvana is described both as a state of unconsciousness and of incomparable bliss.   The practical significance of this contradiction is clear : the Yogin need not, and the average Yogin probably does not seek utter annihilation.   That   which   he   anticipates   is   really   cessation   of suffering and eternal, lethal enjoyment.   Is there a very important difference between this expectation and that of the Christian who seeks the joys of heaven ? Probably not. Let it be remembered in this connexion that the idea of the future life, as it is found among educated Christians, is so vague that nothing specific can be added to the descriptive expression " eternal blessedness."

The effectiveness of the Yoga methods.—The general consideration of the effectiveness of the methods of religious mysticism had better be postponed until after the study of its other forms. We may say here, however, that the final earthly condition of the faithful, uncompromising Yogin, as he appears to the unsophisticated observer, does not seem worthy of man's holiest endeavours. The emaciated, bewildered ascetic, reduced to the dimmest spark of life, equally incapable, for lack of energy, of committing good or evil, is not a demi-god but a shrunken caricature of what man ought to be—so at least does common sense pronounce. The Yogin, as also the user of drugs, may win partial or total unconsciousness and, with it, isolation and peace ; so much must be granted. But that this peace and isolation have the exalted significance attributed to them in the Yoga metaphysics, is quite another matter. We know in any case that he is much deceived in the magical powers he ascribes to himself. His self-deception, the corresponding self-deception of the user of drugs, and, as we shall see, of the classical Christian mystics, constitute one of the most pathetic chapters of human history. To aim so high and to fall so low is in truth both deep tragedy and high comedy. Yet the stupefied Yogin is one of the blundering heroes and martyrs that mark the slow progress of humanity.

We must not fail to remember, however, that those who make the final descent into unconsciousness are fortunately only a small fraction of the followers of Yoga. Most of them never reach that stage. Similarly the final round of the ladder of the Christian mystic is reached only by a few, while millions practise without realizing it, and much to the increase of their peace of mind and moral energy, the initial steps of meditation and contemplation.

Features common to Yoga and to the religious intoxication of the savage.—What features common to Yoga and to the religious intoxication of the savage justify their classification together under the name mysticism ? First of all, the avowed purpose in both is to transcend the limitations of the individual self and to achieve some sort of connexion with the Divine.

This common purpose corresponds to an essential similarity of that which actually takes place under the action of drugs and of

Yoga discipline.   Both achieve a reduction of mental activity that dissociates the individual from the world, and thus liberates him from the pain, distress and effort incident to ordinary life.   Thus, a temporary, if not a final deliverance from physical and moral evil is secured.   In both methods the reduction of mental activity may culminate in complete unconsciousness.

An impression of quickened life and of marvellous, unlimited powers, is also common to both.   It is true that in order to reach the goal set by Yoga (isolation of the self from the world and absorption in the All), it is not necesssary to secure these powers. The acquisition of magical or divine powers in order to control nature is obviously an alien, and, probably, an older element.   If it has remained in Yoga, it is because of the strong appeal it makes to human nature.

Belief in the acquisition of divine or magical knowledge is the last common trait we shall mention.   The idea of " unutterable " revelation that fills so large a place in Christian mysticism, is present both in Yoga and in the lower mysticism.   But it should be recognized that in these three forms of religious mysticism the emphasis is placed not upon knowledge as such but upon knowledge regarded as an instrument for the suppression or the enlargement of the self. This fact is often ignored by the philosopher of mysticism.

CHAPTER IV

CHRISTIAN MYSTICISM

HISTORICAL AND GENERAL REMARKS

THE successive forms of religious mysticism may be regarded as expressions of a gigantic experiential movement aiming at securing in diverse ways an ever fuller satisfaction of fundamental wants. Certain wants and methods conspicuous in the lower forms of mysticism disappear or are reduced to secondary position in the higher; other needs and other methods take their place. The passage from one form of mysticism to another is marked, furthermore, by changes in the conception of the power which is regarded as the cause of the experience.

*　　　*　　　*

Christian mysticism attained full maturity between the sixteenth and the seventeenth century with St John of the Cross, Santa Theresa, Molinos, Mme. Guyon and others. Contemporary Christian mysticism is best represented by the disciples of Fox, known as the Friends or Quakers.

The first formulation of a mystical philosophy and of a system of mystical practice is probably to be found in the sacred books of India. But these have had their own cruder antecedents, such as those considered in the chapter on mystical drug-ecstasy.

What relations have really existed between these antecedents and Christian mysticism, whether the torch passed from hand to hand, continuously from the savage to the Yogin, thence to Greece and to the Christian world ; or whether it was extinguished and rekindled, thus making one or several new starting points, is a very interesting question which it is not our intention to consider. We shall merely remark that, so far as practical Christian mysticism is concerned, there seem to have been present in the Christian attitude towards God and Christ, quite independently of the theories of the pseudo-Areopagite and of those who stood back of him, the elements necessary to its production. If it seems probable that Christian mysticism owes something of its philosophy to India through the intermediary of Greece and the neo-platonists, its practices may well be altogether original with Christianity. Theory and practice need not have had a common origin.

How far the Greek Mysteries may be regarded as mystical in the sense in which we take that term, is an open question. Rhode expresses the extreme negative position when he declares that "*in das Land der Mystik wiesen die Mysterien nicht den Weg*[1]." Others have emphasized the significance of an alleged sacramental meal in which the worshipper, by eating or drinking a divine substance, became of one flesh and blood with the deity. If such a communion as this was really a part of the Eleusinian mysteries, then they certainly included the fundamental mystical purpose. But Farnell and others do not find sufficient evidence of the presence of a communion meal. Nevertheless, Farnell, as well as Foucart, sees in the mysteries aspirations and methods of worship calculated to induce "at least the feeling of intimacy and friendship with the divinity[2]." In Cretan mythology, Farnell finds "glimpses of a communion service in which the mortal was absorbed into the divine nature by the simulated fiction of a holy marriage ; a mystery much enacted by the late Cybele-ritual, which we may believe descended collaterally from a Minoan source[3]." Jane Harrison holds that the cardinal doctrine of Orphic religion was "the possibility of attaining divine life[4]." Immortality was a corollary of that belief.

In any case, whatever may be regarded as mystical in their mysteries, the Greeks placed the emphasis upon a transformation such as would make the worshipper immortal, whereas the Christian mystic sought not primarily immortality but union with God—a union which brings with it immortality, together with everything else that is desirable.

The worship of the Olympian divinities was not at all mystical. The orthodox anthropomorphic religion of Greece "never stated in doctrine, never implied in ritual, that man could become God. Nay more, against any such aspiration it raised again and again a

---

[1] E. Rhode, *Psyche*, vol. I, p. 293. We have already had occasion to quote Rhode's description of the Thracian worship of Dionysus. It brings clearly to light a well marked striving towards deliverance from the limitations of ordinary existence and the attainment of a superhuman state involving an obscuration if not a loss of self-consciousness and at least an approach to divinity.

[2]. Farnell, *Cults of the Greek States*, vol. III, p. 197. Comp. M. P. Foucart, *Recherches sur l'Origine et la Nature des Mystères d'Eleusis, Mémoirs de l'Institut National de France*, Tome XXXV, Part II, p. 52.

[3] Farnell, *The Higher Aspects of Greek Religion*, p. 10.

[4] Jane Harrison, *Prolegomena to the Study of Greek Religion*, Cambridge, 1903, p. 478. See also pp. 571-601.

passionate protest[1]." Taken all in all, it is evident that mysticism played an inconspicuous rôle in the religious life of the Hellenes. The Greek genius loved clearness and self-possession too well to seek the divine in mystical darkness and self-surrender.

In any attempt to trace, however sketchily, the historical connexions of Christian mysticism, the ancient Persian mysticism and its more recent Mohammedan form, so understandingly described by Nicholson[2], should be at least mentioned. With regard to the means of realizing the absorption of the self into the All, Sufism places more reliance than Yoga upon the drug method (wine intoxication) and upon violent rhythmic movements ; this is true at least of the more popular form of Persian mysticism.

The earliest powerful mystical influence within Christianity, after that of Christ himself, is found in the Pauline and the Johannine writings. The mystical character of St Paul's religious experience and teaching is not always sufficiently recognized. His Christian career began with a sudden conversion attended by visions and auditions. He was taken up into the "third heaven," and heard "unspeakable words which it is not lawful for man to utter[3]"; and he spoke frequently with tongues (glossolalia). The Christian life was for him the life of Christ in man. Surely these experiences are of a mystical nature[4].

After the apostolic writings, the most influential events in the history of Christian mysticism were probably the prophetic movement initiated by Montanus (about A.D. 156), and the publication of the *Mystical Theology* of Dionysius the Areopagite (about A.D. 460). Montanus and his followers spoke while in ecstasy, thus distinguishing themselves from the orthodox Christian prophets who communicated their message when they had returned to their senses. The ecstasy of Montanus is said to have been deliberately induced, but we do not know in what way. He regarded himself as a passive instrument, a lyre upon which played the divine plectrum. The prophecies were usually delivered in great excitement and often in an unknown " tongue."

Two features of this movement are of interest to us : the idea of a God communicating himself through the passive instrumentality of the prophet who became the mouth-piece of the Divinity ; and

---

[1] *Ibid.*, p. 477.

[2] Reynold A. Nicholson, *The Mystics of Islam*, London, G. Bell & Sons, 1914.

[3] 2 Cor., xii., 1-4.

[4] The mystical character of Paul's teaching appears in expressions such as these: " He that is joined unto the Lord is one Spirit with Him." (1 Cor. vi. 17); " You are the body of Christ " (1 Cor. xii., 27).

the presence of ecstasy, that is, of an extraordinary rapturous condition involving obscuration or total disappearance of self-consciousness. It hardly need be added that there was nothing essentially new in these two features of Montanism. But as they occurred here within the Christian Church and with striking intensity, their influence upon the Church was very considerable.

Whoever the author of the *Mystical Theology* may have been, it is generally agreed that the treatise was written not earlier than the year 460, and that the Christian doctrine of mysticism is traceable to it. It should be observed that this contribution of Greek thought to mysticism is mainly theoretical. Sharpe, a translator of that treatise, characterizes it as " a kind of grammar of mysticism in which principles alone are formulated, disengaged from the experience and argumentation through which they have evolved[1]."

The substance of the treatise is contained in the following paragraphs :—

" They who are free and untrammelled by all that is seen and all that sees enter into the true mystical darkness of ignorance, whence all perception of understanding is excluded, and abide in that which is intangible and invisible, being wholly absorbed in Him who is beyond all things, and belong no more to any, neither to themselves nor to another, but are united in their higher part to Him who is wholly unintelligible, and whom by understanding nothing, they understand after a manner above all intelligence."

" He is neither one nor unity, nor divinity, nor goodness ; nor is He spirit, as we understand spirit ; He is neither sonship nor fatherhood nor anything else known to us or to any other being, either of the things that are or the things that are not ; nor does anything that is, know Him as He is, nor does He know anything that is as it is. He has neither word nor name nor knowledge ; He is neither darkness nor light nor truth nor error ; He can neither be affirmed nor denied; nay, though we may affirm or deny the things that are beneath Him, we can neither affirm nor deny Him ; for the perfect and sole cause of all is above all affirmation, and that which transcends all is above all affirmation, absolutely separate, and beyond all that is[2]."

---

[1] A. B. Sharpe, *Mysticism : its true Meaning and Value*, London, Sands and Co., 1910, p. 57. Nevertheless, one finds in it such practical directions as the following : " And thou, dear Timothy, in thy intent practice of the mystical contemplations, leave behind both thy senses and thy intellectual operations, and all things known by sense and intellect, and all things which are not and which are, and set thyself, as far as may be, to unite thyself in unknowing with Him who is above all being and knowledge."—*Mystical Theology*, I.

[2] *Ibid.*, pp. 212, 222-3.

The Neo-Platonic influence under which the *Mystical Theology* was written, is revealed best of all, perhaps, in a classical passage of Plotinus, part of which we transcribe: "Now often I am roused from the body to my true self, and emerge from all else and enter myself, and behold a marvellous beauty, and am particularly persuaded at the time that I belong to a better sphere, and live a supremely good life, and become identical with the godhead, and fast fixed therein attain its divine activity, having reached a plane above the whole intelligible realm; and then . . . I descend to the plane of discursive thought. And after I have descended I am at a loss to know how it is that I have done so, and how my soul has entered into my body, in view of the fact that she really is as her inmost nature was revealed, and yet is in the body[1]." To what extent the Neo-Platonic philosophy originated among Hellenes, we do not know; but analogies between the theology of the Areopagite and Hindoo metaphysics are extensive and profound.

The Neo-Platonists doctrine of the nature of God and man was in part derived from ecstatic experiences, nowhere in their writings described with sufficient objectivity. This doctrine, transmitted mainly through the pseudo-Dionysius, exerted upon Christian theology down to the modern period an influence usually regarded as overmastering[2]. In this ancient speculative doctrine, we have but a secondary interest. The first object of this book is the mystical experience itself—an experience which, in Christian practice, is substantially independent of Neo-Platonic teaching. We have just seen that long before the influence of Neo-Platonism could have been felt, ecstatic raptures, mystically interpreted, *i.e.* regarded as union with the divine, existed in Christianity. St Paul and the Montanists were familiar with them and they continued to appear throughout the centuries in virtue of tendencies and of beliefs proper to Christianity. They are the outcome of strivings not chiefly to understand, but rather to enjoy the blessings of the best and fullest life conceivable: the divine life. The completion of our analytical work should place us in a position to pass judgment upon the theories

---

[1] *Enneads*, Fourth and Sixth Books, as quoted in Professor Bakewell's *Source Book in Ancient Philosophy*, p. 386. See also pp. 389-92.

[2] A. Harnack, *History of Dogma*, vol. I. p. 361. "As the writings of this pseudo-Dionysius were regarded as those of Dionysius, the disciple of the Apostle, the scholastic mysticism which they taught was regarded as apostolic, almost as a divine science. The importance which these writings obtained first in the East, then from the ninth to the twelfth century also in the West, cannot be too highly estimated. It is impossible to explain them here. This much only may be said, that the mystical and pietistic devotion of to-day, even in the Protestant Church, draws its nourishment from writings whose connexion with those of the pseudo-Areopagite can still be traced through its various intermediate stages."

derived by the ancients and by the Christian theologians from mystical experiences.

*   *   *

An adequate history of the development of Christian mystical worship from its early beginning to its culmination in the sixteenth and seventeenth centuries, has not yet been written. That task is not ours ; we shall merely jot down a few notes on some of the most salient features of that history. Grand mysticism may be said to have begun in Christianity with the raptures of St Paul and the writings of the Johannine Gospel[1]. Montanus and his followers would provide material for an interesting chapter. About St Augustine little could be said that would contribute anything definite to that history. In one of his last recorded conversations with his mother, he seems to have indulged in the dream of a mystical experience such as has actually come to others : " If the tumult of the flesh were hushed, hushed the images of earth and waters and air, yea the very soul be hushed to herself, hushed all dreams and imaginary revelations, every tongue and every sign ; and He alone speak, not through any tongue of flesh nor angel's voice, that we may hear His very Self without these ;—were not this Enter into thy Master's joy ?[2]"

Hugo of St Victor (1097-1141), sometimes called the " real founder of medieval mysticism," describes the ascent of the soul to God in three stages, *Cogitatio, Meditatio, Contemplatio ;* and this is, so far as we know, the earliest attempt at a systematization of the mystical progress of the soul.

By Bernard of Clairvaux (1091-1153), religion at its best is conceived as a love union. His mysticism appears in lurid colours in the famous interpretation of the Canticles where terms of earthly passion are used without restraint to depict the relation of the human soul to God.

Although St Francis of Assisi (1182-1226) has left no formal description of mystical states, we know that he spent long periods in prayer during which he seemed as in a trance. Not long before his death he withdrew for quiet and contemplation on a mountain, the Verna, in the upper valley of the Arno, as he had already done many a time. Now he desired to prepare himself for death, and he begged his companions to protect him from all intrusion. " His

---

[1] The religious life of Jesus was certainly of a mystical character ; and it included most probably great mystical experiences. The records are, however, not such as can be used by a psychologist.

[2] *Confessions*, Book IX, abbreviated.

days went by divided between exercises of piety in the humble sanctuary on the mountain top and meditation in the depth of the forest. It even happened to him to forget the services and to remain several days alone in some cave of the rock, going over in his heart the memories of Golgotha." As the day of the Elevation of the Holy Cross drew near, Francis "doubled his fastings and prayers, 'quite transformed into Jesus by love and compassion,' says one of the legends. He passed the night before the festival alone in pfayer, not far from the hermitage. In the morning he had a ' vision . . . When the vision disappeared, he felt sharp sufferings mingling with the ecstasy of the first moments. Stirred to the very depths of his being, he was anxiously seeking the meaning of it all, when he perceived upon his body the stigmata of the Crucified[1]." Thus does Paul Sabatier relate the famous incident of the stigmata.

In the situation described above, the essential conditions, psychological and physiological, for the production of a love-trance with accompaniment of visions, etc., seem all present. An eager, sensitive soul, athirst for intimate companionship with the God of Love, weakened by fasting and in the habit of remaining long in silent contemplation before his Lord, might be expected, even without any other tradition back of him than that derived from the New Testament, to fall into ecstatic trances.

With Catherine of Genoa (1347-80) and St John of the Cross (1542-91) we are far advanced on the high road of the great classical tradition, which came to full fruition in Santa Theresa (1515-82), Molinos (died 1697), and Mme Guyon (1648-1717). After these, one meets only with less wonderful types ; and, in so far at least as the general public is informed, the great Latin tradition soon comes to an end. Whatever similar prodigies of the grace of God may exist at the present time, are hidden from the knowledge of the world[2].

The Latin tradition is by far the most spectacular ; it produced what may be called the Grand Mysticism. But England also has had its mystical current. There, however, it ran thin. Richard Rolle of Hampole (died 1349) and his followers[3], chief among whom is Walter Hilton, are the main English mystics until much later when

---

[1] *Life of St. Francis of Assisi*, London, 1894, pp. 295-96.

[2] Flournoy mentions the *Diary of Sister Gertrude-Marie* (1870-1908), published by the Abbey S. Legueu, under the title, *Une Mystique de nos jours*, Angers, Community of St Charles, s.d. pp. xxii+710.

[3] See, for an account of Richard Rolle, *An English Father of the Church and his followers*, edited by C. Hartsman and published as vol. I, of the Library of Early English Writers, etc., 1895.

we come to something different in George Fox and the Friends. Fox is to be regarded not as a continuator of the medieval mysticism represented by the preceding names, but as a relatively new departure. One wishing to know Christian mysticism at its sanest and in its most fruitful form must turn to the tradition of the Friends.

The German strand, with Boehme, Eckhart, Tauler, Suzo, etc., differed from the Latin in being more philosophical[1]. These German mystics were essentially, especially Boehme and Eckhart, speculative minds who preferred to philosophize upon their experiences rather than to foster and carefully describe them.

Within, as well as among these several groups—Latin, English, and German—there were communications; so that the degree of originality of any particular individual is very difficult to establish. Catherine of Genoa was in relation with the Franciscans; François de Osuna and St John of the Cross were teachers of Santa Theresa, and Mme Guyon learned from François de Sales and Mme de Chantal. Molinos who inspired Mme Guyon quotes letters from Santa Theresa and from Mme de Chantal, the spiritual daughter of François de Sales. The torch passed from hand to hand among the Latin mystics. Between the groups the relation is less close; how close, we are not in a position to tell. But this seems incontestable, that wherever there existed a man of the temperament of Francis of Assisi, believing devotedly in the Christian God of love, and in possession of the teachings of St Paul and of the Fourth Gospel, there the essential requirements for the production of ecstasy, mystically interpreted, were fulfilled. A frequent realization of these conditions would explain a frequent spontaneous production throughout Christendom of the core-phenomenon of Grand Mysticism. Much less independence can be expected with respect to the finer elaborations of the Journey of the Soul to God[2].

*   *   *

There are few topics with a literature so vast and elaborate as that of mysticism where the facts which are its occasion have been so persistently slighted. Apart from a few recent publications, there is hardly anything in that voluminous production deserving of the attention of those who wish to know the truth; it is a literature of propaganda and of edification. The basal facts are presented in a

[1] On German speculative mysticism, see, H. Delacroix, *Essai sur le mysticisme spéculatif en Allemagne au XIVème siecle*, Paris, 1899.

[2] On the question of independence, of originality, and of the influence of theories, see Delacroix, *Etudes d'Histoire et de Psychologie du Mysticisme*, pp. 76-80; 345 ff.

fragmentary way and inaccurately, for the purpose of illustrating traditional views or for the solace of afflicted souls. No correct understanding of mysticism may be expected unless it be based upon a detailed and careful study of the mystical experiences. We shall, therefore, introduce the reader to Christian mysticism by means of somewhat detailed accounts of the lives of several of its great exponents : Suzo, St Catherine of Genoa, Santa Theresa, Mme Guyon and St Marguerite Marie. These accounts will not seem unnecessarily circumstantial to those who really care to understand mysticism. We shall then be prepared to consider separately the more important problems of mysticism. In that connexion we shall find occasion to draw confirming as well as new information from a considerable number of mystics other than those just named,—in particular from a protestant, contemporary mystic. Chapters on the Motives and on the Methods of Christian mysticism will be followed by a comparative study of ecstatic trances, within and without religion. The documentary foundation of this study will thus be much broadened. We shall then try to give a psychological account of the beliefs and of the effects of the beliefs connected with ecstatic trance and, in particular, of the beliefs in divine Presence, in divine Union, and in Illumination or Revelation. The two last chapters will be concerned respectively with philosophical implications of mysticism and with practical considerations.

The mystics named above have been chosen for intensive analysis for two reasons : their experiences have been described with a degree of fulness that meets the minimum requirements of a psychological investigation, and they constitute the culmination of a great historical movement and represent Christian mysticism in its most elaborate form.

Against this second reason, protesting voices may be raised. These mystics, it may be said, are not the most worthy of admiration. They are rather extravagant instances, all or most of whom suffered from some form of nervous instability, if not hysteria. This affirmation may not be contradicted ; but it does not constitute a valid argument against the choice of these persons by the psychologist. Why should he concern himself only with the physiologically and psychologically ordinary ? Much rather should he follow the example of the physiologist when, in order to discover the normal workings of the human body, he studies abnormal conditions. Disease, more possibly than health itself, has taught us the nature of the normal processes. Similarly with regard to the mind. The most significant advance in recent psychology is seen, according to William James, in the new conceptions regarding the so-called subconscious.

These, we owe to the investigation of unusual and abnormal mental phenomena. More recently still, important knowledge regarding "suppression" and the active processes of forgetting—knowledge with which the name of Freud is closely associated—has been obtained chiefly again as a result of observations of disorders of behaviour. That which is inconspicuous in a normal organism, attracts attention when it functions in an unusual way. Moreover, the mystics who have given to mysticism its lustre are no other than the extravagant persons we have chosen. *They*, more than any others, have given to Christian mysticism its classic form and they are, as a matter of fact, recognized by either the Roman or the Protestant Church or by both, as true and great mystics.

If these conspicuous mystics stood apart, disconnected from the ordinary Christian worshippers, they would still deserve the attention of the psychologist. But, however extravagant they may be, they express needs and aspirations present in the rank and file of worshippers. The impulses and purposes of ordinary worship are at the root of the behaviour of the great mystics : ordinary communion with God constitutes, as we shall see, the first step on the way to ecstasy. However physiologically unusual and mentally extravagant these wonders of the grace of God may be, the psychologist interested in the understanding of religious life cannot do otherwise than regard them as a most promising source of information.

The significance of this book to the reader will depend largely upon his recognition of the connexion of grand mysticism with the most vital part of ordinary Christian worship. We shall, therefore, indicate briefly that connexion.

When writing upon the higher religions, most authors disregard the manifestations of purely objective religion. They seem to them too insignificant to be taken into account, and so they say of mysticism that it is the very essence of all religion. Although we have found reason to criticize that opinion, we also regard the mystical tendency as characteristic of whatever is best and most vital in religion, and we realize that, among the civilized, objective intercourse with God usually becomes a yearning of the soul for contact with, or participation in, the divine Power and Goodness. This tendency appears with incontrovertible evidence in the forms assumed by Christian prayer. The begging, bargaining, and intercessory prayer occupies clearly a large part even of Christian worship, and yet most writers on Christian prayer almost disregard that form of prayer. They disregard it because it seems to them an inferior kind of prayer and because, as a matter of fact, among educated Christians the first movement of the pious soul on entering a church or in private devotion is to turn away from the complexities of the militant life in order to withdraw within herself, there to hear the voice of God and to feel His loving presence.

In the opinion of enlightened Protestantism, prayer is "the movement of the soul putting itself into personal relation and contact with the mysterious power whose presence it feels[1]." We may, therefore, say with Joseph Maréchal, professor of theology at the Institut Catholique, that "inner devotion, sustained by ritual forms or by vocal prayer, may therefore be considered as a first step on the road to mystical union[2]."

Ordinary prayer, as defined by Protestant and Roman Catholic theologians alike, and the relation with God characteristic of grand mysticism, represent the limits between which move the more vital—the mystical—Christian worship. If, then, most of the ordinary worship is a rudimentary mysticism, much that is to be said of the higher degrees of mysticism finds application to the form of ordinary worship dominant in Christianity[3]. This must now be borne in mind as we proceed to the study of striking instances of the mystical life.

*   *   *

Opinions are strangely at odds as to the social value of the mystics. In 1902, I wrote : "Until recently the few scientists who had cast a more or less disdainful glance upon them, had noted little more than ecstasies, visions, catalepsies, extravagant penances, and they had imagined that the word 'hysteria' explained everything. I do not hesitate to say that despite the naïveté of their admiration, the Christian believers have come nearer a just appreciation of mystical life than the materialistic scientists[4]." During the twenty years that have elapsed since these words were written, the scientific interest in religious mysticism has grown apace and with it a discriminating appreciation of its significance. Professor Royce's high praise would need but a little toning down to express my own opinion : "As a religious teacher he (the mystic) is inspiring, first of all, just because

[1] Auguste Sabatier, *Outlines of a Philosophy of Religion based on Psychology and History*,   New York, J. Pott & Co., 1902, p. 28.   "When in prayer the soul tends to pass into its Master," writes J. Second in *La Prière, Etude de Psychologie Religieuse*, Alcan, 1911, p. 40.

[2] Joseph Maréchal, S. J., *Rev. Philos.*, 1912, vol. XXI, p. 427.

[3] In chapters XV and XVI of the *Religious Consciousness*, Pratt discusses and demonstrates the connexion between ordinary worship and grand mysticism.

[4] From my essay in the *Revue Philosophique*, 1902, Tome IV, p. 1.

he appeals to your own individuality. He breathes the common spirit of all the higher religions when he conceives your goal as an inner salvation, and your search for truth as essentially a practical effort to win personal perfection. It is no wonder then that the mystics have been the spiritual counsellors of humanity." "Mysticism has been the ferment of the faiths, the forerunner of spiritual liberty, the inaccessible refuge of the nobler heretics, the inspirer, through poetry, of countless youth who knew no metaphysics, the comforter of those who are weary of finitude. It has determined, directly or indirectly, more than half the technical theology of the Church[1]."

If there is still in certain quarters a surprising inability to appreciate the profound significance of Christian mysticism, there is in others an equally great lack of discrimination as to who and what among the mystics deserve respect and admiration. It is unfortunate for instance, that a Marguerite Marie Alacoque should have been set up before men as an object of special reverence. And it is also regrettable that it has become a widespread habit to speak of the mystic as of one " in touch with the absolute and eternal," one who " has passed out of the finite into the infinite world," and the like, *ad nauseam*. These expressions do not add anything to our understanding of mysticism, and they betray too clearly a propensity to melodrama and grandiloquence.

*   *   *

As this is not an historical treatise, we shall report little more than the events that may bear upon our psychological problems. Except for the placing of Mme Guyon before St Theresa, we shall take up our instances in chronological order. This inversion is useful for purposes of exposition. Because the documents referring to Mme Guyon and St Theresa are much fuller than those referring to the others, these two will be discussed at greater length. It would be far wiser for the reader to omit altogether the other cases and examine carefully these two, than to skim through all of them ; nothing of great consequence would be missed by following that procedure.

A warning should be added regarding a trait common in different degrees to all our great mystics. Their writings are marred by an inexactness approaching at times deliberate falsehood. This defect is due in the first instance to a strong natural tendency to exaggeration, intensified by hortatory and theoretical purposes. They do not

[1] J. Royce, *The World and the Individual*, pp. 85, 190-1.

write carefully and exactly in the sense in which a scientifically trained person understands these terms. Inaccuracy was facilitated by the long lapse of years which, in most instances, separated the event related from the date of the record.

HEINRICH SUZO[1] (1300-66)

The great mystical tradition of which Germany can boast, is more speculative than practical. Eckhart and Boehme, in particular, prefer to discant upon metaphysical questions rather than to dwell descriptively upon the mystical experience and its practical value. In any case, that which is known about these two philosophers is quite insufficient for the purpose of this investigation. The autobiographical account of Suzo, fragmentary and without chronological order though it is, comes nearer to satisfying our requirements.

Suzo was born in 1300 or a little earlier, on the shores of Lake Constance, in Suabia. Both his father and his mother belonged to the lower nobility. The mother was familiar with religious love-trances and seems to have possessed all the traits that go to the making of a remarkable mystic. The opposition of the father, a child of this world as Suzo describes him, deprived her of any chance which she might otherwise have had to achieve such distinction. The son inherited his mother's delicate and romantic sensibility. He was, moreover, very early introduced by her to devotional religion. At the age of thirteen, he entered the schools of the Dominican Order and was for a time under the direct influence of Meister Eckhart. Nevertheless, until the age of eighteen, his development had been commonplace enough. The adolescent was not at peace with himself and seems not to have known why. Life did not satisfy him. At that age a sudden enlightment marked a step forward in his development. He realized that the main cause of his disquiet was his lovelessness[2]. Suzo was one of those tender creatures whose only reason for existence seems to be to love and be loved.

In entering the Dominican Order he had had to give up the love of woman. He discovered soon that he had to give up his male companions also, for they found pleasure in things forbidden by his conscience. The loneliness of the life-prospect opening before him frightened him. But the Church offers a substitute for earthly love: an incomparable, divine love. The young man resolved to make a trial of it. " See," said he to himself, " whether this great Mistress of whom you hear such wonders would not become your love ; for a young and an unsteady heart can hardly remain long without a personal love " (IV)[1]. For a space of time, exactly how long we do not know, that thought haunted him. At last the day came when he found the heavenly bride. " Then entered into his soul the original source of all good. In it he found everything that is spiritually beautiful, lovable, and desirable." " Should I be," he continues, " the husband of a queen, my soul would find pride in it ; but, now, you are the Empress of my heart, the bestower of all gifts. In you I possess riches enough and all the power that I want. I care no longer for the treasures of earth " (IV).

Thus, Suzo discovered experientially the love of God, and found in it the substitute without which religious life would have been an unacceptable martyrdom. " *Ewige Weisheit*," is the name he gives to his divine love. In his vivid imagination, the Eternal Wisdom is incarnated, according to circumstances, in Jesus or in any saint, but preferably in the Virgin, young and beautiful. Having discovered a way of satisfying his burning heart, Suzo's life enters into a new phase. Temptations still continue to plague him, but he has found his way ; he knows by the strongest of all testimony that he belongs to heaven.

We shall not insist here upon the warmth and intimacy of Suzo's love-relation with the feminine *Ewige Weisheit*. We may, however, transcribe a passage that sets forth in a charming way the knightly nature of his early attachment to his divine Mistress. In his country, there is, he tells us, an old custom. At the beginning of the new year young men go out at night to sing and to recite poetry to their beloved, and the favoured ones receive crowns from them. One year, as Suzo heard the singing of the young men, " His loving heart was so moved that before day-break he[2] went before the image of the pure mother with her tender babe pressed against her heart, knelt and sang silently and sweetly in his soul. He praised her for beauty, nobility, virtue, tenderness, and freedom never without dignity, in which she surpassed all virgins of the world." He told her, " You are the love whom alone my heart loves ; for you I have spurned all earthly love. Therefore, beloved of my heart, let me enjoy thy love and let me to-day receive a crown from thee " (X).

Few Christian mystics have equalled Suzo in the cruel severity and the duration of the torments which he inflicted upon himself. One could wish this tender soul might have been spared the repulsive

---

[1] The Roman numbers in parenthesis after the quotations, refer to the chapters from which they are taken.

[2] Suzo wrote his *Autobiography* in the third person.

pains of extreme asceticism. But the destruction, by torturing the body, of the evil tendencies of the flesh and of the pride of the spirit was an established tradition. By him, as by others, voluntary suffering was regarded in addition as expiation for sin and as visible token of utter devotion to God.

The twenty years during which Suzo persisted, despite the opposition of those about him, in an extravagant ascetism, constitute a period characterized by heroic strivings toward entire inner unification. During a part of that time ecstasies were very frequent. We are told that during ten years they occured as often as twice a day ; they served to sustain and encourage him. Exaltation was not, however, continuous ; it was broken by discouraging moments of " dryness."

The time came at last when the bleeding saint realized that he could not continue. " He was so wasted that his only choice was between dying and giving up those practices." God showed him that asceticism had served as a good beginning, but that now the divine work of sanctification was to continue in another way. Thereupon he threw all his instruments of torture into a stream (XX).

This deliverance marks the end of a period of absorption in himself—" introversion," as the Freudians say—and the beginning of an external activity that lasted to the end of his life. Until then he had refused contact with the World; the walls of the monastery had been his boundaries. Now, he undertook, in the measure of his strength to bring the World to God. From this moment we find him ever in action, on pilgrimages, on errants of mercy, founding monasteries, etc.

In each one of our great Christian mystics we shall note a similar period of inner preparation or introversion, marked usually by severe asceticism, followed by vigorous external activity. It is a fact explicable on the same general principle as the passage from a period of preparation to one of productivity in other individuals. Suzo had achieved to a considerable extent the conquest of the natural man. He was weary of needless self-examination, weary of self-inflicted crosses ; they seemed to have done all they could for him ; his apprenticeship was over. Under these circumstances it is natural that the call to work in the vineyard of the Lord should have rung louder and louder. Yet, after twenty years of cloistered life, he shrank from affronting the World in the quality of messenger of the Lord. A vision encouraged him. He saw a page bringing him a complete accoutrement of knight. The page addressed him thus : "Until now, you have been a servant (*Knecht*) ; from this moment God wants you to be a knight " (XXII).

Suzo differed from certain mystics in that he regarded his active life not merely as a harvesting time, but also as a means of completing his own sanctification (*Gelassenheit*). In the monastery he had been protected as a delicate flower in a hothouse. No wonder that his timid, modest nature shrank in the presence of the World. Would he be able to bear the new scourges that awaited him : ingratitude, deception, calumny, hatred ? These torments would be much more grievous than those he had been in the habit of inflicting upon himself. Would his fortitude be equal to them ? He sought to prepare himself for the ordeal; the ideal of total self-surrender (*Gelassenheit*) developed in his mind[1]. He had to learn not only not to be jealous, not to think evil of others ; but also to bear meekly jealously and calumny. The natural man must die altogether and God alone must live in him.

Poor Suzo's anticipation of calumny was only too completely realized. It may be left to the reader to conjecture the malignity of the accusations that were likely to fall upon a missionary received with open arms in women's monasteries. The success of this poetical and tender soul discoursing upon divine love in terms of human passion, is easy to conceive. But he seems to have come out of every storm unspotted and triumphant.

In this connexion should be noted the presence in his life, as in that of most other great mystics, of an intimate friend of the opposite sex. Elisabeth Staglin, his spiritual daughter, as he calls her, assumed without his knowledge the task of recording his doings and sayings. On hearing of the existence of her manuscript, he commanded her to hand it over to him and burned it. Fortunately she had kept back a portion of it. Later on, Suzo came into possession of that remainder also and used it to prepare the *Life*.

In many passages of that book and of the *Büchlein*, there is evidence of a tendency to ascribe to the final condition of the servant of God characteristics that belong only to the moments of ecstasy and automatism. This is an obvious confusion. The expression, " Total surrender of the self to God," when it refers to Suzo's active life, means something quite different from what it means when used in the description of trance or semi-trance states. And the statement, " nothing is left for man to do of himself, he acts automatically," is literally true not of the final condition of the mystics but only of their brief moments of partial or total loss of self-consciousness and of automatism. Final remarks as to this confusion will be

[1] On self-surrender and passivity, see *Von innerlichen Gelassenheit*, vol. III, pp. 525, 551.

added when we have seen how widespread it is. Here we wish merely to observe that, as Suzo proceeds on his missionary errands, he is obviously in full possession of his critical powers and consciously self-determined—even though he seeks to act in accordance with God's will. His own account of his dealings with the people he meets does not bear any other interpretation.

We have also to remark that St Theresa's elaborate system of gradually developing mystical states, forming a hierarchy, does not apply to Suzo's, nor, as we shall see, to most other mystics. Almost from the first he enjoyed ecstasies which she would have classed at or near the top of her " Ladder of Love," this one, for instance : " It happened that at the beginning (of his converted life), on the day of St Agnes, he went in the choir immediately after the noon meal. He was alone. At that time his trials were particularly heavy to bear. As he was there, comfortless and lonely, his soul was ravished in his body or out of it. Then he saw and heard what no tongue can utter. It was without form or mode of existence, and yet it held all the joy that all existing creatures can hold. His heart was at once yearning and satisfied. He stood transfixed, lost to himself and to all things. Was it day or night ? He did not know. It was an expression of the sweetness of eternal life in silence and peace. He said then, ' if this is not heaven, I do not know what is heaven.' This state must have lasted one hour or a half hour. Whether the soul remained in the body or was separated from it, he did not know. During that short time his body suffered so much that he thought that no man, unless at death, could suffer as much. He came to himself heaving deep sighs and his body sank to earth helpless, like a man who faints " (III). The impression made by this ecstasy was deep and lasting. For a while afterwards he felt as if floating in mid-air ; and, for a long time, there remained "a heavenly taste that made him yearn for God[1]."

Suzo seems to have been familiar with the whole range of the phenomena of Grand Mysticism, not excepting long periods of semi-somnambulism[2] : We have already mentioned moments of discouragement, depression, and barrenness. He was frequently

---

[1] This and similar experiences will be discussed in the sections treating of ecstasy.

[2] The following passage may be interpreted as indicating long periods of semi-somnambulism. " It happened that a great change would come over him, lasting about ten weeks, more or less. Whether in the presence of strangers or in their absence, his senses would lose their natural powers so that everywhere and in everything he could hear only the One and see all things in the One, without any multiplicity or diversity."—*Von innerlichen Gelassenheit*, p. 536.

encouraged and directed by automatisms, mainly visual. A possible aptitude for visual imagery was probably improved by his habit of withdrawing each day to his oratory for rest and meditation. Somnolence would frequently take place and with it hypnagogic hallucinations. Brilliant lights, in his case as in that of others, constituted a striking and frequent characteristic of the visions[1]. He would often come to himself with the conviction that divine secrets had been revealed to him, even though he was not able to give them verbal expression. Once, for instance, "it was somehow shown him in a way that cannot be expressed in words, how God has made angels each different from the others in its nature[2]." He was familiar not only with sensory hallucinations but with those they call "intellectual." With regard to these he speaks, as others do, of an "immediate" view or apprehension (*Schauen*) of the divinity, and thinks that, the less imagery in these experiences, the higher they are and the nearer to absolute reality is the knowledge they impart[3].

*   *   *

Can any periodicity, significant with regard to religious progress, be detected in Suzo's life ? There are prolonged phases of depression and inefficiency, and phases of exaltation and productive activity, and shorter moments of depression (dryness) are interspersed throughout his life, but there is no true periodicity.

For a while, at the beginning, he identified his self both with the worldly and with the godward tendencies. But soon the former were regarded as alien to his self. The remainder of Suzo's earthly journey became a struggle, with the help of ascetic practices, of missionary activities, and of the mystical method of worship, to destroy these disowned tendencies. He was less dependent than other mystics upon external events.

Of his final condition, regarded from a religio-ethical point of view, it may be said that he rose near the top of the class of mystics under study.

---

[1] For instance, the vision recorded in chap. V, p. 28.

[2] *Leben*, chap. XXXVI, p. 149. This is taught by Thomas Aquinas.

[3] In *Leben*, chap. LIV, p. 277, he indicates thus the difference between visions that are pure truth and those that are not : " Contemplation without means (*mittelloses Schauen*) is contemplation of bare divinity and is, without doubt, pure truth ; and the more intellectual a vision is, the more free from images, the nearer it comes to bare contemplation (*bloses Schauen*), the nobler it is."

CATHERINE OF GENOA[1] (1447-1510)

1. *Biographical.*—Catherine Fiesca was born in Genoa in 1447. The Fieschi were the greatest of the great Guelph families of that town. At Catherine's birth, the Fieschi were at the height of their power and splendour. One of her cousins was a Cardinal, and her own father was Viceroy of Naples to King René of Anjou. She was the youngest of five children. " The beautiful, tall figure ; the noble oval face with its lofty brow, finely formed nose, and powerful, indeed obstinate chin ; the winning countenance with its delicate complexion and curling, sensitive, spiritual mouth-line ; deep grey-blue, spiritual eyes ; still more the quickly and intensely impression-able, nervous and extremely tense and active physical and psychical organization ;—all these things we are not merely told, we can still see them and find them, in part, even in her remains, but more fully in her portrait, and above all, in her numerous authentic utterances."

Nothing certain has come down to us concerning her life before the age of thirteen, but between thirteen and sixteen she is known to have been drawn very deeply to the conventual life as she saw it exemplified in her own sister, a Canoness of an Augustinian convent. Before her desire to enter the convent could be realized, her father had died and " a particular combination from amongst the endless political rivalries and intrigues of Genoa soon closed in upon the beautiful girl." She was sacrificed in marriage for a political purpose

---

[1] In this biographical sketch I have relied entirely upon a piece of historical research to all appearances thorough and judicious, *The Mystical Element of Religion as Studied in Saint Catherine of Genoa and her Friends*, by Baron Friedrich von Hugel, London, Dent & Co., 1909, 2 vols.

The biographies of St Catherine and the editions of her works are all derived from the *Vita e Dottrina*, published in Genoa in 1551. " The *Vita* is in its fundamental portions," says von Hugel, " the joint production of her devoted disciples, Cattaneo Marabotto, a secular priest, her confessor, and of Ettore Vernazza, a lawyer, her spiritual son. Its fifty-two chapters are only in small part narrative ; quite thirty-five of them are filled with discourses and con-templations of the Saint, evidently in the simpler of the many parallel versions accumulated here, taken down, at the time of the Saint's communication of them, with quite remarkable fidelity."

If I follow von Hugel, rather than assume myself the task of the historian, it is because of material difficulties, of lack of time, and of the belief that none of the main conclusions is dependent upon the kind of rectification which might conceivably follow a careful reconsideration of the *Vita*. The historical crit-icism seems to have been done by von Hugel with much care and a degree of discrimination unusual in one sympathising so fully as he does with the super-natural interpretation of mysticism. He is familiar enough with the symptoms of certain nervous disorders to discount the naïve admiration of Catherine's biographers for some of the more evidently " physiological " experiences of the Saint. His knowledge in that direction is, nevertheless, clearly insufficient.

In the following pages, the passages in quotation marks, are either from the *Vita*, as quoted by von Hugel, or from von Hugel himself. They are all of them to be found in the first volume of his work, pp. 97-200.

to a man her equal in rank and wealth but profoundly unsuited to her in temperament and ideals. Giuliano, to whom she was married in 1463 at the age of sixteen, was young and rich, "a man of undisciplined, wayward, impatient, and explosive temper, selfish, and self-indulgent." His almost constant absence from home could hardly have been regretted by Catherine. For five years, she nursed her sorrow in seclusion. Then, for several years, she " tried to find relief in worldly gaieties and feminine amusements, short, however, of all grave offence against the moral law. At the end of these experiences and experiments she, noble, deep nature that she was, found herself, of course, sadder than ever, with apparently no escape of any kind from out of the dull oppression, the living death of her existence and of herself."

By 1471 she had become altogether disgusted with the world and with herself. Her sole remaining desire was to die. For two years longer she dragged on along her weary way ; then came a dramatic crisis that wholly altered her existence. The account of this conversion, as it comes down to us through her favourite disciple, Vernazza, incomplete though it is, agrees well with our knowledge of such crises. It had been preceded by a long period of preparation during which glimpses of the saintly life, of God as lover, of the ecstatic gift of oneself to Him, and through Him to humanity, had come and gone. The World had offered her nothing that could content her higher self. But to choose God meant a total renunciation of self. This, even though she would, she could not accomplish. Several years passed. Then, as she was one day on her knees for confession, " her heart was pierced by so sudden and immense a love of God, accompanied by so penetrating a sight of her miseries and sins and of His Goodness, that she was near falling to the ground. In a transport of pure and all-purifying love she was drawn away from the miseries of the world ; and, as it were beside herself, she kept crying out within herself : ' No more world ; no more sins ! ' "

The priest, not noticing the condition of his penitent, withdrew for a moment ; when he returned, she was just able to say, " ' Father, if you please, I should like to let this confession stand over to another time.' And returning home, she was so on fire and wounded with the love which God had interiorly manifested to her, that, as if beside herself, she went into the most private chamber she could find, and there gave vent to her burning tears and sighs. And, all instructed as she had suddenly become in prayer, her lips could only utter : ' O Love, can it be that Thou hast called me with so much love, and revealed to me, at one view, what no tongue can describe.' "

This conversion, like that of Suzo and of our other mystics, was primarily an experience of the " love of God," rather than the sudden triumph of altruistic over egoistic impulses and desires. Progress in these lines was a consequence of the new love-relation established with God. Whether or not her confessor played, in Catherine's instance, a rôle similar to that of the Franciscan monk, and of Father la Combe in the career of Mme Guyon, we do not know. We may suppose that the crisis assumed the more readily the form of a love-storm because of the long sex-repression to which this young married woman had been condemned.

2. *The Phases of St Catherine's Life.*—Hugel finds it convenient to divide Catherine's life into three periods. (1) The first four years after conversion (1473-77), years of extravagant asceticism and penances, of relentless struggle against the egoistic self. (2) The middle period, by far the longest (1477-99), a period of great and beneficent activity, of assured communion with God, and yet not altogether free from temptation and struggle. (3) The eleven years, from 1499 to her death in 1510, characterized, on the one hand, by a permanent breaking down of her health and by much that is mentally abnormal ; and, on the other, by the conviction of the suppression of the natural man and a sense of complete agreement with the divine Will.

Her conversion transformed altogether both her inner and her outer existence. By this time her husband had got his financial affairs into such confusion that they found it advisable to vacate their palace. Their income mounted still to one thousand two hundred pounds a year—a very large revenue for the time ; yet, six months after her conversion, they chose to move into a humble house near a large hospital in which she was interested, in a section of Genoa inhabited by the poor. Giuliano also became a convert, " in his own manner and degree," says Hugel. They lived together, but not as man and wife ; for they had agreed to a life of perpetual continence. He became a Tertiary of the Order of St Francis, and devoted himself together with her to the hospital and a foundling asylum connected with it. In 1490, in the capacity of matron of the hospital, Catherine occupied a small house within its precincts.

During the first period, we find her rivaling the great ascetics in the severity of her penances, wearing a hair shirt, never touching either meat or fruit, fasting often and long, lying at night on thorns, refusing herself even the innocent pleasure of conversation with friends. Six hours a day were spent in prayer. Her life " was a continuous striving to do things contrary to her natural bias and an alert looking to do the will of others." On entering the hospital service, one of her first self-imposed tasks was to get rid of her squeamishness by constraining herself to the most menial and dirty work.

It is not surprising that her health should have suffered. She felt a fire in her heart that seemed to dry up and burn her interior. At times, " so great a physical hunger would possess her that she appeared insatiable ; and so quickly did she digest her food that it looked as if she could have consumed iron." When she walked, it was with the eyes on the ground ; and she spoke in a tone so low as to be barely audible ; " she seemed dead to all exterior things." One need not be a physician to conclude from this report that she was reduced to a very low level of vitality and, during certain periods, made ravenous by partial starvation. All these things she did, or thought she did, for the purpose of self-conquest.

From 1477, the beginning of the second period, the severity of her austerities decreased, and her life gained correspondingly in joy and expansive benevolence. Her relation with God passed more frequently than before into a love-trance. " She would at times have her mind so full of divine love, as to be all but incapable of speaking ; and would be in so great a transport of feeling as to be obliged to hide herself so as not to be seen. She would lose the use of her senses and remain as one dead ; and, to escape the recurrence of such things, she would force herself to remain in company. Even in the midst of her work, " at times her hands would sink, unable to go on, and weeping she would say, ' O my Love, I can no more ' ; and would thus sit for a while with her senses alienated." Usually, however, although she was deaf to intruders, she would hear the call to any duty, however trifling. Whatever sensual indulgence there may have been in the enjoyment of God's favours, she continued faithfully to make them contribute to her sanctification.

In 1490, she became matron of the hospital, and for the six following years was in complete charge of this large establishment[1]. But the work was too much for a constitution undermined by long continued austerities. In 1496, her health having broken down, she was compelled to resign her post and to give up all extraordinary fasts and other ascetic practices.

It frequently happens that persons displaying noble and heroic traits in unusual situations show contrasting defects in the ordinary relations of life. It was not so with Catherine. Her dealings with her wayward husband, for instance, were always patient, generous,

---

[1] The hospital had 130 beds, and the asylum, in which she was also interested, sheltered one hundred girls.

and forebearing, as he himself acknowledged in his will; and her difficult relations with his illegitimate child and its mother were praiseworthy.

The intimate relation of the great mystics with God becomes on occasion surprisingly familiar, as for instance in this incident. Giuliano was suffering from a long and painful illness, in consequence of which he became so fretful and impatient that she feared for his salvation. She cried aloud unto her Love, " O Love, I demand this soul of Thee ; I beg Thee, give it me ; for, indeed Thou canst do so." And having persevered thus for about half-an-hour with many a plaint she was given an interior assurance of having been heard[1]."

And now, for the first time after twenty-five years of Christian life, this self-reliant person felt the need of the kind of comfort in spiritual and temporal matters to be gained from a devoted confessor. She chose a priest, Don Marabotto by name. Never was this good man in any sense her director, but he was " ever gentle, patient, devoted, and full of unquestioning reverence towards Catherine ; naif, and without humor, thoroughly matter of fact, readily identifying the physical with the spiritual." He himself declared that " she was guided and taught interiorly by her tender Love alone, without the means of any fellow creature either religious or secular." To this friend she could report her experiences, communicate her thoughts, and on him she could rely for whatever physical comfort she permitted herself. He became her chief support on this earth during her last years. To him we owe at least half the narrative of the *Vita*.

Is there not a significant discrepancy between the profession made by all the divine lovers that God and God alone is sufficient to them, and the bonds of close friendship and pure love most of them seem unable to avoid with at least some one human being of the opposite sex ?

The Saint enjoyed to the end overpowering manifestations of the love of God. The *Vita* shows us her naïve, miracle-loving intimates endeavouring to get something more than mere ejaculatory accounts of her love-experiences. " Many a time she would say to them, ' O would that I could tell what my heart feels.' And her children would say, ' O Mother, tell us something of it.' And she would answer, ' I cannot find words appropriate to so great a love. But this I can say with truth, that if of what my heart feels but one drop were to fall into Hell, Hell itself would altogether turn into Eternal Life.' "

[1] Giuliano died in 1497.

In the case of St Catherine, as of many another mystic, the friends are chiefly to blame for the extravagant interpretation of whatever seemed unusual to them. They are anxious that God's favours may not remain unexploited. Hugel insists that Catherine discriminated very judiciously between her "physical" and her "spiritual" experiences, between natural disease and divine wonders. We are of another opinion ; but, however that may be, so much is certainly true : she was ever translating her physical disorders and discomforts into spiritual terms, finding in them moral significance and using them as incentives to the perfect life. When, for instance. the internal sensations of burning are pleasurable, they "suggest and illustrate for her the joys and health-giving influence of the presence of God" ; when they are painful, they are turned to account in order to "gain and develop her doctrine concerning Purgatory."

Regarding Catherine's spiritual condition towards the close of her career, it should be noted that two years before her death, in her first confession to Don Marabotto, she declared herself unaware of any sin. "I should like to confess," she says, "but I cannot perceive any offense committed by me." Her meaning, however, does not seem to have been that she was perfect but merely that, as far as her light went, she was not conscious of having committed any sin. Her doctrine was that souls that have already travelled a long way toward perfection may not be aware of the evil remaining in them ; and that, later on, when they have progressed sufficiently to realize these evils, they are no longer guilty of them. There is a healthy self-confidence and frankness in this attitude of Catherine. One prefers it to Santa Theresa's somewhat maudlin lament that, whatever good opinion others may have of her, she is fit only for the company of devils[1].

Catherine's health grew worse and worse. In 1507 life had become so great a burden that she longed to die. She begged her Love, if he would not take her to himself, at least to allow her to go and see others die and be buried. Her Love consented, and so, "for a time she went to see die and be buried all those who died in the Hospital." Unusual nervous disorders multiplied. The Holy Communion exhaled a sweet odour. Thereupon she remarked, "O Love, dost Thou perhaps intend to draw me to Thyself with these savours ? I want them not, since I want but Thee alone and all of Thee."

[1] Of Marguerite Marie Alacoque, his biographer writes, "Her life, pure as it was, horrified her. She would have liked to wash it in her tears, in her blood, track in her veins the last remnant of sin." Mgr Emile Bougaud, *Histoire de Marguerite Marie Alacoque*, 10th ed., p. 139.

" For many days this perfume restored and nourished her body and soul." The simple minded Marabotto, who was going about smelling his own hand and wondering that it had no odour for him, was informed by her that God gives such things " only in cases of great necessity and as an occasion of great spiritual profit."

Comforting and monitory voices were frequent. She suffered for a time from great cöld, not altogether due to low temperature. At other times, great internal heat, skin hyperæsthesia and hyper-algesia plagued her. She could not be kept in bed ; " she was like a creature placed in a great flame of fire, and it was impossible to touch her skin, because of the acute pain which she felt from any such touch." " At times she would be sensitive to such a degree that it was impossible to touch her sheets or a hair of her head."

Much of her suffering took the form of " attacks," the nature of which we shall discuss in another place. She felt great internal heat located chiefly about the heart, stifling sensations, and spasms in the throat. Frequently the seizure would end in a death-like trance. At other times, she would not lose consciousness altogether, but only speech and sight. One day, after they had been bathing her mouth, she exclaimed, "' I am suffocating.' She said this because a little drop of water had trickled into her throat and she could not gulp it down." She would frequently vomit certain food or all food ; yet, she never vomited the Eucharist. These attacks would come and go with great suddenness, and her mood would alter with equal rapidity.

There are in the *Vita* accounts of several visits by more or less distinguished physicians. They never found any trace of organic disorder, and were unable to do anything useful. As to her, she was persuaded that her condition was not one requiring physic, and the medicine she condescended to take was vomited. Shortly before her death, a great consultation of ten physicians took place. They came to the same conclusion as their predecessors and " departed recommending themselves to her prayers." She breathed her last in September, 1510, of a disorder which to the rudimentary science of the time could not easily appear in any other light than that of the supernatural.

Her condition had been aggravated by the conviction, shared by her friends and physicians, that she was the especial object of God's ministrations. One cannot help wishing that this good Samaritan might have been spared the repulsive disorders that disfigured her last years ; or that, at least, she and her friends might have been able to attribute these disorders to natural causes. But, in this failure as in others, they belonged to their age. Had she been able to look upon her disorders as plain, repulsive disease, she would probably have returned to tolerable hygienic habits, and thus made possible at least a partial restoration of health.

The many " wonders " that cast a lurid light upon the last years of Catherine's life may easily produce a distorted impression of her career. It should not be forgotten that until 1499, *i.e.*, during a long period of relative health, her life was one of self-control and admirable self-sacrifice. Her days and much of her nights were given up with unswerving steadfastness to the alleviation of the suffering of the sick and the care of orphans.

*　　　*　　　*

One may, as we have done, divide the life of St Catherine into a number of periods, but there is no real periodicity in it, no rhythmic or cyclic succession of exaltation and depression. Her marriage, which determined the beginning of years of deep misery, followed upon political events far removed from her inner life. When, five years later, she resolved to shake off her gloom and seek in worldly amusements some relief to her conjugal situation, we have a departure again conditioned in part by *external, chance,* circumstances. The sharpest turning point in her career is probably her conversion. It is also chance, and not any particular law of rhythmic development which occasioned that event just at the time it happened. It was, nevertheless, a continuation or rather a culmination of inner struggles. Her zeal in self-sacrifice and the fulfilment of God's Will received at that time a new impetus. The rest of her life may be regarded as a more or less regular progression towards a consciousness of sinlessness which we found her affirming two years before her death.

Ascetic practices began with the conversion-crisis, in response to the then accepted view that in order to be able to perform God's Will the flesh must be subdued and made subservient to the spirit by rigid discipline. A passionate craving to show devotion to the divine Lover and other subordinate motives, intensified these practices ; illness compelled her to mitigate them, and, at the very end, to give them up altogether.

As to those briefer descents of the vital tone below the normal level, familiar to everybody and known to the mystics as states of dryness, if they followed each other according to any particular rhythm, we have no way of finding it out, for the record in our possession is too incomplete.

MME GUYON [1] (1648-1717)

1. *Biographical.*—Although less widely known than Santa Theresa, Mme Guyon is no less interesting to students of human nature. She is more original or, at least, of a more independent temper than her Spanish sister. And, if she describes her ecstasies and trances less minutely, she is less influenced by a desire for systematization and, therefore, perhaps more reliable. Her comparative obscurity is due to the disfavour with which the Church has looked upon her heretical teaching. There were not in Santa Theresa the hard fibres necessary to the composition of a heretic.

Jeanne Marie Bouverie de la Motte was Mme Guyon's maiden name. She was born in 1648 of very religious parents. Her family belonged to the French nobility. She reports that when she was eight years old the Queen of England visited her father and was so charmed by her beauty and sparkling intelligence that she desired to make her a lady of her court. She was of a lively and high strung temperament; wilful, passionate, extremely sensitive and, perhaps most of all, hungry for admiration. These traits are likely to make a person trying even to those who love her.

While still very young, Jeanne was placed in a convent where she passed most of the years that preceded her marriage. The religious ideas and images which haunt the convents impressed her very early. She had hardly reached her seventh year when she dreams of hell and burns with desire to become a martyr. At the end of her father's garden she has a chapel dedicated to the Child Jesus where she performs childish devotions.

At twelve, she is a tall and beautiful girl. It is at this time that, in consequence of a meeting with a priest, she has her first spell of serious devotion. She locks herself in her room, and all day long reads the works of St Francois de Sales and the life of Mme de Chantal. In these works she learns "what it is to make orison," and from now on she practises that form of spiritual exercise. She wishes that she might have the heart of the whole human race in order to love God more. She imitates Mme de Chantal and takes the same vows. In order to satisfy her longing for mortification she performs for her father, in the absence of the servants, the most menial tasks.

[1] The first part of this chapter is a translation, with many changes, of the essay already referred to on a group of Christian Mystics (*Rev. Philos.*, vol. LIV, 1902). The quotations and other information are drawn, unless otherwise stated, from *La Vie de Mme J. M. B. de la Mothe-Guyon écrite par elle-même*, new edition in three volumes, Paris, Libraires Associés. As far as possible I have followed her own phraseology.

This admirable and extravagant zeal lasts a year or two ; but, as she enters womanhood and young people flutter about her, her attention and desires turn from the Creator to His creatures. She exchanges St Francois for romances, which she " loves madly." Then, this girl barely sixteen years old is given in marriage, regardless of her consent, to a man far older than herself, and the tragedy of her life begins in the same way as in the case of St Catherine of Genoa. Her parents had taken pleasure in "showing her off." In her new home it was quite different. " They listen to me," she complains, " only to contradict and blame me. If I talk well, they say it is only for the purpose of showing off. Her new relatives take pleasure in humiliating her. Her pride suffers horribly. Her husband, become gouty, keeps his chamber more and more, and, at last, scarcely leaves it. Behold the young wife transformed into nurse of a jealous husband under the eyes of a mother-in-law, both ill-tempered and envious.

It is under the crushing misery of this unhappy union that she begins to feel an actual need of God. The real world had refused her ; very well, she would return to the ideal world of her childhood, she would become the bride of Jesus. But nature does not easily accommodate itself to this substitution of heaven for earth. It resists ; it demands the usual satisfaction ; long and painful is the struggle.

Three years after her marriage, being still torn between the tendencies of the natural man and an ideal that she could not realize, she consults a Franciscan monk. At their first meeting, he said to her : " Seek God in your own heart and you will find Him there." " That was," she tells us, " the stab of an arrow which quite pierced my heart. At that moment I felt a wound very deep, as delicious as it was amorous, a sweetness which was felt so powerfully by my senses that I could scarcely open my eyes or my mouth " (VIII). This experience opened a period of exaltation ; it constitutes a turning point in her life. Soon after the Franciscan monk became her director.

Nothing, perhaps, arrests the attention so sharply in the *Life* of Mme Guyon as her need for affection and admiration. We read that when she was but a child she could not be happy without someone near her who loved her. Once married, her need of affection became complicated with impulses of an undoubtedly sexual origin. After her meeting with the priest, she would fall into states in which she possesses God " in all his depth," not in her thoughts and understanding, but " in a sweet way as something that one actually possesses as one's own." At times she could not keep from falling into ecstatic trances in which the hours passed as moments. " Love would not give me one moment's rest. I cried : O my Love, this is enough—leave me." She would tell God that she loved Him more than the most passionate lover his mistress. If we put side by side with the preceding passage another one, admirable for its candour, we shall have matter for reflection upon the relation existing between the pleasures of sex and the pleasures of mystic love. Monsieur Guyon found in the never-ending devotions of his wife new cause for discontent. " He said that in loving you so much, my God, I would no longer love him. For he does not understand that true conjugal love is that which you yourself create in the heart that loves you. It is true, O pure and Holy God, that from the first you have implanted in me a love for chastity so great that there is nothing in the world that I would not do to gain it. I am always trying to persuade him of this." This fact, however, did not prevent her from fulfilling her conjugal duties ; but she wishes it understood that here, as in other organic functions, her heart and soul are so completely separated from her body that she does " these things as if she did them not."

Whatever may be the origin and nature of that burning love which dulls all other pleasures, it is a very potent reality. Everywhere in her writings—in the *Autobiography*, in the *Short and Easy Way to Orison,* in the *Torrents*—one feels the ardour of a soul burning with unsatisfied passion. " I crave," she cries, " the love that thrills and burns and leaves one fainting in an inexpressible joy and pain." God answers her cry, sets her aflame with passion, and, after the gratification, still trembling in every limb, she says to him, " O God, if you would permit sensual people to feel what I feel, very soon they would leave their false pleasures in order to enjoy so real a blessing." This characteristic of the religious life of Mme Guyon belongs also, in different degrees, to every other Christian mystic ; we found it in Suzo and in Catherine of Genoa, and we shall find it in the instances that are to follow.

Leaving to a later time a more searching study of the problem of divine love, we pass to another main trait of Mme Guyon's experience. Even during the years of innocent frivolity when she devoured romances by night and rejoiced by day in the admiration of her cousins, she was never able to follow her natural inclinations with complete abandon. Deep down in her heart she despised her coquetry and egoism. She would at times go to church to weep and beg conversion at the feet of the Blessed Virgin.

After the decisive interview with the monk, she appeared, both to herself and to others, a changed being—so, at least, she tells us. She performed her duties without the former reluctance and difficulty, and she saw herself with a keener vision. The loved Master of her heart disclosed to her even the smallest faults; He complained of her every action, of her way of walking, of her penances and mortifications, of her charities, of her love for solitude. Her desire for moral perfection was so great that she imagined the strange internal pains which she felt at various times to be a punishment for her delinquencies.

And although her soul was so sensitive to these pains " that she would have preferred to be torn asunder rather than suffer such torment," she nevertheless submitted to them and did nothing to allay them, either by confession or by penances ; for, they were in her estimation the purifying work of a divine fire. The suffering that came naturally to her seemed not enough. In order more quickly and completely to overcome her bad natural impulses, she invented additional torments. One can scarcely help admiring the heroism with which she seeks to conquer her egoism. Every day this delicate woman undergoes long penances. She wears briers, thorns, and nettles next to her skin ; she puts pebbles in her shoes ; she denies herself everything that would please her palate. When she becomes conscious of a dislike, she has no rest until she has overcome it. She relates, for instance, how she took spittle into her mouth : " One day, when I was alone, I saw some spittle, the most disgusting that I have ever seen, and I had to put my tongue and lips upon it ; the act was so nauseating that I could not control myself, and my heart beat so violently that I thought it would burst every vein in me and that I would vomit blood. I continued doing that as long as my heart revolted ; it was rather long[1]."

The actions of Mme Guyon often take place independently of her will. She speaks in the passive tense, " I was compelled." She ends the passage just quoted with the remark, " I did not do that through habit, or intention, or forethought. You were ever within me, O my God, and you were a master so severe and exacting that you would not let me pass even the least thing. Whenever I set out to do a thing, you stopped me short and made me, without my thinking, do your wishes and all that was displeasing to my senses until they became so willing that they lost all their inclinations and all repugnance." A physician would see here uncontrollable impulses and automatisms.

But if, at first, she tortured herself in order to conquer the natural man, it looks as if she came to love suffering for its own

---

[1] We report further on a similar performance by St Marguerite Marie.

sake. Her " crosses " became her delight. That she exaggerates, is evident and her statements must be taken with a grain of salt. " I submitted myself," she writes, for example, " to all the hardships that I could think of ; but they were not sufficient to satisfy my desire for suffering. I often (sic) had my teeth pulled, although they did not ache. This was refreshing to me. But when my teeth ached, I never thought of having them pulled ; on the contrary, they became my good friends and I was sorry to lose them without pain." Perversion of sensibility is added here to the usual purpose. There is, however, one point of great importance that separates her case from those of ordinary perversion : she never lost sight of the moral goal towards which suffering was to direct her.

During this period, God favoured her more and more frequently with his incomparable presence. At times, against her wish, contemplation turned into a trance. She noticed, for instance, that she was seldom able to hear the voice of the priest during the sermon. " He made such an impression upon my heart and possessed me so completely, that I could neither open my eyes nor hear what he was saying ; " she fell, that is, into a lethargy in which impressions from without were perceived either vaguely or not at all[1]. This somnolence was deliciously sweet to her. Little by little a habit became established and, during certain periods of her life, she would fall into that partial sleep at any hour, wherever she happened to be and whatever she might be doing ; the mere sound of God's name was sufficient to put her to sleep. The rest of the time, she was not always completely awake. One day when her sick husband inquired about the condition of the garden, she went to it, at his repeated request, " more than ten times " without seeing anything !

The condition characterized by an almost continuous conscious-ness of mystical union and an unusual degree of success in suppressing the natural man, lasted for a period of about two and a half years. Then a more usual state of sensibility returned. Union with God no longer came of itself ; she even found it difficult to bring it about at will. If she was now still unable to follow the celebration of mass, it was not, as formerly, because her eyes closed of themselves ; but, on the contrary, because she could not keep them closed ; she could not, even for one moment, compose herself for meditation. Self-mortification had become difficult and unendurable the pains formerly born with pleasure. She complained of dullness, of stupidity, and of an inability to hold her appetites in check : " I could

[1] On attacks of sleep in hysteria, see *Leçons Cliniques sur l'Hystérie et l'Hypnotisme*, A. Pitres, vol. II, pp. 226-38.

not restrain my words, nor refrain from eating what I liked," she writes.

God had forsaken her; or rather, instead of remaining the loving Bridegroom, he had become a rigorous judge. She thought that she had fallen back into the state of the natural man. It was, however, not so much the triumph as the persistent presence of bad inclinations that tormented her. There raged in her soul a continual battle against her selfish nature; the love of ease, of pleasure, and of praise unceasingly came into conflict with her more disinterested impulses. Her husband wished her to wear decolleté gowns, such as other women wore; she herself took pleasure in doing so, but "although her gowns were not nearly so low as those of others," she wept inconsolably because she felt that she had been a backslider. She rebels at her mother-in-law's conduct toward her and afterwards is ready to go to any length to expiate that fault. She goes for a walk, " rather to be looked at than for the pleasure of exercise," and, on her return, she sheds tears of humiliation. " I have within me," she writes, " an executioner who tortures me unceasingly."

He quite fails to understand Mme Guyon who thinks that the discontent which haunted her during this period of depression was entirely the result of a lowered morality. Her conduct is little altered; it is something else that has changed. She no longer, or only rarely enjoys mystical delights; her attention is no longer engrossed by the Bridegroom and she seeks elsewhere the satisfaction of her cravings. But, on returning from innocent amusements, she remembers the caresses of her Lover and cries, " O my God, this is not you. You alone can give true pleasures."

For seven years, that is, up to the year 1680 (she was then thirty-two years old), she was in the condition of "total privation" described above. This expression must not, however, be taken literally; she exaggerates. There were recurrences of a satisfactory affective state; in particular, the five weeks following the dedication of a private chapel and the nine months (or less) of a pregnancy. But for most of the time she suffered either from an ill-defined distress or even from better localized bodily illnesses, at times extraordinarily violent. Throughout that period her physiological energy was at low ebb. Everything conspired, it seemed, to overwhelm her. She lost in rapid succession a son; her father, her only comfort in her wretched family life; a daughter; and, finally, Mother Granger, who had become her chief moral support on this earth. A little later, twelve years after her marriage, as she had just been delivered of her sixth child, her husband also died and she was left alone with her mother-in-law.   She had not even a confessor upon whom to lean, for she had lost the priest who had been the instrument of her conversion; and, since then, no confessor had gained much influence over her. Thus, she arrived at the "state of death"; her life-curve had reached its lowest point.   It seemed to her that she was forever effaced from God's heart and from the heart of all creatures.   She even believed that she was resigned to that condition.

An occurence should be mentioned here which shows the energy, the intelligence, and the practical sense of which she was capable when circumstances demanded.   After the death of her husband she put his complicated and confused business affairs into such good order, in so short a time, that everyone including herself was astonished, because she had thought herself quite ignorant of those matters[1].

Her return to divine favour is bound up in a very illuminating way with the birth of tender relations with a certain Father la Combe. She had made his acquaintance some years previously.   Their first interview had produced a deep impression on both of them.   She said to him things which opened the way to the inner life; he admitted on his side, at a later date, that he had gone away completely transformed.   They lost sight of, without apparently forgetting, each other; for, one day, several years later, she improved an opportunity of writing him concerning one of her servants.   On the same occasion she recommended herself to his prayers.   He comforted her by assuring her that the state of her soul, painful though it was, was nevertheless one of grace.

The Father was then at Thonon, only a few miles distant from Geneva.   Mme Guyon sees in this the hand of God, who, in her opinion set about contriving devices to make her go to that city.   An angel announced to her in a dream that God wished her to be in Geneva, and some marvellous coincidences came about to lead her there. She persuaded herself, however, that she was quite indifferent, that she had no wish in the matter, no desire other than the will of God.

Father la Combe also had "indications."   She had asked him to say mass for her on the day of Mary Magdalen.   During the service, he heard a voice repeat three times with great vehemence, "You shall live in the same place."   That same day Mme Guyon recovered

---

[1] Certain persons who for years had quarrelled with one another had finally come to ask her husband to be their arbiter.   He died before attending to the matter, and they begged Mme Guyon so insistently to take her husband's place that she consented.   For thirty days she closeted herself, going out for mass and for her meals only.   At the end of that time she gave a decision with which every one declared himself satisfied.   This is her own account of the occurrence.

her long lost peace of mind. " It was on that happy day of Mary Magdalen," she writes, " that my soul was completely freed from its pain " ; and she adds, " After the first letter from Father la Combe I began to live a new life."

At the first meeting with the Father after their long separation she was surprised to feel an inner peace and a joy never before felt with any other person. " It seemed to me," she wrote, " that a great wave of grace swept from him to me, passing through our inmost souls, and returning from me to him, so that he experienced the same feeling. But it was a grace so holy, so pure, so clear, that it was as a wave ebbing and flowing and then losing itself in the divine unity." In similar terms she had tried at an earlier time to describe her relations with God Himself.

Her peace was such that she felt the need of a particular word to describe it. She called it the " *Paix-Dieu.*" Why not the *Paix-la Combe* ? Why did she interpret that inexpressible inner state as the " splendid and holy " return of Him she thought she had lost for ever ? For years she had awaited in physical torment and moral desolation the return of the heavenly Bridegroom. He had not come. Now a man, with whom she had at an earlier time exchanged those sentiments which are the harbinger of love, enters her life ; her heart awakes, her soul lives again, and " God's love " manifests itself once more in trances inexpressibly delightful.

These two souls became twin souls, travelling together—one might almost say one in the other—on the same pilgrimage, encouraging, strengthening, counselling, and loving each other so truly that they did not spare themselves the suffering that purifies. La Combe and God became interchangeable. There was, she writes, " complete unity, so that I could no longer distinguish him from God."

Shortly after the renewal of her relation with the Father she entered the Ursiline monastery of Thonon, on the lake of Geneva. She had now achieved her long cherished desire to break with her family in order to join a religious community. From that time, Father la Combe was her confessor and, with the help of Providence and until persecutions threw them into prison[1], they arranged to live most of the time near each other.

Mme Guyon's misery before the advent of Father la Combe had obviously a bodily and a moral cause. The former reacted unfavourably upon the latter and *vice versa :* the ceaseless conflicts within her of contradictory tendencies—of the natural against the spiritual man—exhausted her ; and the aches of her debilitated body

[1] See, for a similar case which, however, ended in immorality, Magnan, *Leçons Cliniques*, vol. I, p. 130.

added themselves to, and intensified her moral torments. She does not clearly know how to account for her condition ; for, on the one hand, she declares an all-embracing guilt ; and, on the other, she recognizes that she does not know of what she is guilty. She is like Bunyan making an imaginary " unpardonable sin " the scapegoat for organic distress. She says, " everything seemed to me full of faults : my charities, my alms, my prayers, my penances ; one and all they rose against me. Either by you, O my God, or by myself, or by all creatures, I felt myself universally condemned." But she adds, " Although the condemnation was so thorough, I could find nothing of which to accuse myself." This pathetic confusion of moral guilt with physiological misery, is responsible for a very large part of the tragic in the lives of our mystics as well as in those of other distinguished religionists. But why did she in the first place lose the delightful and vivifying experiences of " divine " love that began with the visit of the Franciscan monk ? We shall be led to think that this loss was connected with that of this, her first human messenger of divine love.

Mme Guyon had now entered upon the last lap of her earthly course, the end of which was to be the so-called " state of Mystical Death." Already during the long period of depression and despite her own misgivings, some progress had taken place. She had found less and less pleasure in the satisfaction of her natural desires. For example, if she ate something that she craved extremely, she found no enjoyment in it. She was becoming indifferent, submissive, a passive instrument of the divine Will. She tells us that her spirit unresistingly abandoned its own thoughts for the thoughts of others. A gradual death of the natural man was taking place. If, before she had sought " crosses " until she was completely exhausted, now she no longer sought them, nor did she desire them, but received whatever came with an unperturbed spirit. " Formerly the soul saw that nature wished to take part in what was happening, and then she felt it her duty to overcome the desire ; but now nature had learned the lesson of passivity." What was once abhorrent to her, was no longer painful ; she accomplished without complaining the most menial duties : proud Mme Guyon sweeps out the chapel.

We must not, however, misunderstand these statements ; her so-called indifference is not incompatible with incoercible tenacity. We should note, for instance, with what persistence she resisted the efforts of the Bishop of Geneva, and of several other persons in authority, to connect her officially with the religious house in which she stayed at Gex, and also her tenacity in maintaining a morally dangerous relation with Father la Combe.

As to her claim of complete sanctification, it is not borne out by her own account. The following passage, which refers to a late period of her life, indicates the continuation of inner division : " My God became so strict a master that he put me to death whenever I resisted his smallest wish. O God, how clearly did I see then the meaning of the words, ' Who has been able to oppose God and dwell in peace ? ' " Nevertheless her theory is that the conflict between the natural and the spiritual man has ended by the complete elimination of the former ; man and God have become one. This purification and unification of the self is a most significant claim made by the mystics ; we shall have to give to this theory the consideration it deserves.

As the divine ego became established in Mme Guyon, the idea of a mission took form in her mind. At Gex she heard the words : " Thou art Peter and upon this rock I will build my Church." And to Father la Combe came a voice assuring him that it was God's intention to use them both to help souls. It is in the conviction of divine favour and in the consciousness of their moral superiority that the idea of a mission germinates in the minds of the mystics. It is true that there is hardly any profession of moral abjection that they are not willing to make ; nevertheless they realize that the favour shown to them is granted to only a " small number of chosen souls."

Mme Guyon now entered upon a period of feverish activity. She preached moral perfection through passivity—the doctrine known as *quietisme*. She healed bodies as well as souls. Her activity was attended by curious manifestations of automatisms and by the elaboration of strange doctrines. God gave her " I know not what power to bring souls to perfection." She discovered successively the power of *verbal suggestion* and the superior method of *communication in silence*. On the occasion of the illness of a sister in the convent, she found out " what it was to command by the Word and to obey by the same Word." Soon, she noticed that the laying, on of hands was not necessary for the cure of soul or body, the Word alone sufficing. The miracle required only consent, or even only non-resistance, on the part of the sufferer. It was in her relation with Father la Combe that she learned the secret of " spiritual fruitfulness in silence." The method is easy ; she used it systematically. " All those who are my true children have, from the first, the tendency to remain silent while in my presence, and I have likewise the instinct of communicating to them in silence what God gives me for them." Even the presence of the person was not necessary ; the treatment might take place at a distance. In the discovery of these methods, Mme Guyon anticipated the modern treatments by suggestion and even some of the refinements of the latter-day American mind-curists.

Her influence and reputation increased apace. She felt herself invested with an " apostolic state." She had the gift of discerning spirits and a miraculous power over souls. Visitors came to her from near and far. Priests, peasants, and men of the world flocked to her in the hope of being healed in body and soul. This popularity and success continued until her return to Paris. Once in that great city, surrounded by strangers and enemies, her gift lost something of its potency; persecutions brought her thaumaturgic successes to an end.

To the pathological symptoms already noted, there was added during the time of her triumphal public career, automatic writing, a phenomenon of dissociation now well-known to psychologists. She wrote automatically her most celebrated work, *Les Torrents*, as well as the long and fanciful commentary on the books of the Bible. When she took up her pen, she did not know what she was going to write ; " thoughts rose from the depth " and did not pass through her head. When she had finished, she remembered nothing of what she had written.

That she was in a condition of high suggestibility is evident from what we have already related. Father la Combe had only to speak to her or lay hands on her, and she was well. A persistent cough disappeared at his command. One day she fell from her horse. When, despite a bad (?) wound, she mounted again to finish the journey, she felt herself pushed very forcibly towards the side of her fall ; and to keep in the saddle she had to throw herself with all her might in the opposite direction. But in matters significant she is open to suggestions only in so far as they are in agreement with her set purpose. Otherwise, she is both incoercible and non-suggestible. This is an aspect of her suggestibility that must not be forgotten in a comparison of her mental condition with that of ordinary highly suggestible neuropathic or hysterical persons.

She was frequently ill. In 1683 she had a severe attack with contractures, paralyses, hyperæsthesias, etc., during which she returned to " the state of the child." The idea of the Child Jesus, to whom she had bound herself long before by a special vow, effected a surprising transformation in her. Father la Combe would say to her, " It is not you, but a little child that I see[1]."

[1] See, regarding this and other strange phenomena in the life of Mme Guyon and of other mystics, the chapter of this book on " Hysteria and Psychasthenia."

We cannot recount here the persecutions to which she was subjected by the Church. Although from a worldly point of view, it would have been greatly to her interest to give satisfaction to those who accused her of heresy, she, whom we have just found so suggestible, conceded nothing of her claims, nor of what she considered the truth, even before the threats of the powerful bishop Bossuet.

2. *The Phases of Mme Guyon's Life and their Causes.*—The course of Mme Guyon's life, far from resembling that of a stream running smoothly and steadily to its appointed goal, is marked by irregular flowing and ebbing, which divide it in more or less clearly separated periods, themselves broken up by oscillations of minor importance.

Divergent theories have been elaborated to account for these oscillations in the life of the religious mystics. Theologians see in them the mysterious operation of the grace of God in conflict with the human will or the devil. Recent psychological students (Murisier, Godfernaux), pointing to similar oscillations in persons quite free from mystical and even from religious ideas, assimilated them to physiological rhythms, characteristic of a certain type of nervous instability. To later students (Delacroix, Hugel, Hocking), the phenomenon appeared more complex, and they made room in their explanations for influences of a moral order. In that, they were certainly right. Nevertheless, none of these theories seem to us entirely adequate ; they do not follow the facts closely enough. In what respect these later theories are deficient, we shall try to say at the end of the individual studies in which we are now engaged.

First Period (from the age of sixteen to eighteen).—The life of Mme Guyon since her unfortunate marriage may be divided into four main periods. The first would cover the two years immediately following her marriage. These are years of wretchedness, the causes for which have been set forth in the preceding account of her life. She was tormented by the natural cravings of youth, altogether unsatisfied in her new condition. At the same time as this frustration, the call to a holy life was heard again, louder and more insistently than during her girlhood. She could gratify neither one nor the other of these inclinations.

Second Period (from the age of eighteen to twenty-five).—The first period came to an abrupt end with the visit of the Franciscan monk who bade her find God within herself. For the first time she learned what it meant to be caught up in the Lord's embrace. " I felt," she writes, "a wound as delicious as it was amorous, an unction which was felt so powerfully that I could scarcely open my eyes or mouth." Thus began a period of exaltation, marked by moments of veritable ecstasy during which she possessed God " in all His depth." She appeared to herself and to others as an altered being. This alteration manifested itself in three directions : an enjoyment that often flamed up into a burning, passionate love of God ; the performance, without the former reluctance and struggle, of her duties to her husband and to others ; moments of obscuration of self-consciousness, a sort of semi-somnambulism during which someone (God, she thought) acted in her, for her. This period was also marked by sharp pains of obscure origin. But because she regarded them as from God, they had not a depressing effect. Through these pains she was to be purged from the evil remaining in her nature. In order to hasten that purification, she added to the divine pains, ruthless ascetic practices. There is reason to surmise, however, that some of these practices were due to perversions of sensibility ; she found in them some direct sensuous satisfaction, possibly merely a general stimulant.

This period passed gradually into the next. The exaltation of the Second Period well sustained at the beginning, was soon broken by moments of dryness and misery of increasing length, while ecstasy and the moments of the blessed semi-somnambulism noted above became less and less frequent. The struggles with the flesh and the devil increased in number and painfulness. Not only had she to live with an old, invalid husband whom she did not love, a spiteful and jealous mother-in-law, and impertinent servants whom she was not permitted to dismiss ; but now, after an initial period of complete and delightful surrender to God in love-communion, the pride of the flesh asserted itself again. She was forever torn asunder between cravings for human admiration and the stern voice of duty calling upon her to sacrifice all to God. Under these circumstances it becomes possible to believe her when she declares that she rejoiced when, at the age of twenty-two, she saw her beauty destroyed by small pox. By the same disease, and at the same time, she lost her first-born. Two years later her father and another child died, and not long after Mother Granger, who was " after God her only consolation." Her health, always most precarious, seems now almost completely shattered.

Third Period (from the age of twenty-five to thirty-two).— Mme Guyon names the year 1673 as marking the beginning of " total privation." In that state she continued until 1680. But just as the preceding period was not entirely without its dark moments, so the third was not without brief spells of peace and even joy in divine union. Under the very natural desire to make things simple and definite, she exaggerates, when she characterizes these years as a period of total privation of God.

Her misery during these seven years was worse than during the first period. She had now tasted the delights of love-union and the moral unity it implied. The memory of that which she had lost gave her sufferings a peculiar poignancy. It seemed to her that she no longer loved God at all, and that she had returned to the state of the natural man. Her appetite for a thousand things revived. Yet when she ate forbidden things for which she had a violent desire, she found no pleasure in them.

It was during this period, at the age of twenty-eight, after twelve years of married life, that she was at last delivered from the conjugal yoke. But, if God relieved her from that cross, it was only to give her heavier ones to bear. She regarded her two infants, one of them a few months old, as crosses, because they made it impossible for her to withdraw into a monastery. " God," she says, " while freeing me, had nevertheless bound me strongly in giving me two children immediately before the death of my husband " (XXII.)[1]. Her health was unusually bad. Once she was at the point of death during five or six weeks. When relative health finally returned, it did not bring with it moral peace ; she continued at war with herself. It seems that the more completely she thought herself cast away and the more she felt inclinations to lead an ordinary life, the more violent were her yearnings for God. She lost even her former pleasure in good works. At times she cherished such a loathing for herself that she lost all appetite and from sheer exhaustion had to take to her bed (XXV).

Fourth Period (from the age of thirty-two to her death).—It is under the circumstances just related that she had occasion to write to Father la Combe (1680). We have already seen how the sympathy they had felt for each other at their first interview, nine years before, was immediately revived and soon glowed into a warm love. In this spiritual union they continued their earthly pilgrimage until parted by death. The suddenness of her recovery of God when la Combe reappeared is as striking as her original discovery of God when the Franciscan monk directed her to look within. Again now, as during the second period, she enjoyed frequent and inexpressibly delicious ecstasies and peaceful semi-somnambulisms. The struggle

[1] The roman numbers in parenthesis are chapter references to vol. I of the *Autobiography*.

between the natural and the spiritual man ceased, and she passed her days in an atmosphere of love, carrying out, without opposition, the will of her divine Lover.

If one may regard the years between 1680 and her death, in 1717, as constituting a single period, it is not because of entire homogeneity. At first and for several years she was, on the whole and despite marked bodily weakness and disease, in a condition of great exaltation. The love-ecstasies were frequent, as were also automatisms of various kinds and moments of semi-somnambulism. It was also during these years that she suffered the most severe hysterical attack of which she has left any record ; of it she says, " Never was disease more extraordinary or longer in its excess."

We know extremely little concerning her condition during the last thirty years of her life. We may say, however, that gradually the symptoms of nervous instability seem to have abated ; and, with the advent of age, the love-raptures were replaced by a more ordinary communion with God. It is probable that she reached a condition of comparative equilibrium.

These four periods are of very unequal duration and the third has no clearly marked starting-point. That which separates them most conspicuously is, perhaps, the presence or absence of raptures. There are none at all in the first period. The beginning of the second is determined by the first ecstatic experience. For a time frequent and intense, the ecstasies gradually diminish ; and from the third period they are almost entirely absent. Their reappearance with renewed energy and frequency in connexion with the return of Father la Combe serves to mark the beginning of the fourth period. Then again they undergo a gradual, if slow decline.

The passage from one period to the next is characterized also by changes in the dominant affective tone that correspond fairly exactly to the changes in the frequency of the ecstasies. When they are numerous, the dominant tone is pleasurable and optimistic ; in their absence it is the opposite. The production of the ecstasies and the general affective tone have, as we shall see, a common cause.

With ecstasy and buoyancy is associated also the dominance of the godward tendencies. The other impulses no longer manifest themselves or else are easily repressed ; while, with the disappearance of ecstasy and the appearance of depression, the evil tendencies reassert themselves and the subject returns to a condition of painful and exhausting inner struggle.

Finally, a tendency to dissociation manifests itself markedly during the periods of exaltation. Semi-trances and automatisms are frequent, and, so far at least as the information in our possession goes, it is during these periods that the more serious attacks of hysteria take place.

We might have divided the fourth period in two and made of its latter part a fifth period characterized by her activity as missionary, healer, and reformer. But this would have been to separate a part of her life from the rest according to a trait totally different from those we have used in making four periods. Were we to use that trait as a means of division, her life could be divided into two periods only : the years of introversion, that is, of exclusive concern with her own self, during which she was seeking to make herself fit for union with God ; and the years of extraversion, or of her public ministry, a period that could not open until she had undergone the necessary preparation and attained a condition which made it possible for her to regard herself as an instrument of the divine Will.

But when one speaks of periodicity in the life of the mystics, one does not mean something as common-place as the preparation and the realization phases that divide in two the life of almost every-one. The mystics are in no way remarkable in that respect. They might, it is true, have lacked the ambition and energy that made of them at a given moment, social forces, and thus have remained to the end in the preparatory or introversion stage. The probability is that in that case we should never have heard of them. They became great among mystics because, as we have already said, they were personalities remarkable by the energy of their will-to-happiness-and-distinction. Their doctrine of humility, self-surrender and passivity should not blind us to the presence in them of a tremendous energy of self-affirmation. They aim at nothing short of divine perfection and power and, as soon as they have conquered social freedom and won divine partnership, they set out into the world to work in it the divine Will of which they have become, as it were, official instruments.

We conclude, then, that frequent raptures, persistent exaltation, the dominance of the tendencies in accordance with the divine Will, and a proneness to mental dissociation, make up a complex character-istic of two of the periods ; while the total or partial absence of these traits marks the two others. These four periods were not, however, homogeneous throughout their duration ; they were diversified by many irregular oscillations of affective tone and energy-level. The periods of exaltation (the second and the fourth), for instance, were not without moments of flatness and even of depression. Similarly, the two periods of depression were broken by briefer spaces of exaltation.

Causes and occasions of the alternating changes.—Both physiological and psychical causes are to be looked for. It is enough to point to the obvious effects of bad digestion and of alcoholic intoxication to remind everyone of the profound influence exercised on consciousness by physiological factors. Certain forms of insanity, characterized by alternating phases of exaltation and depression, illustrate strikingly how totally independent of moral causes oscillations involving the whole individual may be. Recently acquired knowledge about the action of internal secretions and of drugs upon the psychical life has added much definiteness to our understanding of the rôle played by mere chemical agents in altering the moral self.

We are, therefore, prepared to admit that certain of the psychical alterations we have described may be of purely organic origin, whereas others may be determined by psychical factors, and still others by factors of both classes[1]. An exclusively physiological cause must be ascribed, for instance, to the brief exaltation period which coincided with Mme Guyon's fourth pregnancy. From being depressed, dissatisfied with herself, obsessed with her faults, deprived of the enjoyment of divine love, she became self-confident, able to overcome or at least to disregard her defects, and almost constantly conscious of an overpowering love. That pregnancy may transform the affective state and bring relief from neurasthenic disorders is well known to physicians. Pierre Janet states that more than thirty times he has observed a transformation in his patients at about the fourth month of pregnancy. He records that their obsessions disappeared and adds, " It is well known that the functions of circulation, respiration, nutrition are exalted in that condition, and it is not surprising that a mental disorder that is in relation with cerebral depressions should be favourably influenced by that exaltation[2]."

If, as Janet suggests, the improvement results from increased activity of the great vital functions, why does not every pregnancy produce that improvement[3]? Because pregnancy involves other factors also. Painful physiological disorders may set in ; and moral causes may be added ; for instance, the dislike of having a child. In cases of illegitimate motherhood, the period designated by Janet as one of increased vitality may be one of excruciating torments.

[1] The philosophical reader will observe that I speak here the common-sense language, as indeed I must. No metaphysical theory of the relation of mind and body is to be attributed to me on the basis of these expressions.

[2] *Les Oscillations du Niveau Mental, Rev. des Idées,* 15th Oct.

[3] No similar improvement seems to have taken place during her other pregnancies.

In such cases, dread may override the main physiological effect[1]. In normal conditions, however, the psychical factors make for happiness, and one may very well conceive of a change similar to that in Mme Guyon being due to the mother's happy expectation. But, in the case under discussion, there was no joyful anticipation. We know that Mme Guyon fulfilled grudgingly her duty as a wife and mother. Her children were " crosses " from which she delivered herself as soon as possible. Her euphoric condition must, therefore, have been due to physiological factors.

If physiological causes alone brought about exaltation during Mme Guyon's fourth pregnancy, it was quite otherwise with the brief period of exaltation that followed the dedication of her private chapel. Here, as far as we know, psychical causes and no others determined the change. In a person of her temperament, beliefs, and ecstatic habit, the production of exaltation under the circumstances attending the dedication of a private chapel, is not greatly surprising. To that passionate woman the erection of an altar to her Heavenly Bridegroom at her very door was an inflammatory event.

*　　　　*　　　　*

The characteristics of the first period are accounted for sufficiently by Mme Guyon's temperament, the tendencies and desires of her early years, and the circumstances of her married life. This delicate, beautiful and proud girl divided from her childhood between the World and God, found herself condemned to live with a man twice her age and in ill-health, whom she did not love. The presence in the home of the mother-in-law completed her misfortune. One does not wonder that under these circumstances the Godward tendencies, previously awakened in her, reaffirmed themselves, and that she remembered the saints who had found in God what earth had refused them. Her poor health was aggravated by child-bearing ; two undesired children were born to her before the completion of her nineteenth year. Little imagination is required to conceive the restless, spasmodic yearnings of this poor woman towards the peace and the love offered by her religion. She sought peace in prayerful meditation practised " quite punctually " twice a day ; but found only momentary resignation. Youth would not be denied.

We are to regard her as already a very good young woman ; she did not curl her hair, " or very little," did not powder her face, and looked at herself " very little in the mirror " (VII). Nevertheless

---

[1] The action of fear upon the organism is, of course, to be understood physiologically. See the chapter on fear in W. B. Cannon's *Bodily Changes in Pain, Hunger, Fear and Rage*, New York and London, 1915.

she was engaged in an ever-recurring struggle against commonplace manifestations of pride and vanity.

When the Franciscan monk visited her, she was thus a divided and profoundly unhappy soul. We are told that he produced upon her a deep impression. He did more than that : his advice to seek God within led to the kindling of a sudden flame of love, experienced in a trance. The subject of that love was, as far as she understood herself, God or Jesus—no sharp distinction is made between them. The rôle played by the monk is, however, too important to be disregarded. We are, it seems, justified in thinking that he kindled the divine love and was instrumental in the production of the first love-ecstasy. (Anyone in doubt on this point should re-read the account of the influence upon her of Father la Combe.) In her own eyes and in those of persons about her, Mme Guyon is transformed. It was not a conversion in the sense of a sudden deliverance from bondage to gross evil habits ; it was rather the kind of transformation that would have come had she suddenly fallen in love with her husband. She compares what happened to her to the application of a balm that healed instantly all her wounds. The same thing would have taken place had she lost her heart to her husband ; she would no longer have been plagued by more or less useless struggles with the looking-glass and the extent of her *d colleté ;* nor would she have been made miserable by home duties ; and still less would her self-esteem have smarted from neglect and lack of appreciation. Self-confidence and happiness would have made of her an active, effective and happy wife and mother. It was, however, not the husband but Christ who made her very flesh tingle with love. At one magic stroke, the despised Cinderella became the bride of the King of Heaven. All her starved instincts were gratified. What mattered now slights, repellant home tasks, bodily ailments ; what mattered even rejection by man and isolation ? All these things had become as nothing in the presence of one great, overpowering fact : she loved and was loved by God Himself. A wave of new life reinforced all the impulses and purposes that she regarded as approved of God ; for the love of God when really felt carries with it the triumph of his Will. There is no longer any active suppression of the contrary tendencies ; the energies are, for the time being, drained in the Godward direction.

In short, then, we say that because a genuine love had awakened in her, Mme Guyon passed from a condition of self-division, dejection, and purposelessness to one of moral unity, buoyancy, and activity. No one at all familiar with the miracles of profane love or with the amazing rôle often played by the sympathetic and virile physician who practises among neglected women, psychopathic or otherwise, will wonder at this instance of the effect of love.

The only part of this experience that need surprise is the production of ecstatic love trances. As to that, the only thing we need say now is that her temperament and the circumstances in which she found herself were highly favourable to their production. She knew from her readings and from oral reports that such things were possible ; she desired the event and sought its production by conforming to certain practical directions. Moreover, she did not live a normal sex-life ; she was frigid with her husband. Since her marriage, two years had elapsed, two years of yearning after divine love.

For a considerable time at the beginning of this second period Mme Guyon walked on clouds of glory and passed much of her time in a peculiar absent-minded condition. The trials of her married life seemed insignificant ; she even took pleasure in menial tasks and in multiplying sources of physical suffering ; trials, she thought, would purify her soul as fire purifies gold, and her fortitude would show how great was her devotion to the Heavenly Bridegroom.

. But this extravagant happiness gradually came to an end ; the frequency and the intensity of the ecstasies decreased and then disappeared almost entirely, while the natural man became as obstreperous as ever. A long period of dryness, of complete privation from divine joy, set in.

How is this withdrawal of God to be accounted for ? Several causes present themselves to the mind ; one only, however, do we know to have existed, and that one seems in itself sufficient as an explanation of the passage from the second to the third period. Carnal desires might have drawn her away from God ; the devil, with whom she had only a distant acquaintance, might have taken possession of her. But nothing in the record would justify that hypothesis. No moral deterioration had taken place during these years of depression. On the contrary, she appeared to have made progress toward the realization of the " death of the senses," an expression meaning a condition in which they are " without appetite as without repugnance " (XII). No suffering that promised to further that end seemed to have been too great for her to endure. She was already in disfavour when she finally prevailed upon herself and continued " ever after " to cover her throat entirely with a handkerchief when going out in company, although she was " the only one so fixed up " (XIV). *Décolletage* had been one of the battle-grounds of the natural against the spiritual man. This belated sacrifice was, however, hardly necessary at that time ; for, shortly after, small pox destroyed the beauty that was keeping alive that most tenacious of cravings, the love of admiration. If she felt again with renewed sharpness the goad of pride and the misery of her loveless married life, she was not aware of having yielded to temptation.

May we suppose that the love-trances disappeared because of a return to a more normal physiological condition ? This would involve the assumption that health runs counter to the unusual phenomenon regarded by the mystics as union with a God of love. That assumption also is unsupported by facts. What we know about her health between 1666 and 1673 does not indicate an improvement. Her behaviour during that period of extravagant happiness was so strange and uncomfortable for those who lived with her, that the petty home persecutions became increasingly bitter. Caring for ought but the solitary enjoyment of God, she managed to keep herself much of the time in a condition that looked like imbecility ; the work she was doing would fall from her hands ; she would sit in company without seeing what was going on. She was furthermore often sick ; her life seemed to hang on a thread. The death of her husband, in 1676, did not restore her to health or happiness ; for four years longer she continued without God.

If it was not return to physiological health that lost her the entrancing communion with God, one might suppose that the loss was the result of increasingly bad health. This conjecture again is not altogether supported by the facts known to us. Her worse hysterical attack coincided with the exaltation at the beginning of the fourth period. Moreover, the conjecture appears superfluous in the presence of an event in itself sufficient to explain a return to the distressing condition which preceded the advent of the Franciscan monk. That fateful event is the passing out of her life of that very monk. He had become her confessor. We do not know how long that happy relation lasted, nor why it ended. Mme Guyon is much too discreet in her report of her relation with him. We know only that in 1672, or shortly before, a certain M. Bertot had become her director. We know furthermore that they never became friends. She could not " open " herself to him. The lack of understanding between them went so far that, according to her own testimony, she never spoke to him of the favours she had received from above. He pressed upon her directions that she could not or would not follow. She tried to obey him, but " found it entirely impossible." One may surmise that he did not regard her mystical theories and practices favourably. However that may be, they did not get along together. At a certain juncture, he even dismissed her, probably because she refused to follow his directions. Later on he took her back but without better results. He was " of little use " to her, although she yearned desperately for someone upon whom to lean.

Our surmise is, then, that the Franciscan monk to whom, " after God," she says she owed her love-ecstacies, took them away with him, together with a moral support they and his own presence provided. This opinion is confirmed in an almost irrefutable manner by what happened when Father la Combe, in his turn, appeared upon the scene. Then a new period of exaltation (fourth period) opened. We know that they had met many years before and had felt in sympathy with each other. His coming into her life in 1680 determined almost instantaneously overpowering love-ecstasies. She lost so completely her heart and head that she was hardly able to separate the Father from God. Thanks to his encouragement and support this eager soul, in the prime of life (thirty-two years old), whose life-energies had been baulked for so long could now throw herself headlong into the holy life as she had conceived it.

Her dependence upon the Father appears conspicuously, some would say shockingly, in her pursuit of him. At one time she appeared suddenly at Verceil where he was. She relates naïvely that the Father was " strangely annoyed " at her arrival. As a matter of fact, evil rumours were already abroad, and he was afraid for their reputation. Nevertheless, she made a prolonged stay. When at last she left for Paris she was not alone, the Father accompanied her the whole way, by order, she says, of one of his superiors!

The first part of the fourth period was marked by striking manifestations of various forms of dissociation, by automatisms, and high suggestibility, as well as by love-ecstasies. It is during these years that took place the most violent disorders of an hysterial nature or semblance of which she has left any record.

The absence of true periodicity.—The information contained in the preceding pages makes it quite impossible to regard the four periods into which Mme Guyon's life divides itself as the expression of any natural rhythm. The first was due to a combination of complex physiological and psychical causes ; on the one hand, her temperament, her education, and mainly, perhaps, the mystical ideal implanted in her very early in life ; and, on the other, her abnormal moral and physiological conjugal relation. The third period was in substance a return to the situation characteristic of the first ; it was due to the disappearance of that which had for a season (the second period) lifted her out of the misery of moral rejection and isolation into the fulness of a glorious love.

The beginning of the two periods of exaltation (the second and fourth) was occasioned, according to our explanation, by circumstances entirely external to herself, namely the coming into her life in one instance of the Franciscan monk and in the other of Father la Combe. One may wonder whether, in the absence of these two men, she would have spent her whole life in the darkness of the first and third periods. This question gives us the opportunity of stating formally what has been throughout implied ; namely that Mme Guyon's exaltations, as well as her depressions, were due primarily to what she was, and only secondarily to outside influences. These two men were little more than stimuli that brought out prepared responses or sparks that set fire to combustible material. It cannot be said that in their absence no other men could have taken their places, nor that a solution independent of the assistance of particular human individuals was impossible. It remains, however, that the most remarkable aspect of the " dealings of God " with Mme Guyon is the rôle played by these two persons of the male sex. We shall see in the next chapter that the love they kindled was no ordinary platonic love.

3. *Did Mme Guyon attain her ethical goal ?*—Two of her fundamental cravings were undoubtedly gratified during the periods of exaltation : her need for tenderness and for recognition. But what of her struggle for the suppression of the natural man, the absorption of her will into the universal, divine Will ? According to her understanding of it, every scene in the divinely guided drama of which she was the centre found its meaning in progress toward that goal[1]. A judgment passed upon the social value of the great Christian mystics would have to be based primarily upon their conception of the divine Will, the contribution they have made to methods of realizing it, and the extent to which they themselves have done so.

Hugel draws a careful picture of the character of the unregenerated Catherine of Genoa—a picture which would need little if any retouching to be also that of Mme Guyon and of Santa Theresa :

" A great self-engrossment of a downrightly selfish kind ; a grouping of all things round such a self adoring *Ego* ; a noiseless but determined elimination from her life and memory of all that would not or could not, then and there, be drawn and woven into

---

[1] It is interesting to observe how relatively insignificant in Mme Guyon's life was the influence of the idea of heavenly salvation. She, of course, believed in heaven and hell but no deferred heaven would do for her ; she wanted salvation here and now in the form of a fulfilment of the dominant requirements of her nature.

the organism and functioning of this immensely self-seeking, infinitely woundable and wounded, endlessly self-doctoring ' I ' and ' me ' ; all this was certainly to be found, in strong tendency at least, in the untrained parts and periods of her character and life[1]."

We are not sufficiently well informed to be able to say how far the saint changed in the course of her intimacy with God. In the case of Mme Guyon we can speak both as to the degree of completion of the union of her will with the divine Will, as she conceived of it, and as to the relation of the exaltation periods to her moral progress. Was it during and in consequence of the ecstasies that the lower, egoistic, self-centred impulses disappeared ; and was that disappearance final ?

At the beginning of the two periods of exaltation, and as long as they were at their height, she was indifferent to the admiration as well as to the ill-will and criticism of men. But this lofty detachment, appearing as the accompaniment of a peculiar love-relation with God, may hardly be taken as a sign of a character transformation, of a genuine increase in altruism and self-control. How could one who had become the favourite of the most High be disturbed by withheld human admiration ? How easy for the bride of the Almighty to bear slights and sneers ; how impossible for her to be jealous of a mother-in-law !

In other respects her conduct during the first exaltation period raises grave doubts. When her husband tried to limit the length of her prayers by not permitting her to get up at four but only at seven o'clock in the morning to perform her religious duties, she secretly defeated his purpose by doing her devotions on her knees, in bed. And when he forbade her to go to mass as often as she desired, she devised ways of attending without his knowledge. The Lord made himself her accomplice in these deceptions ; he worked miracles in her behalf ; he held back the rain and kept her husband asleep in the morning so that she might not be discovered. She corresponded secretly with Mother Granger. Thus, for many years of inexpressively sweet converse with God, she lived on earth in an atmosphere of concealment and deception. Nothing seemed to have been further from her thoughts than to seek normal, honest relationship with her family and society by making the sacrifice of her extravagant devotions. The divine Will never demanded renouncement of ecstatic love-enjoyment in order that she might comply with the wishes of her family, turn her attention to her children, and perform whole-heartedly her duties of mother and wife.

[1] Friedrich von Hugel, *The Mystical Element of Religion*, vol. II, p. 37.

The divine honeymoon passed, restlessness and discontent returned. When out of the divine embrace, she spent her time grieving for the loss of it, unable to exist without that incomparable enjoyment (XIII). Virtue, so easy to practise before, demanded now the most painful effort. During the period of complete " dryness," when the ecstasies had ceased, she continued to yearn after God without feeling His love. Her heart, formerly occupied with God alone, was now filled chiefly with worldly concerns (XXI). Her appetite for a thousand things came to life again. When at mass, she was inattentive. In order to punish herself she would go to a second mass and then to a third. " But," she writes, " it was always worse. My eyes which formerly closed of themselves, in spite of myself, would now remain open, and I was able neither to keep them closed nor to withdraw within myself for a single moment " (XXI).

The affirmation that her inclination to all evils was irresistible (XXIII), must, however, be interpreted in the light of utterances such as this : " I had an inclination to all sins, without, however, committing them ; and these inclinations seemed in my mind to be realities, because I felt my heart filled with worldly concerns " (XXIII). As far as there is backsliding during this long period of depression, it amounts merely to a return of the impulses of the natural man and not to a yielding to them. The worldly desires that had for a time ceased to manifest themselves, because the root instincts of her nature were satisfied to repletion by God's recognition and love of her, now again afflict her.

When Father la Combe appeared on the scene everything changed once more as by magic. Again love freed her from promptings against which she had been fighting. Her husband was now dead, and the young children whom God had added to her troubles, were growing up. She found it possible to fulfill her long-cherished desire ; leaving her only remaining son behind and taking along her five-year-old daughter, she entered a religious house. It is not without pain that she parted from her son, but (her own words deserve quotation) " the confidence I had in the Holy Virgin to whom I had devoted him, and whom I regarded as his mother, quieted all my displeasure." Of the death of her youngest child from small-pox, she writes : " The spirit of sacrifice possessed me so strongly that although I loved him tenderly, I never shed a tear when I learned of his death." And of the loss of a daughter and of her father, she says, " My heart was not shaken " ; " I mourned no more the daughter than the father." The sufferings of a daughter placed in a convent brought out the only sign we have noted in her *Life* of real parental affection and of remorse for non-fulfilment of duty.

If we compare Mme Guyon's state as it appears at the beginning of the first exaltation period or a few years after, when " dryness " was setting in, with her condition about ten years later when she entered the monastic life, or twenty years later when in the middle of her great missionary activity, we find no clear evidence of important moral improvement. At the earlier of these last two dates, despite her teaching on mortification, she refused to bear the " crosses " that had come to her in the course of a grudging discharge of conjugal duties. Enticed by the prospect of freedom for her devotions, she parts from her young children. And despite her ceaseless discourses about the death of the natural man, not even under risk of ruining his reputation is she able to resist the attraction of Father la Combe.

Regarding her later condition one might point, in support of an accusation of uncurbed self-will and pride, to her stubborn refusal to yield to the authority of the Church in the controversy about quietism ; to her belief in her possession of marvellous gifts, that, for instance, of discerning without external signs what passed in men's hearts and minds ; and to the extravagant dream of a great religious order of quietists, of which Fénelon should be the General, and she, by the grace of God, the inspiring and directing power[1]. One might also draw attention to many of the petty incidents she thought it advisable to record in her *Autobiography*—a work written when she thought herself emptied of the natural man. In the account of her childhood, we find this passage : " It happened that the Queen of England came to our house while I was present. My father told the confessor of the Queen that if she wanted to enjoy herself she should talk with me and ask me questions. He asked me several questions, and some very difficult ones. I answered them with so much *à propos* that he took me to the Queen " (III). Poor Mme Guyon had no more been able to do away with her little proud self than to part with her own shadow ! In this instance as in a host of others she displayed her cleverness for the admiration of the whole world, not only when she was a child, but when in old age she wrote down her biography.

There is, however, one important achievement to set down in an account of her moral development. Before her marriage, she not only felt urged by evil promptings but she identified herself with them. From the advent of the first exaltation period, whenever she recognized the natural man, she steadfastly disowned it and identified herself exclusively with the godward tendencies ; the others no longer belonged to her. This achievement took place as early as her

[1] See her letters to Fénelon in *Fénelon and Mme Guyon*, by Maurice Masson.

first ecstatic union, when she was but nineteen years old. It was her real conversion, her turning to God.

SANTA THERESA (1515-1582)

1. *Biographical*[1].—A similarity of temperament and of education make moral replicas of Suzo, St Catherine of Genoa, Mme Guyon and Santa Theresa. They all pursued, and by the same method, the satisfaction of the same fundamental cravings.

The judgment of the Church upon Santa Theresa is, according to Bouix, her translator, that "even at the time of her greatest waywardness, she was a model of virtue." She, herself, could say, " There was in my nature a happy inclination to virtue " : " I have never felt the slightest attraction for anything that might have withered my innocence, because I held in invincible horror all things dishonest." When, nevertheless, she accuses herself, as other mystics also have done, of being the blackest creature alive, deserving " to live in hell with the devils," we must remember that we are dealing with persons given to extravagances and passing readily, in their writings as in their lives, from one extreme to another ; and that they, especially Santa Theresa, wrote their biographies in order to magnify the goodness and the power of the Lord. It will not betray any uncharitableness on our part if we add that that is a way of vicariously setting forth their own.

Her repeated affirmation that she was cherished "wherever she went," need not, however, be discounted. As a child she was happy at home and, in the convents and monasteries where from the age of eighteen she passed her years, she was loved and admired. Her life, despite the impression that the *Autobiography* may leave, ran on the whole a fairly even course. Its ups and downs were not so pronounced as in the case of Mme Guyon.

She belonged to a family where religion was practised. When still a mere child, she built a hermitage in the garden and indulged

[1] We have used the French translation by Marcel Bouix of the Saint's *Autobiography*, Paris, 1857. The roman figures, in parentheses after the quotations, refer to chapters of that book.

The *Autobiography*, or the *Life*, was not all written at the same time. The first twenty-two chapters date from 1562. She was then forty-seven years of age. The last eighteen chapters were added between 1563 and 1566.

The *Book of Foundations* continues the *Life*, and relates in particular her activity as founder of monasteries. It was written in 1567.

The *Interior Castle* or the *Castle of the Soul* dates from 1572.

There are, in addition, three volumes of letters, also translated by Marcel Bouix.

An excellent critical study of Santa Theresa's life may be found in the *Etudes d'Histoire et de Psychologie du Mysticisme*, by Henri Delacroix, Paris, 1908.

with her numerous brothers in dreams of pious heroism. When she was twelve years old, her mother died. With the advent of womanhood her life took for a while the usual direction. She found pleasure in dresses and ornaments, enjoyed the company of cousins of the opposite sex, and behaved sufficiently like ordinary young people to deserve, she thinks, the accusation of frivolity. In order to give another direction to her thoughts, her father placed her at the age of sixteen in a convent where she soon found life enjoyable. A year and a half later a serious illness brought her home and led to the first religious crisis of her adolescence. It was not on a very high spiritual level. She tells us that servile fear, more than love, impelled her to the religious life. The question was, shall it be heaven or hell ? (III). For three months she underwent a severe struggle, and then, against the determined will of her father, she entered the convent of the Incarnation at Avila. She was eighteen years old. In this convent she remained as sister for twenty-five years and subsequently ruled it as prioress.

She was now at peace, happy to be safe, with Jesus as Bridegroom. " The first year was spent in purity, almost without giving any offence to the Lord (IV). But ill-health soon compelled her to travel in search of a cure. It is during that time (in 1535), after a sustained effort of nine months' duration, that she discovered the delights and comforts of orison[1]. She owed the discovery to the *Third Abécédaire* of François de Osuna, lent her by an uncle. For a while her illness grew worse and her life was despaired of. In 1537, she suffered a severe attack of something that seems very much like hysteria (VI)[2]. In the same year, she returned to the convent, weak and partially paralysed; but, thanks to St Joseph, she soon recovered the full use of her limbs.

The rule of the convent, in which she had found protection against a threat of perdition, was not severe. The sisters enjoyed considerable freedom of relation with the outside world, so that God was neglected and Theresa's love of worldly intercourse and friendship was largely gratified. In the seventh and eighth chapters of the *Life*, there is drawn a picture of her moral condition which, she thinks, " will wither the soul of all her readers " : " During almost twenty years I crossed a sea full of storms and tempests. I fell, I rose, and fell again. . . . I did not enjoy God, and I found no pleasure

---

[1] She defines " orison " as " an intimate, friendly intercourse with God, in which the soul expresses her love freely to Him who loves her " (VIII). It does not involve a trance. Under orison, she includes only the first degrees of the mystical Ascent of the Soul to God.

[2] For a study of her illnesses, see the chapter on " Hysteria and Neurasthenia."

in the world." " I wanted, it seems, to combine these two opposites : spiritual life with its delights, and the life of the senses with its pleasures." For a while ashamed of approaching God, she gives up orison entirely and limits herself to the vocal prayers prescribed by the rule. She adds, " I must, nevertheless, admit that during these years there were months and even one entire year of generous faithfulness (*fidélité généreuse*)[1]. Giving myself up to orison, I avoided with the greatest care the least fault and I took serious precautions against giving offence to the Lord " (VIII).

Taken as a whole Theresa's account would show that during these twenty years of ups and downs, she lived quite up to what was expected of her, even by her confessors ; and that she did not suffer very great inner qualms. There were not in her case the causes of wracking misery present in the life of the unhappily married Mme Guyon.

Throughout her adolescence, and at least up to her forty-third year, she continued in that condition, never conforming completely to that which she felt God required of her. What she reproached herself for was mainly the pleasure she found in the admiration of her fellowmen. There was in particular a visitor, precious beyond all others. Who he or she was, she does not say. Perhaps the worst of the misdeeds she reports is letting her father believe that she had given up orison because of ill-health. But that deception does not seem to have troubled her.

In 1555 two events stirred her to the depth and led her one step nearer to the goal. The first was the sight of a statue of the Saviour covered with wounds. " The wounds of the Divine Master seemed so recent ; it was a representation so moving and so vivid of that which He had endured for us that, seeing Him in that condition, I was completely unnerved " (IX). She fell on her knees, shed torrents of tears and begged Him for strength never to offend Him again. Thanks to the help of St Madeleine, she did not cease from that day to make " rapid progress in the inner life " (IX).

The second memorable event was the reading of the *Confessions* of St Augustine. It produced in her a tempest similar to the one just described. She " was overpowered by the anguish of a most bitter sorrow." From that moment she sought God more diligently and became aware of a desire to remain longer with Him in orison and to keep away from the causes of her dissipations.

In spite of their intensity, these experiences of her fortieth year do not divide her life in two parts widely separated ; they mark no more than steps forward towards the goal she had set for herself

---

[1] She refers probably to the first year of her monastic life.

long ago when she resolved to withdraw from the world. When she refers to the period preceding these events as " her own life," and the one following them as " the life of God " in her (XXII), she greatly exaggerates. Almost in the same breath she admits that she is still attached to the World by interests which, though not very bad in themselves, nevertheless compromise the progress accomplished (XXIII). One sacrifice she could not yet make : " It was the giving up of certain friendships, very innocent in themselves, but for which I cared much " (XXIV). One may well suspect an attachment to a person of the opposite sex, more profound than she admits, deeper perhaps than she knew.

The help of St Madeleine being insufficient to break her chains completely, she sought the added guidance of a saintly man. He also proved inadequate. Then God himself came again to her assistance, in a wonderful manner : he granted her a rapture (*ravissement, i.e.,* ascent to the fourth degree in her scheme of the Ascent of the Soul), the first she had ever experienced, and said to her : " I do not want you any longer to converse with men but only with angels." Fear, which at first had seized upon her as life seemed to withdraw, vanished before the assurance of God's Love. After this new favour she thought herself altogether transformed : " From the day when God in one moment changed entirely my heart, my resolution to give up everything for His sake became unshakable " (XXIV). This statement should not be construed as signifying that self-regard and pride never again asserted themselves and led her astray, but only that she gave up the relations that had been the source of many of her shortcomings. In order to estimate correctly the potency of the alleged divine intervention, one should recall that Theresa had reached her forty-third year. At that age, particularly in sunny Spain where women bloom early, little remains of the pride of the flesh ; pride, however, may have found refuge elsewhere.

Until this momentous rapture the Spanish saint had known only the first three of the mystical states described in the *Autobiography*, and visions and auditions had been extremely rare when compared with their frequency afterwards. The complete surrender of her to God's will, following upon her total possession by him in ecstasy, marked the beginning of the period of the great love-trances, of the monitory and premonitory visions and voices, and of persistent external activity in the foundation of reform monasteries.

The most peaceful years of her life were those spent in the newly-established monastery of St. Joseph ; never before or since, did she enjoy " so much sweetness and repose." And yet she was not altogether contented. Now that inner conflicts had ceased, that she was a unified soul possessing in safety God's favour and trust, she was thinking of new worlds to conquer : " I seemed like a person who guards a great treasure and desires to share it with all the world, but whose hands are bound to prevent him from distributing it too generously. For my soul was as if thus bound, and the great blessings which God had given me seemed ill-used, shut up within me¹."

An authorization was obtained, and she entered into an indefatigable activity as a founder of monasteries with a stricter rule than the one then common in Spain. In the face of violent attacks from within her own order, she founded altogether thirty-two monasteries. In that work she demonstrated rare abilities as an organizer, manager and diplomat. During these years, even more than before, she was guided and supported by automatisms, usually in the form of voices.

* * *

2. *The Phases of Santa Theresa's Life.*—Three dates would claim the attention of anyone wishing to divide Theresa's life into periods : her decision in 1533 to embrace the monastic life, the two memorable events of 1555 described above, and the first rapture in 1558.

The first period would then extend to her entrance in the convent of the Incarnation at Avila where she took the veil. Her motives in consecrating herself to God were, as we know, mainly to secure her heavenly salvation. Convent life, such as it existed in many places in Spain, was not without its own charm even for those who craved social intercourse Taking the veil did not mean burying oneself alive.

The second period would last from 1533, for about twenty-two years, and end with the moving incidents that led to the making of new resolutions of complete surrender to God. It was not a homogenous period. It began with a year of great faithfulness to the Lord. Then, she again heard and yielded to the call of the World. At various times she reined herself in and remained for a space closer to God.

One might be tempted to make a separate period of the first year of her monastic life, when, under the impetus of a fresh decision to lead a holy life, of the impressive ceremonies through which she had just passed, and of the new surroundings into which she had come, she gave herself up whole-heartedly to the service of God. But, even then, she was not altogether faithful. And there were later on brief periods of probably equal faithfulness which it would be impossible to date.

¹ *Livre des Fondations*, chap. I.

From 1555 to 1558 might be regarded as a third period, although no very marked changes distinguished these years from the preceding.

In 1558, a definite step forward took place : she at last succeeded in breaking entirely with worldly friendships. This event might serve to date the beginning of a fourth and last period.

The events used in order to divide Santa Theresa's life in periods are mere incidents in a development determined essentially but not exclusively by a logical inner growth. There is no evidence in support of the opinion that she would not have attained an equal degree of self-renunciation and faithfulness to God in the absence of the sight of the statue of Christ with the wounds and of the reading of St Augustine. It is that which was already passing in her that gave to these incidents their significance. Since the moment of their appearance depended upon chance events, these periods do not, any more than those of Mme Guyon, indicate any natural rhythm. Her forward course traced an irregular zigzag line, the exact turning points of which were determined by accidental, external circumstances.

*   *   *

Divide her life as you may choose, Santa Theresa's development was a fairly regular one. There is no particular moment at which one may say that a profound moral transformation took place. Her determination to enter the holy life did not involve a moral rebirth. The long second period, extending to 1555, was one of moderate oscillations. Despite certain statements about the tortures she endured during these years because of unfaithfulness—statements made many years later when writing her biography with a pious purpose—there was little of the tragic in her career. She suffered, as we shall see, periods of dryness ; but they do not seem to have been frequent during these years. She was a general favourite both with the Sisters and with the many visitors, and she endured with much fortitude the sense of her waywardness. Towards the end of that period, however, her burden seemed to have increased. She became seriously distressed. A vision of Christ with " a very severe face," interpreted by her as displeasure at her " vanities " (VII), indicates a grave inner conflict. Then came the statue of Christ with the wounds, and the readings of St Augustine's *Confessions*, with new resolutions as consequence. But no great transformation followed. The chains that kept her attached to the World were not yet broken.

Three years later, in 1558, a new experience—a rapture— occasioned the giving up of the worldly friendships. Nearly all her life she had been flirting with the World from behind the nun's veil, getting what satisfaction she might from her youth, feminine charm, and intellectual cleverness. Why did success come at this time ? The particular occasion for the rapture, we do not know ; but this we do know : she was now forty-three. Age must have materially abated the cravings of the natural man ; and, as they weakened, her other tendencies became more insistent in their claim for realization.

With this surrender, she found herself on terms of perfect trust and understanding with the Lord. Until then, her allegiance had been divided and her energies dissipated in inner struggles. Now there was no other way for her to gratify her aggressive and conquering soul than to place at the service of God whatever ambition and energy she possessed. And so her life ends, like that of Suzo, of Catherine of Genoa, of Francis of Assisi, and of Mme Guyon, in constructive activity, potent enough to overcome every obstacle put in its way.

We have already said in connexion with Mme Guyon why we do not make of these active years a distinct period. Our purpose is to indicate the main phases of a moral development. What happens when that development has reached its end cannot be regarded as constituting a period in that development. From another point of view, however, St Theresa's action as reformer and founder of monasteries evidently constitutes a well-defined phase of her life.

Her moral development resembles very closely that of Mme Guyon. It is less smooth in the latter, and the incidents that mark her movements forward are more dramatic. On the whole, the moral development of the Spanish Saint was as evenly graded as that of most persons, and it followed the course one would expect in a person of her early education and tendencies and breathing the particular religious atmosphere surrounding her.

*　　　　　*　　　　　*

Santa Theresa has described with considerable minuteness, under the general name of " dryness," a variety of closely-related states of lowered vitality. These minor oscillations vary greatly in duration and amplitude. They last one, two, three weeks, " perhaps longer." From the data at hand, it would not be possible to establish a chronological table of them ; but they do not, any more than the longer phases, seem to have followed any rhythm.

Her descriptions bring out the following features : doubt, scruples, frivolity, restlessness, mental dispersion, inertness, irascibility, discouragement, inefficiency ; and, in the realm of feeling and emotion, displeasure, boredom, fear, and anxiety. Doubt of one's salvation, of the love of God, of the divine origin of the raptures, are horribly tormenting ; while mere indifference or the frivolous activity of a mind unable to fix itself, are not sharply painful. We add in a footnote three instances of dryness to illustrate the diversities produced by various combinations of these traits[1].

In chapter XXXVII of the *Life*, she refers to a week just spent in dryness. She was then in the neighbourhood of fifty years of age : " I could feel neither a sense of my obligations toward God nor remember His favours ; my mind was powerless. I had, in truth, no evil thought ; but I felt myself so incapable of good thoughts that I smiled at myself." And here she breaks out in the following amazing speech to her Lord. " What ? Is it, then, not enough that you should keep me in this miserable life ; that I should submit for the love of you. Must you also hide yourself from me ? How can that be reconciled with your compassion ? How can your love for me tolerate that ? Lord, were it possible for me to hide myself from you as you do from me, your love, I feel sure, would not tolerate it. Such ungratefulness is too cruel ; consider, I beg of you, that it is not fair towards the one who loves you so ardently." The astonishment with which one reads this passage is not much relieved by this explanation : " Often, love moves me in such a way that I am no longer master of myself ; then it is that with the greatest freedom I dare to address such plaints to our Lord, and He is gracious enough to tolerate all this " (XXXVII)[2].

It will be granted, we think, that the presence of these minor oscillations of the psycho-physiological level does not call for any

---

[1] " All the favours ever granted me by the Lord were swept out of my memory. My mind was so greatly obscured that I stumbled from doubt to doubt, from fear to fear. I believed myself so wicked that I regarded my sins as the cause of all the evils and of all the heresies that afflicted the world " (XXX). In that false humility induced by the devil, the soul thinks of God as a stern judge only, ready to destroy. " Faith and compassion remain to the soul, it is true, because no effort of the devil could take these away ; but this ray of faith, instead of consoling, only increases the torments of the soul, in that the greatness of its obligations to God is made clearer " (XXX).

" The devil filled suddenly my mind with things so frivolous that at other times I should simply have laughed at them. In that condition one loses neither faith nor the other virtues, but faith sleeps, and the soul becomes the prey of I know not what anguish and torpidity : knowledge of God and of the truths of religion seem a mere dream coming from afar. When the soul wishes to find solace in reading, it gets as little comfort as if it knew not how to read. One day I read four or five times four or five lines of it [the life of a saint], without understanding them "(XXX).

" I find myself at times in a very singular state of stupidity. I do neither good nor evil ; I walk after the others, as the saying is, experiencing neither pain nor consolation, indifferent to life as to death, to pleasure as to sorrow ; in a word nothing matters to me " (XXX).

[2] It is impossible fully to understand certain aspects of the religiosity of Santa Theresa and the likes of her without realizing their familiarity with God. Similar conversations with God may be found in Suzo's *Leben*, chap. XXXI, pp. 121-2, and in our account of Catherine of Genoa.

explanation on the part of the student of religious life, for they are phenomena in no way peculiar to religion. Moments of staleness, doubt, self-distrust, inertia, and general discomfort, morbid or not, are by no means rare outside of religion ; most people are familiar with them. Many an artist, not to speak of more ordinary persons, could match Santa Theresa with regard to recurrent moments of self-doubt, of fretfulness, of flights of shallow uncontrollable thoughts, of sterile dullness, of vacant distress. Oscillations of the psychical level, universal in their minor manifestations, constitute, when much exaggerated, specific forms of mental disorder—the so-called cyclical insanity, for instance, in which periods of great excitement follow upon periods of deep melancholy.

How insignificant psychical influences may be in the production of these conditions is obvious. In later life, St Theresa herself became clearsighted enough to recognize that " at times poor health was for a large part the cause " (XXX) of her periods of dryness. It is one of the pathetic fruits of human ignorance that the unfortunate who suffers from depression physiologically induced, should add torment to misery by interpreting the depression as divine chastise-ment or, even, permanent rejection. To Bunyan, it meant the unpardonable sin ; to Mme Guyon, final reprobation (XXVII).

*   *   *

3. *Did Santa Theresa attain her Ethical Goal ?*—The answer is substantially as in the case of Mme Guyon : she was mistaken when she thought she did. She is frank or naïve enough not to hide the proofs of her imperfection. At fifty years of age she admits that she still feels springing up in her vanity and other defects (XXXI). The account she gives of a long visit, under order from her superior, to a lady, " one of the first of the kingdom," who had recently lost her husband, is an excellent example of self-complacency, aggravated by extravagant professions of humility and wickedness. " Extreme sorrow " is alleged at the thought that the good opinion they had of her decided her superior to send her to the lady. She makes difficulties about going on the ground of her unworthiness. Yet she did not refrain fr.m penning these lines : " During my stay in that house, all those who lived in it made progress in God's service, thanks to His blessing " ; and concerning the lady herself, she says, of the time she spent with her, " Her soul expanded from day to day " (XXXIV). On many occasions she speaks with obvious pride of her influence upon various persons. But it is especially in the way in which she proceeded in the matter of the foundation of her first monastery that she reveals her common humanity. All her immediate superiors opposed or discouraged her. Humility and

obedience prevented her neither from thinking she knew better nor from persisting in her intention. For many years she bided her time, quietly pulling wires. Finally, by dint of persistent secret diplomacy and disregard of her immediate superiors, she succeeded in obtaining a permission from higher authorities.

Those about her accused her of seeking her own gratification ; the town objected for other reasons and carried its opposition to the council of the King. In the end, however, she triumphed. At the first celebration of the mass in her new monastery she exulted ; it was to her " a foretaste of the glory of heaven " (XXXVI). But she did not escape remorse : " Three or four hours after this ceremony the devil stirred up in me a conflict. He suggested to me that perhaps I had offended God in doing what I had done, and that I had failed in obedience in establishing this monastery without the order of my superior." These and other reasons for blame came to her mind, but she dismissed them all as the devil's work !

The conviction of her greatness welled up more than once, but never so baldly as in the vision in which she saw herself being clothed by the Virgin Mary, assisted by St Joseph, with a gown of dazzling whiteness. They decorated her with priceless jewels and told her that she was altogether free from sin (XXXIII).

The significance of this incidence lies not in the dream itself ; for the ethical, hard-won self is not responsible for dream-elaborations, they are the creation of older strata of the mind. It is the Saint's failure to reject the dream as the devil's own that gives to it its significance. Instead of being inexpressibly shocked by this lurid burst of pride, she complaisantly and unhesitatingly accepts it. It would not be sufficient to urge in her defence that she was in the habit of regarding dreams populated by angels, the Virgin, and other inhabitants of Heaven, as sent from God. That she could regard that dream as sent from God is a material fact in the evidence to be adduced against her perfect humility. Her saintliness was shot through with an ambition and a pride that death alone could subdue. We may repeat here that the ambition of our mystics soars so high that nothing short of divine power and glory satisfies them

*   *   *

St Marguerite Marie[1] (1647-90)

This contemporary of Mme Guyon was beatified in 1864 and recently canonized. She offers really nothing new to the student of the preceding biographies. The same dominant tendencies and the

---

[1] Unless otherwise stated the quotations are from the *Histoire de la Bien-heureuse Marguerite Marie et des Origines de la Dévotion au Cœur de Jésus*, by Emile Bougaud, Bishop of Laval, Paris ; Poussielgue, 1900, pp. 365.

same general environment produced results of the same sort. But she lacked the superior intelligence of her great predecessors. Intellectual inferiority, combined with a powerful sex-impulse, early awakened by religious symbolism and directed to Jesus, make of her a link between the great, accepted mystics and a class of mystics with whom the Church will have nothing to do. If, despite her mental inferiority, the *Dévotion au Cœur de Jésus* grew out of her " revelations " and she was canonised, it is thanks to others who saw in her visions an opportunity of fortifying the Church of Rome. The worship of the Sacred Heart of Jesus spread rapidly, acquired vast proportions, and continues to wield great influence in France and in other countries.[1]

Marguerite Marie Alacoque was born in 1647 of humble parentage. When eight years of age, on the death of her father, she was sent to a convent where she seems to have been profoundly impressed by the continual prayers and the midnight devotions. She made her first communion at the early age of nine. Soon after she suffered a serious illness and was withdrawn from the convent. During that long disease she was powerfully attracted to orison. Already then a consuming desire to love God, to suffer with him and for him, and to absorb herself in him, tormented her. The amusements and diversions of her age had lost their attraction.

At home she was miserable. Her uncle, who had become the head of the household, treated her badly. She found refuge more and more completely in God, subjecting herself to austere penances, fasting, iron chains, sleeping on a board, and spending nights in prayer.

Under these conditions she continued to live until the age of fifteen. It is at that time that God began to appear to her. She repeats on almost every page of her *Memoirs* that her Sovereign Master had taken possession of her soul and directed her in everything. It seems as if she had already attained the complete surrender of her will to God. During her devotions she gets into a state of absorption or trance, as the following quotation indicates. " As soon as she had a moment to spare she would run to church. She

---

[1] " The revelation of the Sacred Heart," writes Mgr Bougaud, " is, without doubt the most important of the revelations which have enlightened the Church after those of the Incarnation and of the Eucharist. It is the greatest illumination since Pentecost." Over against this opinion may be placed that of another of her biographers, " The devotion of the Sacred Heart created by Marguerite Marie Alacoque, or rather founded upon her hallucinations, should be abolished as a religious aberration unworthy of humanity."—" Marie Alacoque," by Dr Rouby, *Revue de l'Hypnotisme*, vol. XVII, 1902-3, pp. 112, ff. ; 150, ff. ; 180, ff. ; 373, ff. This study written from the standpoint of the alienist is based upon the *Journal* of the Saint, as published by Mgr Languet in 1827. The edition that I have used, first published in 1876, is not in complete agreement with that of 1827.

could not remain in the nave, love carried her to the foot of the altar.
She was never near enough the tabernacle. ' I could no longer pray
vocally before the holy sacrament,' she would say. 'I could have spent
there days and nights without food or drink. I did not know what
I was doing there, except that I was being consumed in the presence
of God like a burning holy candle ' " (73).

As she reached the age of seventeen her home situation changed.
Her brothers, now of age, assumed the leadership. Their financial
situation was now good and the household was happy and gay.
She responded to the new surroundings. " I began," she says, " to
see people and to adorn myself in order to please, and I sought amuse-
ment so far as I could " (80).

But God did not let her go. She describes thus her experiences
on coming back from an evening's entertainment : " At night, when
I took off these cursed liveries of Satan—I mean these worldly
trappings, my Sovereign Master would appear to me as He appeared
at His flagellation, all disfigured, and would reproach me strangely,
saying that my vanities had led Him to this state, that I was betraying
Him, persecuting Him, Him who had given me so many proofs of His
love. In order to punish myself for the injuries that I had done Him,
I would bind this miserable criminal body with ropes full of knots,
and I would draw them so hard that I could hardly breathe and
eat " (81-82). She adds that the ropes remained on her so long
that she could not remove them without tearing off bits of her
flesh. On another occasion she engraved with a pen-knife the
name of Christ over her heart. The wound was not deep, for at
her death no scar was visible.

Her mother, who was not happy in her sons' house, was in
haste to see her married in the hope of finding a better home with her.
But Marguerite Marie was haunted by the vow of chastity made in
infancy and the thought that, if she broke it, she would be punished
by " frightful torments." Thus for four years, from 1663 to 1667,
she struggled between her love of the World and her love and fear
of God. As she approached her twentieth year her desire to be a
nun grew so fervent that she resolved to realise it " at any cost."

During these years she had read the lives of the saints, including
probably much mystical literature, and had spent much time teaching
children in her own room and visiting the poor. Her passionate love
of Christ had apparently been growing. She felt that he was urging
upon her the fulfilment of her vow. He said to her : " I have chosen
you as my bride ; we promised each other faithfulness when you
made me a vow of chastity. I pressed you to take that vow before
the world had any part in your heart, for I wanted it altogether pure,

untainted by any earthly affection " (88). " One day, after holy communion, He showed me that He was the handsomest, the richest, the most powerful, the most perfect and accomplished of lovers ; and demanded why it was, since I was promised to Him, that I wanted to break the engagement " (92). Thereupon, she renewed her vow of chastity and definitely refused to marry.

Three years later, at the age of twenty-three, she entered the monastery of the Visitation, founded by St. François de Sales at Paray. " Seventeen months later she lay down on the pavement of the church, the sheet of the dead was spread over her, and she rose again, radiant, for she was henceforth to be dead to the world."

It must be said in praise of the good sense of the monastery that during her noviciate much was done to put an end to her ecstasies and her excessive asceticism. The extraordinary graces that she enjoyed were under suspicion. The monastery demanded the plain Christian virtues : obedience, humility, brotherly love. She declared herself willing and desirous to obey ; but, as in the case of St Theresa, encouraging visions and ecstasies continued to appear.

In order to assuage the consuming fires of love, the Mother Superior sent her to the garden to take care of an ass and her colt. This remedy proved ineffective ; the company of the asses did not restrain her from seeking and finding that of God. But presently the sisters not only became accustomed to her visions and revelations, they grew proud of her ; and, as revelations followed fast upon each other, she came to be looked upon as appointed of God to perform a great task.

Her behaviour impressed her associates as perfect, says her biographer. A Mother Superior declared that during the six years that she had known her she had not once failed to live up to her promise to make God rule in her before all, above all, and in all. She herself was not quite of that opinion. One comes frequently in her *Memoirs* upon passages of this tenor : " On another occasion I spoke of myself with some vanity. O God, how many tears this fault caused me ! For when we were alone together He reprimanded me with a stern countenance, saying, ' What have you, O creature of dust and ashes, of which you can boast, since you are but Nothingness ? In order that you may not forget again what you are, I will show you a picture of yourself,' and immediately He made me see in miniature what I am. This picture awakened hatred of myself and desires of vengeance against myself " (145-6).

She seems to have suffered in common with other mystics from attacks of sleep. Her biographer finds pleasure in quoting attestations of her companions from which it appears that she would forget herself for indefinite periods while on her knees before the altar, remaining all the time perfectly motionless. Everyone wondered how she could stay so long in the same attitude. They described her as filled with God, motionless as marble, with eyes closed and an expression of ecstasy on her face. At times, however, things took another turn. While on her knees in the choir, she would suddenly faint and then " she had to be carried out, trembling and burning. Her face was flaming, her eyes in tears. She could not utter a word."

She was subject to sensory automatisms and to imperative impulses. We have already met in the lives of several mystics incidents similar to this one : " I was so sensitive that the slightest dirt gave me nausea. He (God or Christ) found fault with me on that score so strongly that once while cleaning up the vomit of a patient, I was not able to refrain from doing it with my tongue. He caused me to find so much delight in that action that I should have liked an opportunity of repeating it every day. In order to reward me, the following night He held me at least two or three hours, the mouth glued upon His sacred heart[1]." One may suppose that the " delight " involved in that repulsive action was merely relief at having yielded to an imperative impulse. Resistance to imperative ideas is known to cause at times anguishing pain. In another connexion she reports that resistance had no other effect than to make her suffer.

Her love for Jesus was at times so intense that it became an excruciatingly delightful pain : " When I have received Jesus, I feel quite done up, but filled with a joy so intense that at times for a quarter of an hour everything is silence within me except for the voice of Him whom I love." " The longer she lived," writes her biographer, the " more the love of God consumed her. Her frail and delicate constitution could not resist such emotions. Emaciated, pale, with transparent flesh through which shone as it were, the flame of the spirit, she realised more and more the song of her noviciate :

> " I feel myself a harassed doe
> Wounded and panting for water ;
> The dart of the huntsman has pierced to my heart,
> His hand has compassed my slaughter[2]."

Once as the bridegroom was crushing her by the weight of his love and she was remonstrating, He said : " Let me do my pleasure There is a time for everything. Now I want you to be the plaything

---

[1] Quoted by Dr Rouby, *loc. cit.*, p. 180 ; and also more briefly by Mgr Bougaud, p. 172.

[2] pp. 173-4.

of my love, and you must live thus without resistance, surrendered to my desires, allowing me to gratify myself at your expense[1]."

The *Apostolat du Sacré Cœur*, by which, according to her biographer, the Church was revivified, is the outcome of a series of revelations vouchsafed her during the cataleptiform attacks described above ; of their puerility the reader will be able to judge for himself. She was commanded to put these revelations in writing. She obeyed, blotting the pages with tears. Only one of her note-books now remains. She states that nothing but her vow of obedience would have made possible to her this task, so much did it outrage her sense of humility. Nevertheless, she was evidently deeply impressed by the glorious rôle to which her visions called her. They are of Jesus and of His heart, of flames issuing from it, and of her being drawn upon His bosom—of this and of little else. The time came when " every first Friday of the month the sacred heart of Jesus would appear to me as a sun shining with a dazzling light. Its rays struck perpendicularly upon my heart which was set afire and threatened to be consumed to ashes " (322). The heart of Christ appeared at times pierced through and torn by blows ; at other times pressed upon by a crown of thorns and bleeding. Whatever the vision, there was always the thought of ardent love attracting the soul. Like other mystics, she usually felt that her descriptions did not do justice to the revelations.

The tablet commemorating the Devotion of the Sacred Heart bears this quotation from her *Memoirs:* " My Sovereign Master made me repose long upon His divine breast, and discovered to me the marvels of His love and the inexplicable secrets of His sacred heart which He had so far hidden from me. Jesus said to me : ' My divine heart is so filled with love for all mankind and for you in particular that it is unable to contain longer within itself the flames of its burning charity ; it must spread them abroad by your means.' After these words He asked for my heart, and I begged Him to take it ; this He did, and placed it in His own adorable heart."

The following information concerning the scenes that attended the ceremonies of the beatification of Marguerite Marie and the miracles alleged to have signalized them, deserve perhaps a place here as documents revealing the utterly pre-scientific attitude of a large part of the contemporary population of civilized countries.

In 1824, one hundred and thirty-four years after her death, Pope Leo XII, in response to the appeals of the sisters of the Visitation, took the first steps

[1] " Je veux que tu sois maintenant le jouet de mon amour, et tu dois vivre ainsi abandonnée à mes volontés sans résistance, me laissant contenter à tes dépens." This passage, the translation of which I give above, is taken from the *Memoirs* of Marguerite Marie (Edition Languet) as quoted by Dr Rouby. In the edition that I have elsewhere followed the meaning has been modified.

toward her canonization and proclaimed her " Venerable." Six years afterwards, the apostolic delegates appointed by the Holy See to investigate the " heroic virtues " of Marguerite Marie arrived in France. Her tomb was opened in the presence of the diocesan bishop, a large number of priests and monks, and four physicians. They found within " only the bones, but these exhaling the aroma of immortality. The bones were dried, and all the flesh consumed ; the brain alone remained intact ; that alone, O wonder of wonders ! had resisted corruption. This part, so soft, so delicate, which so rapidly wastes away, which is the very first to decay, was there, after a hundred and forty years, in all its former freshness. One could scarcely credit the evidence of his own eyes : the miracle was overwhelming."

Fourteen years more were found necessary for examining the virtues of the " Venerable." " Everything was analysed, studied, discussed, with that exactitude, that deliberateness which characterizes the irrevocable acts of the court of Rome. The Congregation of Rites had just reported favourably on her heroic virtues, when Gregory XVI died, leaving to Pius IX the glory and joy of proclaiming them." This, Pius promptly did ; but not until twenty-four years later, in 1864, was the final decree of beatification promulgated. Its celebration began at Paray by the re-opening of the tomb for the final removal of the sacred relics which were to be placed " on the altar of St. Peter to receive the first homage from the Pope and the Church." The chief magistrates of the town and more than three hundred priests accompanied the sacred remains where they were to be examined. A moment of tense anxiety prevailed as they waited to discover the condition of the brain, which in 1830 had appeared quite free from corruption : " In what state was it going to be found ? Would God have preserved this sign of life in the dry bones ? The bishop lifted the skull. ' Behold, behold the sacred sign ! ' In vain had thirty-four years slipped past ; in vain the opening of the casket and the exposure of the brain to the air ; it is intact, though slightly hardened and shrunken. The crowd prostrate themselves and adore ; they recount to one another similar happenings, and all hearts beat high with a holy enthusiasm." (444-58 abbreviated.)

These extraordinary scenes took place not in the Dark Ages but in the latter half of the last century ; and the author of this account of them was a bishop of the Roman Catholic Church. In 1900 his book had reached its tenth edition.

CHAPTER V

THE MOTIVATION OF CHRISTIAN MYSTICISM

WHAT do the Christian mystics want ? Were we to ask them that question, they would give us the traditional answer. But it should not be assumed that it would name fully and exactly the forces that drive them on. The motives assigned for action are often mere justifications for promptings very imperfectly understood. We are all distressingly like the unfortunate asylum patient impelled in and out of season to wash his hands. He washes them " because they are dirty." Yet, the psychiatrist is aware of other promptings hidden to the patient.

The mystics say that they want " God." That is a convenient traditional way of naming their goal. But what is it that urges them on, what do they really want when they want " God " ?

That is our present problem. We began to seek an answer to it in the first chapter where we inquired into the effects of drugs used by the non-civilized to make him divine. We shall continue in the present chapter, and here with special reference to Christian mysticism.

*   *   *

The behaviour of the mystics, like that of everybody else, is instigated by innate tendencies to action and by needs[1] that express themselves in forms determined mainly by experience. The tendencies and needs that come to expression with especial intensity in our group of mystics may be listed as follows :

1. The tendencies to self-affirmation and the need for self-esteem.

2. The tendencies to cherish, to devote oneself to something or somebody. These tendencies come to their most perfect expression in the parents' relations with the utterly dependent child but, strange as it may seem, they appear even in man's relations with God.

---

[1] " Tendency to action " means here an impulsion to behave in a particular way, while the term " need " is used to designate a striving restlessness without specific direction. Experience soon teaches us, however, how our ordinary needs can be relieved, and, then, definite tendencies become connected with them. The feelings due to lack of nourishment and to moral isolation constitute respectively the need for food and the needs for social relationship.

3. The needs for affection and moral support.

4. The need for peace, for single-mindedness or unity, both in passivity and in action.

5. "Organic" needs or needs for sensuous satisfaction (especially in connexion with the sex-life). If the mystics profess disdain for the body and its pleasures, it is not because they are indifferent to sensuous delight as such, but because they see some incompatibility between the pleasures of the flesh and the soul's welfare. When they are not aware of the bodily origin of sensuous enjoyment, they give themselves up to it with great relish and complete abandon.

There is nothing singular in the existence in the mystics of these springs of action; they are present in every civilized individual. It is the energy and tenacity of certain of them, and, more especially, the method used to gratify them that distinguish the mystic.

Whatever particularity marks the mystics off from other persons is due to their education as much as to their temperament. Each one of those we are considering fell very early under the influence of two great ideals of monastic Christianity : self-surrender to God's Will and chastity. These ideals might not strike very deep roots if the Church did not present them not only as good in themselves, but as conditions of securing the highest imaginable good—divine love. One of the effects of that belief is that chastity does not appear merely as an abstention, a negative virtue ; it leads up to a most intense love. Our mystics were taught furthermore that the only means of adequately realising these two ideals are to be found in the Christian scheme of salvation.

The ideals of self-renunciation, of chastity, and of surrender to a loving and righteous God constitute the essential acquisitions of their early years. It can be said of these ideals that they represent the potency of medieval Christianity.

Suzo, guided by his pious mother, entered the Dominican Order at the age of thirteen, and, a little later, came under the direct influence of Eckhart. In early childhood Catherine of Genoa was extraordinarily moved by a picture of the dead Christ in His Mother's lap ; it " seems to have suggested religious ideas and feelings with the suddenness and emotional solidity of a physical seizure[1]." Between

---

[1] Von Hugel, *loc. cit.*, vol. I, p. 28.
We are told of Catherine of Sienna that when six years old, she saw above the Church of San Dominico " Christ seated on an imperial throne, clad in the papal robes, and wearing the tiara. He smiled upon her and blessed her and the girl became absorbed in ecstasy until her brother, calling and pulling her by the hand, brought her back to the sounds of earth (Gardner, p. 8). From that moment she began to do penance and to constrain herself to ascetic practices.

the ages of thirteen and sixteen, influenced by her confessor and her sister, the Canoness of an Augustinian convent, she desired to enter a monastery. Santa Theresa was familiar from early childhood with religious devotions. At seven she ran away with her brother, Roderick, to seek martyrdom among the Moors. At sixteen, she was placed in a convent. Mme Guyon spent in a convent most of the years that preceded a very early marriage. At the end of her father's garden she had a chapel dedicated to the child Jesus where she performed her childish devotions. At twelve, under the influence of a priest, she had her first spell of intense piety and learned to make orison. At eight years of age, St Marguerite Marie was sent to a convent. At nine, she made her first communion. She had already lost taste for the pleasures of her age. Very soon after, she was able to " absorb herself in God."

One might continue through the list of the great mystics and show how their imagination, heart and conscience became very early possessed by the ideals of the Christianity of their times.

In the only instance we shall consider of a Protestant modern mystic (Mlle Vé), the idea of self-surrender to God's will was also implanted early as well as the ideal of chastity ; this last was trans-mittted to her in the form common in Protestant Christianity where virginity is not regarded as superior to the married state.

Fear is a relatively insignificant factor in the lives of the great mystics. It is often entirely absent, and it is only in early life that it is ever present as a fear of divine punishment on earth, or of hell-fire hereafter. The only two noteworthy instances of this fear appear in Theresa and in Marguerite Marie. When the former embraced the holy life, she was aware of the fear motive. The second was restrained from breaking her vow to remain a virgin, by fear of the wrath of Christ, her Bridegroom. Later in the career of each, fear vanished altogether. There is no place for that emotion in the intimate love-relation they maintained with the heavenly Powers. Not even during the periods of dryness does fear of hell reappear ; the fear of which they may speak at those times is the fear of having offended and lost God.

Thus our mystics were placed very early in life in the presence of a dilemma : two roads opened before them, one leading to the World, the other to Heaven. The advantages of the holy life were kept before their eyes during the most impressionable years, by the matchless prestige and the powerful means at the disposal of the Church of Rome. The World appeared full of dangers mortal to the soul, and offered at best inferior satisfactions, while Heaven involved a renunciation of the cravings of the natural man. But this sacrifice was to be rewarded after death with an eternal life of bliss ; and, on this earth, with an incomparably delightful love-relationship with God and Christ.

But even the Church influences, powerful as they were, seem to have been, in the majority of our instances, insufficient to compel the choice of the road ultimately followed. Nothing less than a peremptory rejection by the World was necessary in order to bring them to the other alternative. It was not until finally spurned by the social group in which he was ambitious to move that Francis of Assisi turned to Christ. If in the case of Suzo it cannot be said with assurance that the World rejected him, it seems that his native disposition and the quality of his religious ideal made it difficult if not impossible for him to accept the love of woman as adequate. In the absence of a maiden's love, he sought the divine Mistress ; and, having found her, never could or would leave her for any mortal.

St Catherine of Genoa met with the most grievous disappointment that can befall a woman of delicate sensibility and ethical refinement. Scarcely out of childhood she was married to a man quite unworthy of her. Love was baulked of its dues perhaps even more completely in the instance of Mme Guyon. These two women were thrown into the arms of the divine Lover by an unbearable earthly situation. We do not forget that in similar circumstances other women seek worldly compensations ; they find love outside the marriage bond and regard their lot if not as satisfactory, at least as tolerable. The mystic differs from these persons by the presence in him of the high ideals we have mentioned and by the belief that the holy life is more than an acceptable alternative to earthly love.

The case of St Marguerite Marie is also quite clear. She was somewhat inclined to marry and would, it seems, have done so had she not bartered away her freedom when a mere child. Repeatedly she had vowed to keep herself a virgin for Christ's sake, and she had early tasted the incomparable sensuous delight with which he rewards some of those that give themselves up to him. There is something clearly morbid in her relation with Christ, both with regard to love and to the fear of his wrath should she break her vows of virginity. Mlle Vé also suffered, and in a marked degree, from unrealized love-aspirations and unsatisfied sexual need.

Not one of the prominent representatives of mysticism lived a normal married life[1]. The kind of love bestowed by them upon God and Christ is apparently incompatible with normal conjugal relations. Anticipating a later section, we may say already now that many of the curious phenomena to which most great mystics owe in part their

[1] George Fox is no exception to this rule.

fame or notoriety are due to perturbations of the sex function consequent upon its repression.

*   *   *

The saying that reciprocated love brings with it everything that the heart desires is true, if at all, only when the object of love is perfect in goodness and power. The mystic seeks, and, as he thinks, finds union with a loving God, the embodiment of all perfections; or, rather, he seeks that which the divine Presence would bring in the way of peace, affection, self-assurance, self-respect, etc. To realize the presence of the God of Love is the mystic's method of securing the satisfaction of his essential wants.

In mystical ecstasy, that Presence is secured in a peculiarly concrete—one might say, sensuous manner. In another connexion we shall have to consider the cause of that concreteness, and we shall learn that the relation of certain classes of patients to their physicians and its practical results, especially when they hypnotize their patients, is in a surprising degree similar to the relation of the mystic with his God and to its results.

But trance ecstasy is rare and not vouchsafed to all those who seek and find the companionship of a loving God. Also at other times the mystic may be conscious of the nearness and love of God, feel him by his side, walk, as it were, hand in hand in blessed companionship with him. The following analysis of the boon of divine Presence refers, therefore, to the experience of all those who enjoy, in various degrees of intimacy, personal relations with the Christian God.

For the purpose of exposition it will not be advisable to follow the order in which the significant springs of mystical life have been listed above. A number of them will be grouped under the heading " Universalization or Socialization of the Individual Will." The discussion of that topic and of the sex impulse will demand most of the space occupied by this chapter.

*   *   *

1. *The Tendencies to Self-affirmation and the Need for Self-esteem.*

To be loved means to be esteemed and admired beyond all others; it is an acknowledgment of one's worth. The greater and better the lover, the more complete the satisfaction. Thus, to be loved by God gratifies in a perfect way the need for self-respect and the tendencies to self-affirmation.

Certain aspects of the behaviour of the great mystics, especially their professions of humility and obedience and their apparent readiness to suffer anything, however offensive, has led to an altogether wrong interpretation of their character. They have been assimilated with the humble and purposeless. This is a misunderstanding; they are, on the contrary, determined not only to be worth while but also to be recognized as such; they will not tolerate the "inferiority complex." Their light shall not shine under a bushel. They show the firmest purpose and accept no influence that does not lead where they want to go. The reader will recall how forcibly their relations with their directors illustrate this point.

Francis of Assisi may be taken as a representative of the group in point of ambition. He is pictured by his biographers as a wild youth, consumed with a desire to shine. The son of a merchant in the little town of Assisi, he must needs keep company with the gilded youth of the place and squander with them the hard-earned money of his father. His extravagance gained for him some local celebrity. " To his fancy, life was what the songs of the troubadours had painted it; he dreamed of glorious adventures and always ended by saying : ' You will see that one day I shall be adored by the whole world[1].' " He was " tortured with the desire for that which is far off and high[2]." But his position among the favourites of fortune was precarious; he had to swallow many a bitter rebuff. After a most painful experience[3], his pride wounded past healing by the contempt of those of whom he thought himself the equal, he made a *volte-face*. If the World would not feed his ambition and appease his aspiring heart, the Church and God would. He soon came to be of the opinion that the holy life had provided him with grander triumphs and greater love than the World could have offered him.

Similarly with Ignatius Loyola ; when, in consequence of the loss of a leg, a glorious career in the armies of his earthly sovereign had become impossible, he sought and found compensation in the service of God and the Church. With the consent of the Pope, he made himself the General of an army before which both satanic and earthly powers trembled. The reader will recall that the desire to attract attention and to play a distinguished rôle is written large in the autobiographies of Santa Theresa and of Mme Guyon.

It is hardly necessary to add that, after all, humility, in the sense of a genuine rejection of admiration, is not possible to man and that no sort of greatness can be achieved by one devoid of ambition and of moral energy. Moral worth is not measured by the absence of these traits but by the purpose which they serve.

*　　　　*　　　　*

[1] Paul Sabatier, *Life of Francis of Assisi*, London, 1894, p. 13.
[2] *Ibid.*, p. 9.
[3] *Ibid.*, pp. 17–20.

2. *The Dread of Isolation; the Needs for Moral Support, for Affection, and for Peace in Passivity and in Activity.*

Man is just as dependent upon friendly association with his kind for his mental well-being as he is upon food for his bodily health. To be shown the cold shoulder by everyone, to be despised and rejected, is so abhorrent as to make one shrink from the very thought of it. Isolation entails not only unbearable misery, but inevitable deterioration[1].

But the enjoyment of any company and the possession of the esteem of any kind of persons is not sufficient for the highest happiness. Association with those that are regarded as the best and highest is alone entirely satisfying. The divine Presence, constant and intimate, is necessary to the entire and highest satisfaction of this aspect of human nature—that, in any case, is the mystic's opinion.

Much of that which comes to man in the divine companionship may be designated as *peace*—the peace of repose and the peace of single-mindedness in activity. By peace of repose we mean that which is experienced when the mind, relieved from impulses and desires, ceases to strive. It is relaxation, rest, passivity—the Nirvana for which thirst all the sons of man when the pace has been too quick, the problems of life too complex, and even when the ordinary day's task is done. This peace, man must have at more or less regular intervals. It is such an essential, natural want that he could not get along if nature had not provided relief for it in the automatic subsidence of self-consciousness into sleep. But to that automatic relief he has added others of his own finding. The use of narcotics is largely a response to the demand for relief from tension, perplexity and worry; and worship is a device for producing, among other things, the same result. The Bishop of Puy in a speech to crusaders under the walls of Antioch tells them that "he who shall die, shall have his bed prepared in Paradise." "To conquer a bed in Paradise was to be the goal of all good knights[2]." Thus is expressed, in its crudest form, the desire for the peace of passivity. That peace is a

[1] The fear of isolation, expressed in its simplest form in the herd instinct, assumes a very different form in men of high intellectual culture. In an essay on immortality, C. F. Dole writes, " I own that the more I know about life, the more I desire to discover rationality in it. I had rather be a citizen for even a brief period in a significant and intelligent world than to live forever in a meaningless world . . . . I cannot help this kind of bias." An irrational world would mean to this writer intolerable isolation. In order to be happy, he must be able to think that the Universe is, like himself, rational. This assurance would bring him, if not all, at least some of the essential stimuli found by the mystic in the divine Presence.—*The Hope of Immortality*, Ingersoll Lecture, 1906, p. 4.

[2] Léon Gauthier, *La Chevalerie*, p. 99.

boon so great that millions of men look no further : the consumma-
tion devoutly to be wished is, for them, the attainment of permanent
Nirvana, that is, of peaceful oblivion. Mystical worship offers a
remarkable and effective method of obtaining moments of perfect
peace in passivity.

But the temper of the people who have produced or accepted
Christianity, is one that sets the *peace of action* above that of
passivity. It is not that they disregard the latter ; but that,
instead of setting it up as an end in itself, as Buddhism does, they
regard it merely as a preparation. What they want is not subsidence
of the personality into an impersonal All, but fullness of individual
existence. Refreshing and blissful moments of passivity are
merely a condition of effective and undistracted activity. In the
religions possessed of that ideal, God has been conceived accordingly,
and worship has taken a form conducive both to the peace of
passivity and to the mental unification and vivification required for
success in the struggle for a more satisfying life.

The need of realizing, in the interest of efficient action, a
condition of mental harmony, appears with startling vividness in
persons particularly lacking in energy, in victims of irresolution,
doubt and worry. These people illustrate in a sphere other than
religion, the need of what we have called the peace of activity, and
also the surprisingly powerful influence of a personal relation of
admiration and trust.

Dr Paul Farez writes of a neuropathic woman afflicted by
obsessions, " Mme C. has been for a long time under the care of one
of the most sought after physicians of Hospital staffs. She visits
him on an average once a month. If he receives her well, she enjoys
good health for a month ; if, from the slightest indications, she
gathers that he is preoccupied, apprehensive, tired, she is ill during
the whole following month.

" Although he does not consciously hypnotize, this physician
exercises upon his patients a considerable psychical influence. When
in his presence, Mme C. is, as it were, drowsy, and can hardly speak.
She recovers her thoughts only when she is again outside ; but the
hand that he has shaken remains warm ; she feels stronger,
encouraged. She has found in her physician the guide, the moral
support, the director of thoughts whom she needs[1]."

Similar observations will be found in the writings of every
physician who has practised among sufferers from this form of mental
insufficiency. But no one has understood this aspect of human nature

---

[1] Dr. Paul Farez, *Stigmates de Dégénérescence mentale et psychothérapie,
R v. de l'Hypnotisme*, April, 1901.

and the rôle of the physician as "*directeur*" more completely than Pierre Janet. His works contain many illustrations of what he ventures to call the *maladie de l'isolement*. Gièle insists upon her need to give herself up to another, to abandon herself, to sacrifice her personality in order to live in something superior. She has always felt "an impulse to cuddle up[1]." Nadia declares : "Life is nothing if I have not someone to admire, to listen to. It seems to me that the one I love is like a solid rock to which I am tied in the midst of a raging sea[2]." These needs are universal. Everyone of our mystics expresses them in words and deeds. When Mlle Vé attempts to state her chief needs, she writes, "Nothing makes me more unhappy than not to have anyone who interests himself in a particular way and sympathetically to what goes on in me[3]." In the loved presence, we know how to act, we are relieved from tormenting uneasiness, hesitations and scruples.

"Many of these psychopaths do not realize the nature of their disease, and do not go to a physician ; but they nevertheless find a person whom they entrust with the direction of their minds. B.K., twenty years old, daughter of an epileptic and alcoholic father, had had hysterical seizures and contractures. She visits the chaplain of the hospital, who admonishes and advises her. She feels happy and in better health, and so she returns to him and asks advice concerning even insignificant actions. She goes to see him every day. Her parents, who look upon these visits with suspicion, do not succeed in reducing their frequency. From the day when she first saw the priest the hysterical manifestations ceased ; and, yet, he certainly did not hypnotize her, nor did he make use of suggestion in any form[4]." Did not something similar happen to Mme Guyon when she met Father la Combe, and, in general, to those who live in the divine Presence ?

A young woman, twenty-three years old, "falls sick, shows a beginning of hysterical manifestations, because her husband who is compelled to go to work away from her leaves her alone several days a week. She says : I had merely a mechanical life ; I would dream wide-awake ; I was like a somnambule, as if I were tipsy. When, under these circumstances, she takes a lover in a quite haphazard fashion, it is, I believe I have the right to say, not under the stress of a physical need, but because of the moral need for some one near her

[1] P. Janet, *Les Obesssions et la Psychasthénie*, Paris, 1903, vol. I, p. 388.

[2] *Ibid.*, p. 389. See also by the same author, *Les Médications Psychologiques*, Paris, Alcan, 1919, vol. III, pp. 386-93, and the following sections.

[3] *Une Mystique Moderne*, p. 153.

[4] P. Janet, *Névroses et Idées Fixes*, vol. I, p. 458-9.

who would make her obey. As a matter of fact, the hysterical manifestations disappeared immediately[1]. Isolation is, according to Janet, the chief factor in many psychoses, particularly in serious cases of aboulia. He has gathered many instances of young wives tormented by fixed ideas, by the doubting mania, by hypochondria, by hysterical manifestations, because their husbands have not known how to assume the rôle of directors of their minds. " They are people who feel an instinctive horror of isolation and make desperate efforts to keep some one near them[2]."

However insufficient when inhibited, scattered, and divided against itself the energy of the patient may be, it becomes relatively adequate when stimulated, organized, and directed under the influence of a trusted friend. That is precisely what is accomplished in the preceding instances : thus the peace of activity is secured.

The relation of two persons to each other when one controls and guides the other by means other than rational persuasion, is seen in its most complete example in hypnotism. The French word, *rapport*, has become the technical term for the designation of the relation of the hypnotized person to the hypnotizer. If the reader will turn to the account of Mme Guyon's life, he will observe that, between her and God the relation is essentially that of the hypnotic *rapport*. God, she says, prevented her from acting or prompted her into action without her will taking any part. In ordinary mysticism the relation with God, although still of the same type, is nearer to that formed between friends, when one is greatly dependent upon the other.

It would not be necessary to insist upon the profound effect of human relationship if the influence of God upon man did not continue to appear to many as of another order. The frequency with which a human being is utterly dependent upon an intimate companion might be illustrated by a long list of lovers who have pined away when the loved one had disappeared. In chapter XI (The Sense of Invisible Presence and Divine Guidance) will be found a striking instance of the dependence of a man of high intellectual distinction, John Stuart Mill, upon his wife, even after her death.

Intellectual activity itself is fertilized by such a happy companionship as Mill enjoyed with his wife, not only by direct contribution of the beloved to the solution of the common problems, by the

---

[1] P. Janet, *Névroses et Idées Fixes*, vol. I, p. 465.

[2] *Ibid.*, p. 465. When considering the hallucination of presence, we shall have occasion to return to the influence of God upon the believer. In his last work *Les Médications Psychologiques*, vol. III, chap. V, *La direction morale*, P. Janet discusses again and more fully the problems of isolation and of direction.

stimulus of discussion, and by the desire to please her and to enhance oneself in her eyes, but in still another way: her presence and even the *mere thought* of her presence clarifies the mind and purifies the will by calming fretfulness and eliminating the lower greeds. One of my correspondents (No. 52) who complains of being "too often mentally cross-eyed," observes that when in the presence of God his vision is clarified and that he sees things in their true proportions. Thus, by the establishment of what we have called the peace of activity, if in no more direct way, the friendly presence contributes to intellectual productivity and to moral guidance. Of all the methods of suppressing evil complexes, the exorcism effected by a loving presence is the ideal one.

That the blessings secured by rare human friendship may come, in as full if not fuller measure still, through the feeling of the presence of divine personages, has been abundantly illustrated in the preceding biographies. We may bring this subject to a close with two brief quotations expressive of the peace, of the guidance, and of the power that is sought in God and Christ by Christians who do not belong to our group of great mystics. Almost any Christian prayer may serve our purpose—this one by Cardinal Newman especially well : "Teach me, O Lord, and enable me to love the life of saints and angels. Take me out of the languor, the irritability, the sensitiveness, the anarchy, in which my soul lies, and fill it with Thy fullness. Breathe on me with that Breath which infuses energy and kindles fervour[1]." Pusey's supplication differs but little from the preceding : "Let me not seek out of Thee what I can find only in Thee, O Lord, peace and rest and joy and bliss, which abide only in Thine abiding joy. Lift up my soul above the weary round of harassing thoughts to Thy eternal Presence, . . . That there I may breathe freely, there repose in Thy love, there be at rest from myself, and from all things that weary me; and thence return, arrayed with Thy peace, to do and bear what shall please Thee[1]." John Stuart Mill found in a woman, and after her death in the memory of her, what these persons sought in God.

*   *   *

[1] Mary W. Tileston, *Great Souls at Prayer*, London, 1904, p. 35. In an interesting "Study of the Psychology of Prayer," Walter Ranson, in the *Amer. Jour. of the Psychol. of Relig. and Educ.*, vol. I, emphasizes the "unification of consciousness through æsthetic contemplation of God." The very remarkable success of "Christian Science" is mainly due to the skillful use made in it of means of producing the peace of quietude and of action. Mrs. Eddy's cult addresses itself in a business-like way to the elimination of anxiety, worry and other negative attitudes, and fosters mental peace, self-confidence, and optimism.

3. *The Universalization or Socialization of the Individual Will.*

Mental unification, a condition of joyful effectiveness in the struggle for life, is the outcome of a double process : elimination of the elements of discord and organization of the others. This process includes what may be called the universalization or socialization of the individual will ; it is commonly spoken of among Christians as purification, sanctification, the death of the natural man, etc. Its social significance is so great and it occupies a place so conspicuous in the consciousness of our mystics, that we must submit it to some scrutiny.

The mystics have frequently written as if the elimination or the limitation of the egoistic tendencies was merely a condition of drawing near to God in order to enjoy divine union. Thus, the best known of the works of Ruysbroeck, the *Ornements des Noces Spirituelles*, begins with twenty-two chapters describing the virtues, the " ornaments," needed by the soul that wishes to meet the Bridegroom. He is exacting : he wishes the bride to know how to suffer in patience, to be humble and obedient. She is not to be attached to any individual, above all not to herself ; she is to be ready for all sacrifices and services. She must be sweet and full of compassion, generosity and gentleness. Calm in all things, she will meet anger with loving looks and words and deeds of mercy. At the same time, she is to be modest and temperate, and pure in body and soul. " Purity of heart signifies that in all physical temptations or in any prompting of nature, man unhesitatingly turns to God, abandoning himself to Him with a new confidence, . . . for, to consent to sin or to a desire of the body, as an animal, is a separation from God[1]."

But, taken by themselves, passages such as these do not fairly represent the mystic's attitude towards the problems of conduct. Sanctification is not to be achieved only because it is a condition of the divine embrace. The mystics realize, with various degrees of clearness that that would be only another form of selfish indulgence. Since God, their divine model, is in their eyes the embodiment of all perfections, likeness to him implies the elimination of all selfishness. Thus, sanctification is both a part of the ultimate end and a condition of meeting God face to face and enjoying his love.

There is at bottom entire unanimity among our mystics with respect to the ethical goal and to its place in the scheme of things. And the reader who may care will easily find in the preceding biographies and in that of any other Christian mystic, utterances paralleling the following of Santa Theresa : " True perfection consist in the love of God and of the neighbor. . . . Our rules

[1] *Noces Spirituelles*, from Maeterlinck's French translation.

are only means to attain better that end[1]." "Let it be clearly known that the true love of God does not consist either of sweetness or of that tenderness which we ordinarily desire because it consoles us, helps us to serve the Lord in justice with a manly courage and humility. That our Lord should lead by the path of the inner pleasures weak women lacking courage like myself, well and good, it may be fitting. . . . But that servants of God, staid, learned, high-minded men, should feel so much pain when God does not give them any pleasurable experiences, this indeed disgusts me." That she loves visions for the enjoyment that they give her, is evident ; but she approves of them because they contribute to her moral growth. She never tires of showing what high practical value can be derived from these divine favours. In the light of ecstasy, she discovers "not only the beams, but also the motes." In visions God gives her advice and comfort. The impress of the ineffable beauty of the Man-God remains in her soul, and her disposition is purified. Then, heroic promises and resolves spring up. When she wants to justify her high opinion of " the most sublime " of all her visions she says, " its effects are admirable ; it purifies the soul marvellously and robs sensuality of almost all of its power[2]."

St Theresa is no exception. Whatever the mystics may say that seems to subordinate unselfish activity to the passive enjoyment of God is belied by specific passages such as the above, by the general trend of their writings, and still more convincingly by their lives ; all of them, so soon as unity was established in their consciousness, have spent themselves without stint in the service of their fellowmen. The delight of the ecstatic trance is for them, in final instance, God's way of encouraging them to greater effort towards saintliness, of clarifying their moral vision, and of making of them more useful instruments of divine action.

Both the primacy of the ethical purpose and the thoroughness with which it must be carried out, come out in high relief in the sermons of Tauler. He seems to have enjoyed ecstasy a few times only, nevertheless, and quite properly, he is generally accounted a great mystic. The ever-recurring theme of his sermons is the replacement of the egoistic, individual will by the divine Will. Union with God means to him, as to most Christian mystics, opening a source of energy to be used in the service of humanity[1]. He is very severe for those who seek first the pleasures of devotion : " We must regard the search after warmth of heart in devotion . . . as a lack of

---

[1] *Inner Castle*, 1st Dwelling, chap. II.

[2] *Vie*, p. 414. Comp. François de Sales in Fortunat Strowski's *Saint François de Sales*, Paris, 1898, p. 263, ff.

spiritual chastity." And, of the Beghards, who called themselves "Contemplators of God," he says, "They may be recognized by the carnal peace which they obtain in making an emptiness in their souls, believing that to be union with God."

There are few chapters in the history of humanity more profoundly significant than those relating the heroic effort to set aside the "natural" man, and to establish in his place the divine Will or, in modern language, the effort to make perfect social beings out of creatures with an animal ancestry. That effort in behalf of the universalized will has appeared in no uncertain manner in everyone of the preceding biographies.

There is a story of a moral crisis, falsely reported of Tauler, which we shall nevertheless transcribe because it brings out excellently the ethical ideal pursued by the great mystics.

The *Friends of God*, a sect influential in Tauler's time along the Rhine valley, remarkable for the purity of their lives and the simplicity of their worship, regarded him as their spiritual father and leader. Yet, according to some of them at least, he was still far from the spiritual goal. A certain Nicholas of Basle, who was of that opinion, made a moral diagnosis of the great preacher and bluntly communicated it to him. Here it is in brief: "You are trusting to your own knowledge and your own talents. Instead of loving and seeking only God, you are seeking your own will. You are attracted to the creature and especially to a certain person whom you love immoderately. You will find in yourself vanity and love of ease. You have wasted your time in living for yourself."

On hearing these accusatory revelations, Tauler is pictured as throwing himself on his accuser's neck, crying out: "Thou hast held a mirror before my soul, my son. Thou hast unveiled all my faults; thou hast told me what was hidden within me, even that I am attached to a creature. But I tell thee truthfully that I myself did not know it, and I do not believe that any other human being could know anything about it. I see quite clearly now that I am a sinner and I am resolved to mend my ways, though it cost me my life." And he, the Master, placed himself under the direction of him whom he called his son.

The task of Nicholas is to bring about in Tauler a radical transformation: the replacement of the primary, self-regarding tendencies by a higher principle of life. Tauler must learn to converse, smile, keep silence, study, preach, in a word *live*, without aiming at personal success, without consulting his pleasure, moved by the sole desire to make the divine Will triumph. To this end, Nicholas puts him under strict discipline.

The soul of a hero was indeed needed to endure voluntarily for two years the continual humiliation of the purifying regimen prescribed for him. Before a year had passed, his convent friends had come to despise him, and he had been abandoned by his spiritual children. Finally, after a crisis that need not be related here, Nicholas assured him that he had at last received the real divine Grace, and added, " Your teaching, which formerly came from the flesh, will proceed now from the Holy Spirit."

The universalization of the individual will is, after all, the root of the ethical purpose of Christianity. It is more than that : it is a tendency generated in man in virtue of his nature and of the circumstances of social life, and, therefore, it transcends Christianity. It appears everywhere, in all human communities, in and out of the religions. The special contribution of the great mystics to the socialization movement consists in having taken certain Christian principles literally, without the compromises and approximations so dear to the practical man. They have believed that the ideal could become the actual ; and relentlessly, heroically, they have striven after complete universalization. Their undertaking may be regarded as a daring experiment in ethical radicalism.

Nothing in conduct is to them insignificant : everywhere they perceive the manifestation of one of the two opposed forces respectively personified as the Evil One and God. Seen from this naïve point-of-view certain incidents in the lives of our mystics, which might appear puerile or absurd, assume the importance which they themselves ascribed to them. Mme Guyon was not tilting at windmills when she put herself repeatedly in a passion of remorse because she had yielded to her desire and that of her husband to go out in a décolleté gown. A trifle such as this assumes the proportion of a tragedy for him who makes of it a contest between the flesh and the spirit. The triumph of that desire would prove the subjection of the spirit ; it would be a first step towards surrender to the devil. Similarly, perhaps, of the strange scene in which the same person takes sputum into her mouth[1]. The repulsion she felt at the sight of it, hit her as a condemnation. It meant the dominance of the flesh, and she could rest satisfied only when she had proved to herself the mastery of the spirit.

*　　　　*　　　　*

[1] That, and other similar performances, had something irresistibly alluring for the more unbalanced of the mystics. St Marguerite Marie seems to have found a perverse enjoyment in them. One should probably relate actions of this sort to the irresistible impulsive ideas that appear in certain classes of mental disorders.

The Christian mystics are often accused of having exerted an anti-social influence. That judgment is based upon three related characteristics. (1) They lived separated from the rank and file of their fellow men and in celibacy. (2) They prepared themselves not for life on this earth, but for its continuation in heaven. (3) They sought the means of salvation not among men but in God. In this unfavourable judgment the fact of primary importance to which the preceding pages are devoted is left out of consideration : The mystic's preparation for heaven consists essentially in making themselves worthy of it. There was no question among them as to whether salvation was by faith or by works. Salvation began on this earth ; it involved the transformation of the earthly into a divine man ; i.e., the replacement of the egoistic individual will by the universal Will. And they were not satisfied with the practice of this theory in cloistered seclusion. When they felt themselves prepared, they sallied forth as apostles of this eminently social gospel and spent the remainder of their days preaching the love of the All-Father and universal brotherhood. No group of men have loved or tried to love according to a more radically social theory.

The adequacy of their conception of the divine Will and the possibility of realizing it, are questions of ethical appreciation and, as such, fall outside our purpose which is the psychological investigation of mysticism *as it is*. We shall remark, however, that the mystical ideal of Nicholas of Basle may seem unrealizable, but that no one who takes the teaching of Christianity seriously may call it absurd. In a preceding chapter we came without surprise to the conclusion that, despite the drastic methods to which they had had recourse, Mme Guyon and St Theresa never reached their goal, and that the degree of sanctification attained by them did not seem to have been greater than it is in thousands of other inconspicuous Christians and non-Christians. The energy of self-assertiveness to which they owe in part their fame was the main obstacle to the elimination of self-seeking. Not only did they not reach their goal, but they were not morally clear-sighted enough to be aware of their failure.

The Analysis of the Morally Imperative Impulse, and the Conditions of its Production.—From the point of view of human development, the most remarkable aspect of the movement we are studying is that it does not seem to tend to a better adaptation of the individual to society as it is, but rather to an ideal community. The accredited theory of development sees in what is called " progress " an increasing adaptation of the individual to his surroundings. It is undeniable that the ordinary man swims complacently with the current ; his concern is adaptation to the existing social order. Here and there, however, one meets with a man or a group of men who, instead of supinely yielding to external pressure, stand up against it. The behaviour of these people appears to be controlled by a creative urge that sets them in opposition to the existent order. Hardly condescending to accommodate themselves to physical necessities, they endeavour with relentless tenacity and indomitable energy to establish a new type of society. This creative force comes to expression in every society and with particular, although perhaps morbid, intensity in grand mysticism. It is a phenomenon that deserves the attention of the philosopher who would know the forces that are fashioning human society.

The mystic's life and death struggle against the natural man is in part conditioned by the belief that in order to enter into a blessed relationship with God he must accept his Will as his own. But the depth of the problem does not appear until we ask how he came to think that God demands of him something so alien to the more obvious aspects of his nature as sanctification—something impossible of complete attainment ; and how he came to believe so profoundly in that ideal as to regard no effort leading to its realization as too great or too painful ? A phenomenon powerful, persistent, and universal as this one, must, it seems, be an expression of something fundamental to human nature.

Custom and reverence for holy things have tended to keep the psychologist away from the consideration of this most interesting problem. It was supposed to be sufficient to say that man was driven by the " Voice of God," or that in this respect his behaviour was an inscrutable expression of " Universal Reason." Science is now in a position to remove this phenomenon from the position of splendid isolation it has too long occupied and assign to it its proper place in human psychology : its psychological origin, the conditions of its production, and its development can be traced.

* * *

Insistency and imperativeness are traits belonging not only to moral but also to certain non-moral tendencies. Illustrative of the latter class are such teasing experiences as the prompting to get out of bed in order to see whether the gas is properly turned off. You have just put it out and you know that you have done so, nevertheless an impulse to get up in order to verify the fact reappears as often as you dismiss it ; until finally, in order to havepeace, you get up and do the imperative bidding.

In explanation of that type of non-moral imperative tendency, a Freudian might look for suppressed, subconscious factors. The probability is, however, that in most cases a purely physiological cause should be sought. Just as a particular bit of skin may be in a state of irritation, and, therefore, produce a more or less continuous tendency to scratching movements, so one may suppose, in the central nervous system, groups of neurones in a state of abnormal irritability or which have become open channels of discharge. Thus, in the absence of any logical cause, a tendency to a particular action and a corresponding system of ideas might recur insistently.

But the tendencies with which we are concerned are not only imperative and insistent, they possess also another quality : they are approved of, they carry with them the sense of duty, of oughtness. The essential fact is that whereas in the case of non-moral imperatives, the subject is aware that the prompting is absurd or unnecessary ; when the moral imperative is felt, the action appears as required : it *ought* to be performed. The non-moral and the moral imperatives may be equally insistent and may both seem the expression of an external will ; but the second alone receives the subject's allegiance. Without it, a prompting is not felt as morally imperative.

Before we attempt to state the conditions under which an insistent impulse is felt[1] as morally imperative, let it be definitely understood that we are not concerned with the conditions of rightness, considered objectively, but only with those producing the *conviction* of rightness. This difference is a familiar one. That which appears as a duty to a person at a particular time, may not appear so to another, nor even to the same person on another occasion. It is with rightness as with truth ; the conditions that produce, in any particular situation, an assurance of truth are not necessarily sufficient to insure the discovery of the truth.

The specific qualities of the feelings of rightness and of oughtness are, of course, undescribable. One may seek to determine the conditions of their production, but the feelings themselves are simple, immediate data of experience.

An illustration will help us to realize the nature of the situation which might give rise to a feeling of moral obligation. Let us suppose that, at night, I am awakened by the coughing of my brother lying ill in the next room. My first movement may be to go to him in order to do something for his comfort. But before that action is carried out, and following upon a more or less obscure apprehension of the

---

[1] We are not concerned with moral judgments in which a course of conduct is merely classified as belonging to a class we have learned to regard as right.

discomfort of getting out of bed in the middle of the night in a cold room, an antagonistic impulse, i.e., a shrinking from getting out of bed, arises. The shrinking has hardly subsided before a chain of considerations, each with its own tendency to action, may pass through my mind : My brother might be in real need of assistance ; if I do not go to him, serious consequences might result ; it is selfish of me to let myself be stopped by the apprehension of discomfort ; and yet, if I rise, I might catch cold, and colds are not to be trifled with ; etc., etc. The discussion may be brought to an end by a categorical imperative : " You ought to get up."

It might happen that, moved by a sympathetic impulse, I rise and go to my brother before I have heard the categorical command. In that case, my kind behaviour would not possess the quality of a moral imperative. It would be merely an impulsive behaviour—just as my action in remaining in bed when I shrink from getting up. An original sense of duty is felt only if the consequences to myself and to my brother, both of my going and of my not going to him, are passed in review and brought to a conclusion.

When the consideration of the consequences of the performance, as well as of the non-performance of the action, is complete, the resultant tendency to action does necessarily feel categorically imperative. The expression " complete " does not mean that every consequence must have been thought of and properly evaluated—that would be possible only to an omniscient being. It means merely that the discussion was not prematurely brought to an end by an emotional wave, but had been permitted to develop in an atmosphere of dispassionateness, of objectivity, of universalized purpose[1].

If, instead, my intention in the deliberation had been to ascertain what would most advance my own interest and to ignore or slight other motives for action—altruistic motives, for instance—the outcome would not feel morally imperative : I should not have the conviction that it is the one thing to do. The vaguest awareness

[1] When a dispassionate consideration does not end in a tendency to a specific action, we are left in doubt as to the path of duty. But we are now concerned with deliberations issuing in a clear and specific impulse.

The outcome of a dispassionate deliberation which should include only selfish interests, i.e., which should coolly weigh against each other all the selfish aspects of a problem, in so far as the subject was aware of them, would be categorically imperative *provided it were the resultant of the whole man*. But this hypothetical case could hardly be realized in a civilized society, for it is incredible that any one should be able to consider dispassionately a course of conduct and not be aware at some juncture or other that the interests and the rights of others constitute elements of the problem. There are in the human individual innate tendencies making for self-sacrifice and regard for others that could hardly remain entirely unfelt during a dispassionate consideration of prospective conduct.

of something suppressed is sufficient to take the sense of duty away from the decision.

We say, then, that the feeling of moral obligation necessarily accompanies any tendency to action which is the outcome of a deliberation from which no impulse has been excluded, i.e., a deliberation representing the whole man. When this is realised the resultant prompting cannot feel otherwise than as *the one thing to do*, since it is a resultant of all the tendencies present to consciousness.

The quality of the moral imperative decision described by the traditional expression, " the still, small voice," and the attribution to it of an origin external to man, result naturally enough from the circumstances of its production ; it lacks the loud, fleshly quality of decisions taken in the stress of passion ; and it seems external to the individual, in part because of its dispassionateness and in part because it proceeds from a universalized purpose. It may well be called the voice of Universal Reason.

*　　　　　*　　　　　*

But the felt duty may not be performed. Why is it that the conclusion of a dispassionate consideration is not always carried out ? During the deliberation which may end in a moral imperative, the contending forces are not present with their full conative and emotional energy ; they are merely represented. The representation disregards the intensity of the impulses and desires and takes into account only their quality, their worth ; it is a qualitative not a quantitative representation of conative forces. Hence the decision, when it comes, is not of might, but of right.

The nature of these representatives, bearers of the qualitative value of impulses and emotional forces, constitute a difficult problem to which we are not now able to give a solution[1]. We must rest content with the affirmation, borne out by introspection, that to reflect upon a course of conduct with the intention of determining what ought to be done, implies the endeavour to discover and to evaluate all the thinkable results of the possible lines of action with respect to everyone affected. Such appreciation is possible only when, assuming a universalized point of view, the individual enjoys the freedom and the fairness that come with the silencing of the passions, and this is equivalent to a displacement of the energy of the tendencies by their quality-value.

Now, these qualitative substitutes, although not without some motor energy of their own, are very weak when compared with the

[1] The speech mechanism is assuredly included in the mechanism of that representation.

power of the impulses and desires they represent. Nevertheless the decision would usually be carried out if the subject remained in the attitude of dispassionateness long enough for the purpose. Unfortunately in most men that state of integration is highly unstable; it is very easily broken down by any stimulus that sets in activity some particular tendency. And so it very frequently happens that before the command can have been executed, the state of dispassionate deliberation has given place to the ordinary condition in which some particular prompting or group of promptings lead to action without reference to other promptings.

In order to be carried out, dispassionate decisions must usually be backed by some of the primary forces of human nature. When they point to self-sacrifice, they may be supported by those original, innate, altruistic tendencies most powerfully expressed in the relation of parents to their children, and by the self-regarding sentiment in the form which it assumes in civilized persons. In the course of social development the individual comes to prize the good opinion of his fellowmen and, therefore, to seek it. For people of high culture it is the good opinion of only a small class of distinguished persons that matters; and, for those of the highest development, it is, above all, self-approval that is sought—an approval that can be won only by conforming to an ideal of the self. Action in accordance with the dispassionate decision is a developed form of self-affirmation[1]. Aspirants to spiritual perfection are actuated mainly by the thought of moral defeat or victory; while, at a lower level of development, one may be moved to action by the thought of physical defeat or victory.

In persons imbued with the Christian beliefs, the idea of God comes to play in the moral life a rôle of capital importance. It is in the last instance the approval of God that the Christian seeks. How powerfully the idea of God may influence human action when he is regarded not only as Lawgiver and Judge, but also, and primarily, as the loving Companion, is proclaimed by the lives of all the great Christians.

*   *   *

It has already been remarked that the inner compulsion to socialization so dramatically expressed in the lives of our great mystics, is in disagreement with the overt requirements of society. In this respect their lives, as also that of all those who feel keenly the moral imperative, does not conform to the current law of

---

[1] For a presentation of the nature and the formation of the self-regarding sentiment and its function, see Wm. McDougall's *Introduction to Social Psychology*, chaps. VII, VIII, and IX.

development by adaptation to the *milieu*. It is rather an adaptation to inner conditions.

We understand now that what we have called " inner adaptation " consists in a specific organization of the tendencies present in human nature. So that from a first stage of mutual independence, and a second stage of conflict, they become in a third and final stage functionally organized and unified on the basis of their social values. The resultant promptings to action are, then, expressions of a unified personality in functional relation with an ideal society. This work of unification cannot be regarded merely as an adaptive response to external stimuli ; it betrays the presence of inner constructive forces—forces which result in an alteration of the social order.

*   *   *

4. *The Sex-Impulse.*

Sex which, with food and self-affirmation is man's chief concern, could not in principle remain disconnected from religious life since the religions are methods of maintaining and enhancing life. They separate themselves from secular life not so much by their purpose as by the means they use in order to realize them. That which secular life would obtain by natural, human means, the religions seek by appealing to superhuman, divine agents.

The more striking of the many historical connexions of sex with religion are these three : (1) In early religions the procreating power is worshipped in gods regarded as its embodiment. (2) Virginity is sacrificed to gods in order to secure their favour. (3) Virginity and continence are enforced either, again, as a sacrifice pleasing to the gods or because indulgence in the pleasures of the flesh is regarded as the root of great moral evils.

From these connexions of sex with religion a great variety of ceremonies and customs, some of them abhorrent to the civilized conscience, have developed. Sex factors are sufficiently in evidence in religious life to have led careless or ignorant writers to affirm that the whole of it is of sexual origin. It would not be any falser to say that the only need of man is that of sex.

We are concerned in this section with the sexual instinct as it manifests itself in Christian mysticism only. The recognized connexion of that masterful instinct with Christian mysticism is twofold : the Christian God is conceived of as a God of love, and chastity and continence are regarded as states of perfection. The conjunction of these two beliefs leads of necessity to conflicts which can be kept within bounds only in normal, well-balanced persons.

A discussion of sexual matters in connexion with religion may be offensive to some readers ; and yet, there is no avoiding it in a study of grand mysticism. These readers may in the end find themselves in possession of valuable light ; in any case our task is clear, and all that may be asked of us is that we should not unnecessarily insist upon certain unpleasant facts which have to be mentioned in order to make clear the rôle of sex in mystical religion.

The theses which we shall maintain is that the delights said by our great mystics to transcend everything which the world and the senses can procure, involve some activity of the sexual organs. In order to establish that thesis we shall have to show among other things that there exists a connexion between the emotions of affection and love, on the one hand, and sexual activity on the other ; and that the sex organs may be aroused to a considerable degree without the person becoming aware of their participation.

The connexion of affection and love with organic sex activity.—(a) We shall begin with the formulation of what is held in common by practically all the specialists in sex psycho-physiology. The theories of Joanny Roux, of Albert Moll, of Havelock Ellis, and of Sigmund Freud agree together and differ from the popular view in that they give to the sexual impulse a basis much wider than the sex organs proper[1]. According to these theories, the original source of that impulse comes from the organism as a whole. As the body matures, and especially at the time of puberty, it becomes more and more narrowly connected with the organs of reproduction.

The facts which have led to this conception are numerous and in no way equivocal. Many of them have been known for centuries. Here are the most noteworthy of them : the removal of the ovaries in women does not usually do away either with sexual desire or sexual pleasure. In some instances these are increased by that operation. Frequently also the sexual impulse persists after the menopause. There are, furthermore, a number of cases on record in which, in the congenital absence of all the sexual secretory organs connected with the sex functions, the sexual desire has nevertheless appeared[2].

In man the facts are quite parallel : the removal of the testicles after puberty does not take away either sexual desire or enjoyment. The earlier the castration, the less marked the sexual desire ; but even when castration is performed in early infancy sexual desire may develop. It is also well-known that voluptuous feelings are experienced by young children long before puberty, and that the

[1] A fuller discussion of the theories of Moll and of Ellis may be found in the latter's *Studies in the Psychology of Sex*, vol. III, section I. For Freud's theory see *Three Contributions to the Theory of Sex*, New York, 1916. For the theory of Roux, see *Psychologie de l'Instinct Sexuel*.

[2] Cases observed by Colman, Clara Barrus, and others, are reported by Ellis, *Ibid.*, pp. 11-2.

evil of abnormal sex gratification extends to children hardly out of the cradle[1].

The preceding information indicates that the sex-impulse has a much wider origin than the one ascribed to it when it is regarded as attached exclusively to the function of the essential organs of procreation. According to this view the sex-impulse, the *libido* of the Freudians, is originally a function of the whole body. Even when, in the course of animal development, it becomes especially connected with certain parts of the body, it remains nevertheless, in some degree connected with the whole organism. It is with sex very much as with hunger. At the beginning of animal life, no specialized organs of nutrition exist; every part of the body absorbs and digests food. Gradually, these functions are surrendered to specially adapted organs from which now proceed the more obvious hunger-sensations. Nevertheless the rest of the body has remained to some extent sensitive to the need for food and may, up to a certain point, be satisfied without the intervention of the special apparatus provided for the purpose[2].

(b) Sexual excitement appears primarily as a consequence of internal bodily activity and of external stimulation (contact, odour, sight). In civilized man, however, sexual desire is almost as effectively aroused by representations and ideas as by actual sensations. And, because of the richness of his mental associations, the number of objects perceived, or merely thought of, which can lead to thoughts of sex, is almost unlimited.

(c) Ideas are not only sufficient in man to awaken amorous desires, but they may adequately replace the physical stimuli and lead to the orgasm itself. That which has happened to nearly everyone in sleep, is a familiar instance in point. There are persons in whom, even in waking life, the sexual orgasm takes place in the

---

[1] In *The Sexual Life of the Child*, by Albert Moll, are found these statements: "The voluptuous acme may occur in children in the absence of spermatozoa and ova" (even before seven years of age) ; " It may be regarded as definitely established that the equable voluptuous sensation, and more particularly the voluptuous acme, may occur at an age at which, at any rate, secretion does not yet exist in sufficient quantity to be expelled from the urethra, and the existence of such secretion is therefore not unequivocally manifested." pp. 58-9.

[2] Comp. Joanny Roux, *Psychologie de l'Instinct Sexuel*, 1899, p. 22, ff. Similar analogies exist with every one of the specialized functions originally belonging to the whole body. Jacques Loeb and others have shown how, especially in lower animals, before the nervous system has reached a great complexity, the nervous fibres are not necessary for the transmission of the stimuli. They merely facilitate conduction and direct the nervous stimuli to sharply defined points of the body. But when the nerve elements are removed, movements in response to external stimuli continue nevertheless.

absence of any appreciable external physical intervention. Ellis reports the case of a man of fifty-seven, a somewhat eccentric preacher : " My whole nature," writes this man, " goes out so to some persons, and they thrill and stir me so that I have had emission while sitting by them with no thought of sex, only the gladness of soul found its way out thus, and a glow of health suffused the whole body. There was no spasmodic conclusion but a pleasing, gentle sensation as the few drops of semen passed." Ellis suggests that it was not semen, but prostatic fluid. " This man's condition may certainly be considered somewhat morbid ; he is attracted to both men and women, and the sexual impulse seems to be irritable and weak ; but a similar state of things exists often in normal women probably because of sexual repression, and in individuals who are in a general state of normal health. Schrenck-Notzing knows a lady who is " spontaneously sexually excited on hearing music or seeing pictures without anything lascivious in them ; she knows nothing of sexual relationship. Another lady is sexually excited on seeing beautiful and natural scenes, like the sea. . . . Such cases are far from rare[1]."

A sufficient acquaintance with facts that come to the knowledge only of diligent students of the sexual life establishes the conviction that the sexual organs respond in some degree to all tender thoughts, with a certainty and delicacy which will appear impossible to those not well informed. Even the most chaste thoughts of love, those of the mother for her infant and the pressing of it to her breast, awaken the activity of the sexual organism. There are, however, very great individual differences in the intensity of that reverberation. This statement may be made more credible by the mention of experiments[2] in which Mosso demonstrated that, in a normal person, almost any perceived stimulus, and invariably those producing

[1] Havelock Ellis, *Auto-Erotism : a psychological study, the Alienist and Neurologist*, April, 1898.
A case similar to the above is reported by R. Dupouy in the *Jour. de Psychologie Normale et Pathologique*, vol. II, 1905, 421-3. Before she had become a kleptomaniac, Hélène M. had found an increasing pleasure in handling large sums of money, depositing it in the bank or spending it. Her husband was in business. She would beg of him not to pay by cheque in order that she might not lose the delicious shock of counting out the money—a delight which became each day more exquisite. She came to experience the same delight later on, after the loss of her husband and of her fortune, when she had become kleptomaniac. On stealing, for instance, a piece of lace she would feel a great satisfaction, her heart would beat violently and her respiration be impeded. She compares her sensations to the great joys of former times when paying large bills. This person was aware of the participation of her genitals in her enjoyment.

[2] *Clark University Decennial Publications*, 1899, pp. 396-407. Reprinted in appendix to H. Goddard's *Psychology of the Normal and Subnormal*.

emotion, caused contractions of the bladder, contractions of which the subject was unaware.

(d) The subject of the voluptuous excitement may not be aware of the participation of his sex-organs and may, therefore, regard his delight as " spiritual."

Very coarse manifestations of sex regarded as " spiritual happiness " may be witnessed in persons mentally deficient. For several years Pierre Janet had under his observation a remarkable psychopathic woman in whom this connexion was evident. She enjoyed frequent ecstatic trances, described by her in terms customary with the great mystics; I have " enjoyments which, outside of God, it is impossible to know. . . . Earth becomes for me in truth the vestibule of Heaven, I enjoy in advance its delights. . . . I would like to be able to communicate my joy. . . . My impressions are too violent and I find it difficult to hold in check my happiness[1]. . . ."

" In many hysterical and psychically abnormal women," writes Ellis, " auto-erotic phenomena and sexual phenomena generally, are highly pleasurable, though they may be quite innocent of any knowledge of the erotic character of the experience. I have come across interesting and extreme examples of this in the published experiences of the women followers of the American religious leader, T. L. Harris, founder of the ' Brotherhood of the New Life.' Thus, in a pamphlet entitled *Internal Respiration*, by Respiro, a letter is quoted from a lady physician, who writes, ' One morning, I awoke with a strange new feeling in my womb, which lasted for a day or two ; I was so very happy, but the joy was in my womb, not in my heart.' ' At last,' writes a lady quoted in the pamphlet, ' I fell into a slumber, lying on my back, with arms and feet folded, a position I almost always find myself in when I awake, no matter in which position I may go to sleep. Very soon I awoke from this slumber with a most delightful sensation, every fibre tingling with an exquisite glow of warmth. I was lying on my left side (something I am never able to do), and was folded in the arms of my counterpart. Unless you have seen it, I cannot give you an idea of the beauty of his flesh ; and with what joy I beheld and felt it. Think of it, luminous flesh ; oh, such tints, you never could imagine without seeing it,' etc.[2]"

---

[1] *Une Extatique, Bull, de l'Institut. Psychol. International*, 1901, p. 230. The sexual connexion to which I allude above was mentioned to me by the author himself.

[2] *Auto-Erotism, ibid.*, pp. 20-1 of reprint.
We call attention, in the last two quotations, to the sensuous beauty that seems to invest most objects. It is a phenomenon not infrequent after intense

Among my correspondents, an unmarried woman (No. 120), reports that feelings connected with her love-affairs, regarded at one time as religious, she now knows to have been of sexual origin. She was assisted in that discovery by the reading of various women mystics and especially by Maudsley's *Mind and Body*. At first, she was " rather horrified," but now she is not only reconciled to that connexion, but thinks it natural and beautiful.

The preceding instances show what degree of blindness may normally exist in women regarding the participation of sex in matters of religion. Should one be tempted to ascribe to profound stupidity the failure to recognize the sexual connexion of certain " spiritual transports," the case of Mlle Vé (soon to be set forth)[1] would be enough to undeceive. The participation of the senses, though obvious when once recognized, may be overlooked even by persons of keen intelligence given to the habit of self-observation, as was Mlle Vé. In men there are evident physiological reasons that render the participation of the senses more difficult to overlook.

(*e*) Before passing to the application to our group of mystics of what we have just learnt, it remains to be said that auto-erotic phenomena are obviously much more likely to occur in persons deprived of normal sexual satisfaction than in others. The opinion of specialists in this matter is that, barring an extremely small number of abnormal persons, when the free play of sexual impulses is restrained, " auto-erotic phenomena inevitably spring up on every side[2]." " Such manifestations are liable to occur in a specially marked manner in the years immediately following the establishment of puberty[3]," and with greatest frequency in young girls innocent and unperverted[4]. They are, indeed, clearly enough aware of some need, of something lacking ; but what it is, they know not—not

---

emotional seizures ; we shall have occasion to mention it again when considering the impression of illumination or of revelation in ecstasy. The following information may be added here. " It is well known also that both in men and women the vibratory motion of a railway-train frequently produces a certain degree of sexual excitement. Such excitement may remain latent and not become specifically sexual." Ellis, who makes the above statement, adds, " A correspondent to whom the idea was presented for the first time, wrote, ' Henceforth I shall know to what I must attribute the bliss—almost the beatitude—I so often have experienced after travelling for four or five hours in a train.' "—H. Ellis, *ibid.*, pp. 120-1.

[1] See chap. IX, of this book.

[2] Ellis, *Auto-Erotism*, p. 39. See a similar statement in *Studies in the Psycho. of Sex : Modesty*, etc., p. 113.

[3] *The Sexual Impulse in Women*, p. 5.

[4] *Ibid.*, p. 6.

even when they call it love. Amiel, the philosopher, suffering from the gnawing of dyspepsia, thought it meant the absence of God. Similarly do the mystics and many others, urged by a starved body, cry to Heaven for solace and peace.

Auto-erotism in grand mysticism.—The great mystics united in themselves all or most of the conditions which we have just seen to be favourable to the induction of auto-erotic phenomena. They were young and had either never become acquainted with the sexual relation, or, after a brief and unsatisfactory if not frigid practice of it, had lived in abstinence. At the same time, and without being aware of it, they were sexually excited by their " spiritual " love for Jesus or the Virgin Mary ; and also, in most cases, for persons of the opposite sex. St Francis was attached to Santa Clara ; Suzo to Elizabeth Staglin ; François de Sales to Mme de Chantal ; Mme Guyon to Father la Combe ; etc. Moreover, their temperament favoured the appearance of auto-suggestive phenomena.

The intensity and the concreteness of the felt presence of the divine object of their love should not be lost sight of in this connexion. Jesus or the Virgin were not to them simply ideas ; they acquired at times, in particular during the ecstasy, the concreteness of a bodily presence.

The quality of Suzo's relation with the *Ewige Weisheit* appears in this account of a memorable evening spent with " spiritual daughters " in the seclusion of a monastery. He was discoursing with them on the ordinary theme ; and, as he says in his quaint speech, " Eternal Love was making love to them." " As they left him, his (Suzo's) heart was, I know not how, heated by his yearning discourse upon divine love." And, as he was in meditation upon this matter, he lost his senses and had a vision : " A stately youth from Heaven led him by the hand upon a beautiful green meadow. Then the youth brought forth a song in his heart, so winsome that it deprived him of all his senses because of the excessive power of the beautiful melody ; and his heart was so full of burning love and yearning for God that it beat wildly as if it would break, and he had to put his right hand on it in order to control it, and tears were rolling down his cheeks." At the same time, " he saw the Mother with her child, the Eternal Wisdom, against her heart ; and he saw written this word : *Herzentraut*, i.e., ' Beloved of my Heart[1].' "

---

[1] *Leben*, chap. XLIII, p. 205-6. Suzo writes of himself in the third person. If it were accessible to investigation this experience would constitute very interesting material for psycho-analysis.

Most people are familiar with the extravagant carnal imagery used by the mystics to describe their intense enjoyment of divine love. Make whatever allowance seems proper for the accepted habit of speaking of sacred things in terms of profane love ; yet, this query remains : Is the flesh likely to remain unmoved when continence is combined with familiarity with a loved woman and with indulgence in the imagery dear to the libertine ?

Santa Theresa relates that she wrote her *Memoirs* against her inclination, at the direction of her ecclesiastical superiors. How much she and they suppressed is not known. There remains, however enough to indicate, it seems to us, the participation of the organs of sex in the extraordinary enjoyment of union with the heavenly Bridegroom. On several occasions she had the vision of an angel who "held in his hands a long golden dart, tipped with fire." She relates that "from time to time he would plunge it through my heart, and push it down into my bowels. As he withdrew the dart, it seemed as if the bowels would be torn away with it ; and this would leave me aflame with divine love[1]." This voluptuous pleasure was associated with a strange pain ; it was both an "indicible martyr" and "*les plus suaves délices.*" "It was not a bodily, but a spiritual pain, although the body participated in it to a high degree. There takes place, then, between the soul and God such a sweet love-transaction that it is impossible for me to describe what passes[2]." The experiences reported above, of members of the "Brotherhood of the New Life," do not differ materially from those of Santa Theresa.

She was not only surprised at these experiences, but she feared that they were not what she had taken them to be, and she tried, but in vain, to eliminate them : "I saw that in spite of my effort I was powerless before these great love-transports, and they became for me an object of fear. The pleasure and the pain they gave me simultaneously was for me a mystery. My reason was baffled by the conjunction of a spiritual pain so excessive and a happiness so ravishing[3]." When, however, Peter of Alcantara assured her that these experiences were from God, she gave herself up to them unreservedly.

This mixture of exquisite pain with incomparable delight is usual in mystical love-ecstasy. The pain, as much as the pleasure, indicates

---

[1] *Life*, p. 354. The French word translated here as " bowels " is " *entrailles.*" I do not know what the original Spanish word is.

[2] *Ibid.*, p. 354.

[3] *Ibid.*, p. 357.

most probably, as we shall see, the participation of sex organs tormented by an insufficient stimulation.

Of Catherine of Genoa it is related that, when at prayer, " she received suddenly a love-wound in her heart that put her beside herself ; she was like a crazed person seeking relief for the ardour of her wound. And, one day, astonished and afraid, having asked God for the cause of this wound that burned her heart, she felt herself tenderly drawn upon the bosom of Jesus crucified, and there she learned that it was from the sacred heart of Jesus that issued the flames that were consuming her own heart¹."

St Marguerite Marie provides as lurid a picture as can be imagined of a virgin sexually excited from childhood by repeated vows of chastity to Christ, her bridegroom, and by the constant consciousness of his loving presence. Her case is clearly one of erotomania. God rewards her for a repulsive act of self-mastery by keeping her mouth " glued to his sacred heart during two or three hours of the following night." There was no rest for her, day or night, from divine love. " The more she progressed, the more this love of God consumed her. Her delicate constitution could not endure such emotions. Lean, pale, almost transparent, as if through her flesh one could see the flame of the spirit, she realized more and more the song of her novitiate :

> " I am a harassed doe,
> Ardently seeking cool waters.
> The hand of the hunter has wounded me ;
> The dart has reached to my very heart²."

In the intensity of a tormenting love-passion, Mme Guyon does not remain far behind the worse examples of the " love of God." She would tell God that she loved him " more passionately than the most passionate lover ever loved his mistress³." Made frantic by excess of love, or, rather, not obtaining full satisfaction, she would at times, cry out : " Oh, my Love, this is enough—leave me³." Mean-while, she was insistently trying to persuade her husband " that true conjugal love is that which you yourself, O God, create in the heart that loves you³." The husband remained incredulous. Throughout

¹ Quoted in *Histoire de la Bienheureuse Marguerite Marie Alacoque*, by Mgr E. Bougaud, p. 201, 10th edition.

² *Ibid.*, pp. 173-4. Mgr Bougaud states that he wrote this account from autobiographical notes. The same author draws from official documents information concerning various sisters of the monastery of Paray that would indicate the breaking out among the holy sisters of an epidemic of erotomania (pp. 125-6).

³ These quotations are drawn from chap. X of the *Life*.

her writings, one feels the ardour of an unsatisfied passion. "I crave," she exclaims, "the love that thrills and burns and leaves one fainting in a inexpressible joy and pain[1]." And, after God's response, still trembling in every limb, she would say to him, "O God, if you would permit sensual people to feel what I feel, very soon they would leave their false pleasures in order to enjoy so real a blessing[1]."

It may cause some surprise that a woman frigid with her husband, as was Mme Guyon, experienced, nevertheless, the voluptuous sensations she describes. Her irresponsiveness to the conjugal caresses might appear as an argument against the sexual nature of her delights. But it is one of the facts well established by the literature on sex that frigidity in the normal sex-relation does not preclude intense enjoyment in consequence of other than normal exciting causes. Enough has already been said in this chapter to satisfy the reader on this point.

The obvious rôle played by persons of the male sex in the production of her love-trances makes the case of Mme Guyon particularly useful for the elucidation of the topic under discussion. We have already sufficiently stressed the conjunction of her first love ecstasy with the visit of a sympathetic Franciscan monk, and that of her second violent outbreak of love-passion with the renewal of her acquaintance with Father la Combe. She was rapt up in him to the extent of finding it impossible to live away from him. In her devotions, la Combe and Christ became one ; it was this dual being that was present in her amorous trances.

The only fact which we shall add to the preceding in order to complete the demonstration of the participation of sex in the spiritual enjoyment of God is provided by Mlle Vé, a contemporary of Protestant belief whose experiences have been admirably described by her and commented upon by Th. Flournoy. Despite the deepest aversion she had to recognize the participation of sex in ecstatic trances which had been for her a revelation of the love of God.

The life of Mlle Vé was a long, secret tragedy—the tragedy of the woman with irresistible sex and parental instincts who is denied the satisfaction of marriage. At fifty years of age, her trials almost over, she wrote these revelatory lines : "The beast is not altogether dead in me ; despite my fifty years, she breaks out still, with some violence. To say the truth, I am not reconciled at reaching the end of my life without ever having had 'my day,' the day of happiness and enjoyment to which, it seems, every human being has a

---

[1] These quotations are drawn from chap. X of the *Life*.

right[1]." "I can appreciate the attraction that the theory of the right to sexual satisfaction has for so many women (a theory detestable in principle) ; but it is not merely a question of pleasure, it is one of the legitimate satisfaction of an instinct the more powerful that it is bound up with that of maternity. There are moments in my life, when I cannot take in my arms a little child without risk of breaking into sobs. There is in the contact of the little trustful body, the caresses of the little hands, a something which reawakens in me a passionate sorrow[2]."

If Mlle Vé discovered what others do not suspect, it is perhaps because her sexual life was more intense, because she was more enlightened than the mystics of the past, and especially perhaps because she was superior to them in scientific curiosity and independence of judgment.

Despite the best and firmest principles and intelligent efforts to live according to them, her sexual impulses found throughout her life objectionable expressions. One of her adventures not only illustrates but also throws light upon the relation between sexual vice and religion, a relation about which much has been written : " I have been very much concerned with the relation, still so strange to me, between the religious emotion, very pure, very lofty, and sexual excitation. A page of my life striking in that respect came back to me. In 1892, shortly after my return to my native country, the moral and religious life reawakened in me with great intensity. During several years I was interested in religious subjects only, finding all my pleasure in religious meetings." At that time, she formed a friendship with a former schoolmate, who was soon carried away by "the same religious whirlwind" as herself. An intense interest in missions spread among the young people of her circle. She decided to offer herself for service in India. Her friend was the sole confidant of her intention. " The anticipation on an imminent and perhaps final separation brought to a paroxysm our passionate attachment. It became a real debauch (*débordement*). I gave up the project, for it seemed to me impossible to go so far away from her. It was not long after that we felt the fearful moral danger in our affection ; our special religious point of view led us to see in our intimate relation a monstrous sin. . . . Horribly miserable one

---

[1] Th. Flournoy, *Une Mystique Moderne, Archives de Psychol. de la Suisse Romande*, vol. XV, 1915, p. 149.

Mlle Vé's account is fearlessly frank. She was writing to one whom she regarded as her moral director. He obtained permission to offer this moral nude to the attention of the scientific world. I transcribe parts of her confession the more willingly that it may help to produce a compassion and a helpfulness greatly needed.

[2] *Ibid.*, p. 188.

in the other, and yet absolutely incapable to part, the winter was, for us, one of suffering and humiliation, as well as of intense enjoyment. I do not remember exactly how that phase of our intimacy ended; but it gradually became normal again and survived the storm that might have destroyed it[1]."

Many years later, she became entangled in a friendship with a married man. It had begun quite honorably, but her heart and her senses had gradually become engaged until she felt herself powerless to resist longer. It was in the hope of help in this situation and also in a search for deliverance from attacks of auto-erotism that she appealed to Professor Flournoy.

We shall reserve for another place the account of the origin of her religious ecstasies. It will be sufficient to say here that although not naïve in sex-matters, she remained for a while unaware of the connexion existing between her ecstasies and her sexual cravings. She realized very early, however, and with much surprise, that the terms fitting best these experiences were those used for human passion. Describing the Ninth Ecstasy, she says : " A kind of languor coursed through my blood (I was going to use the term voluptuousness, but it has a carnal meaning which I dislike). . . . I felt most of all my weakness, my powerlessness, and the uselessness of any attempt at resistance[2]; and also that curious impression of being surrounded by something at once violent and tender. I understood now that the mystics of the Middle Ages could compare their ecstasies, altogether spiritual, to the enjoyment and the embraces of human love. Those are certainly the symbols (could I bring myself to use them) which best fit, not the experience at the moment of contact, but the sensations that follow or precede it and that ultimate impression of the aim reached, of fulfilment (*point final*)[3]."

Not long after writing these lines the participation of sex in what she had thought " altogether spiritual," forced itself upon her reluctant observation. In the Twelfth Ecstasy, the beast, " the creature made out of passion never satiated," broke her chain with consequences that could no longer be overlooked; " I hardly dare put this down," she confesses ; " I do it only because of the engagement I made with myself to be entirely truthful in these descriptions[4]."

[1] Th. Flournoy, *Une Mystique Moderne, Archives de Psychol. de la Suisse Romande*, vol. XV, 1915, p. 188-9.

[2] The uselessness of resistance is mentioned by several mystics. See, for instance, Santa Theresa, *Livre des Fondations*, Paris, 1869, p. 82.

[3] *Une Mystique Moderne, ibid.*, p. 81-2.

[4] *Ibid.*, p. 94.

Nevertheless, on a subsequent day, she sought to escape from the, to her, dreadful significance of the fact she had observêd. She wanted, at any cost, to keep the precious " experience of the divine," pure from every sensual admixture. But the fact, once seen, could no longer be concealed. In the end she did as our correspondent quoted above but without so good a grace, for she was of a puritanic temper : she accepted the fact as a mystery of human nature[1].

With this connexion made manifest, Mlle Vé's interest in her trances decreased. When, in addition, she realized clearly that the Power revealed to her was not the divine, *personal* being she needed, her extraordinary trances soon came to an end. She returned to a more ordinary form of piety, i.e., to the fellowship with God usual among devout Christians.

Cursed as she was by that which in a normal life would have been a blessing, she nevertheless did not bring religion to shame as so many others less intelligent and of coarser fibre have done[2].

* * *

The excruciatingly delightful pains and other pains.—The reader can hardly have failed to notice with surprise the presence in the divine love-ecstasy of "supremely delightful pains." This phenomenon can be understood only when the share taken by the sexual organism in the divine union is recognized. But we must separate from these curious pains, bodily pains that bear no relation to the love-ecstasy.

In hysterical attacks and in attacks simulating hysteria, there appears frequently more or less well localized and violent pains. St Theresa, Mme Guyon, St Catherine of Genoa, St Marguerite

---

[1] *Ibid.*, p. 187.

[2] The history of religious aberrations due to the sex-impulse is a long one. At puberty, the period of most frequent conversion, the newly awakened sex-impulse, prevented in civilized countries from running into the natural channels, assumes readily enough the religious form ; i.e., it is directed to ideal personages, to the Virgin Mary, Jesus, God. Religious revivals produce usually a crop of sex-delinquencies. Jonathan Edwards became aware of the danger of permitting certain expressions of holy love : " Mutual embraces and kisses of persons of different sexes, under the notion of Christian love, and holy kisses, are utterly to be disallowed, as having the most direct tendency quickly to turn Christian love into unclean and brutish lust."—From *Narrative of Many Surprising Conversions*, Johnathan Edwards, Worcester, 1832, p. 292, as quoted by Schrœder.

The life of *Mathias, the Prophet,* is a good instance of what becomes of religion in the life of weak-minded persons with strong sexual instincts. See "Matthias the Prophet," by T. Schrœder, *Jour. of Relig. Psycho.*, vol. VI, 1913, pp. 59-66. Many a Christian clergyman of a tender and weak nature, unwittingly stoking the fires of lust by thoughts of " divine " love, has purged in prison the guilt of his incontinence.

Marie, and others, complained at divers moments of intense pains apparently belonging to that category. The first mentions, for instance, during her first great illness, " pains about the heart so acute that it seemed at times as if it was being torn to pieces by sharp teeth." She suffered also from an " internal fire," and from " contractions of the nerves so intolerable " that she had rest neither day nor night, etc.[1] Pains much less intense and not definitely localized are experienced also during the period of dryness. One should, of course, not confuse these " physical " pains with painful conditions of psychical origin—for instance, the distress of thinking oneself abandoned by God.

The mystics were at a loss to describe the other pains, those that are a constituent part of the love-ecstasy. They possess apparently contradictory qualities : they are *delightful* pains. After what we have learned, we shall have little trouble in recognizing their source in an insufficient, tantalising, sexual excitement that does not come to a head, does not reach the " *point final,*" to use a significant expression of Mlle Vé. In *Inner Castle* St Theresa describes the experience thus : " Often when the soul least expects it, our Lord calls her suddenly. She hears very distinctly that her God calls her, and it gives her such a start, especially at the beginning, that she trembles and utters plaints. She feels that an ineffable wound has been dealt her, and that wound is so precious in her sight that she would like it never to heal. She knows that her divine Spouse is near her, although He does not let her enjoy His adorable presence, and she cannot help complaining to Him in words of love. In this pain, she relishes a pleasure incomparably greater than in the Orison of Quietude (a lower stage in the Ascent of the Soul, i.e., a condition less removed from normal consciousness) in which there is no admixture of pain. The voice of the Well-Beloved causes in the soul such transports that she is consumed by desire, and yet does not know what to ask, because she sees clearly that her Lord is with her. What pain could she have ? And for what greater happiness could she wish ? To this I do not know what to answer ; but that of which I am certain, is that the pain penetrates down to the very bottom of the bowels and that it seems that they are being torn away when the heavenly Spouse withdraws the arrow with which he has transpierced them. As long as that pain lasts, it is always on the increase or on the decrease, it never remains at the same intensity. It is for that reason that the soul is never entirely on fire ; the spark goes out and

---

[1] See the case of Father Surin, in Delacroix, *loc. cit.*, pp. 328-31. These and other violent pains are common in hystero-epilesy. In certain mystics of little significance suffering of this sort is prominent.

the soul feels a desire stronger than ever to endure again the love-pain she has just experienced[1]."

We must surrender to the evidence: the virgins and the unsatisfied wives who undergo the repeated " love-assaults of God " until they are, in their own extravagant way of speech, " on the point of death," who complain that it is enough and beg of him to let them go for a while[2], suffer from nothing else than intense attacks of erotomania, induced by their organic need and the worship of the God of love[3].

The production of an inordinate degree of sexual excitement is greatly favoured by the semi-trance condition during which it happens. The more or less considerable obfuscation of self-consciousness deprives the organism of the higher mental control. The subject is in a condition similar to that of sleep when instinctive activities are left in a large measure to their own doings, and thoughts which could not abide the full light of consciousness are in possession of the mind.

If, in his Assent to God, and while only partly self-conscious, the very mechanism of procreation is aroused unknown to himself, the mystic can hardly be blamed. The very mystics who have suffered violent sexual excitement have spoken with a convincing naiveté against fleshly indulgence. On this point we have already quoted

---

[1] *Inner Castle, Sixième Demeure*, chap. II, pp. 413-5, abbreviated. Comp. chap. XI, pp. 497-8. H. Delacroix has understood these pains in another way. See *loc. cit.*, pp. 65-7. He deals with *Les Peines Mystiques* in chap. X of his book.

[2] See, in this connexion, the biographical sketch of Saint Marguerite Marie, in this book.

[3] The presence of these excruciating pains of suspense and non-fulfilment, points to a possible connexion between pathological anxiety and disorders of the sex-function. When sexual excitement is frequent, and does not reach its acme, and, with it, peaceful contentment, there exists a situation that may conceivably give rise to anxiety neurosis. For the pains of which we speak include an element of expectation—the expectation of the sequence and *point final*. And, painful expectation, under high tension, never fulfilled, may easily enough be transformed into anxiety.

It may interest the reader to see St Theresa's lame attempt to separate the excruciatingly delightful pain of ecstasy from " natural " pain :—(a) " The pains from which the devil is the cause are never pleasant like those of which I have just spoken. He may indeed mix with them some satisfactions which seem spiritual in their nature ; but to join to a pain so great, peacefulness and pleasure, is beyond his power which extends only to the external : and so the pains which come from him will never be sweet and peaceful, but distressing and full of trouble."

(b) " This tempest which fills the soul with such sweetness comes from another region than the one where this unhappy spirit exercises his power."

(c) " The soul secures from this pain great advantages " of a moral nature.—From *Inner Castle*. VI. II.

St Theresa and also Tauler, whose sentence against carnal indulgence in religious worship may be repeated here : " We must regard the search after warmth of heart in devotion . . . as a lack of spiritual chastity[1]." The great preacher of Strasburg did not, probably, recognize that the connection between so-called platonic or Christian love and sex-love is an expression of human nature itself : affection and devotion have developed together with or, rather, had their cradle in sex-love and the care of the young.

The wonderful transforming effect of a lofty interpretation should not be overlooked in this connexion. No pleasure is in itself base or debasing. It is only through its direct effect upon the body or through the meaning or significance ascribed to it, that it may become so. In so far as a pleasurable state is interpreted as an effect of the divine Presence, it becomes a source of moral energy even though it should arise from the stimulation of the sex-organs.

The great mystics have been in respect of love, as also in other respects, daring experimenters. And here, as with regard to moral perfection, and just as unavoidably, they have partly failed. Their aim involved the separation of organic sex activities from feelings and behaviour originally linked with them. In this attempt they were following a tradition older than Christianity. The Greeks had already sought to divorce what has been called platonic love[2] from sex satisfaction. That effort marks one of the most significant trends of modern development. It constitutes a part of a general effort to transform original, " animal," man into a higher, " divine," being. It manifests itself with respect to all the primary instincts. With regard to fear, for instance, humanity is engaged in an effort to eliminate or, at least, to control the original instinctive reactions to danger in order to be able to treat each particular danger in a fitting way. A being as intelligent as man is, can do better than meet every kind of danger in the uniform, blind ways of the animal, i.e., either by running off in a panic or by turning to stone on the spot. Therefore he endeavours to free himself from the undesirable parts of

---

[1] Comp. utterances of Molinos on this subject in the *Spiritual Guide*, pp. 76, 86-8. Edition without date or name of publisher.

[2] Although the expressions platonic and Christian love, are not exactly synonymous, their meanings seem sufficiently similar to permit here an interchangeable use of them.

In an appendix to *God in Human Experience* and also in *The Meaning of Mysticism as seen through its Psychology Mind*, vol. XXI, N.S., pp. 57-61, W. E. Hocking discusses my understanding of the relation of sex-love to the love of God, as set forth in my article on the Christian Mystics in the *Revue Philosophique* for 1902, pp. 459-68. A part of his disagreement with me is due, it seems to me, to a misunderstanding which the preceding pages, will, I trust, dissipate.

'the original reaction and to remain mentally alert so that he may best adapt his conduct to the particular danger to which he may find himself exposed.

Pleasure and happiness in mystical ecstasy.—The preceding pages are not to be understood as meaning that the delights experienced by the mystics are all of sexual origin. Pleasure has other sources besides that connected with sex. One should in particular separate happiness from pleasure, for these words designate affective experiences possessing altogether different significance.·

The sensory pleasures are at the bottom of the scale. Some of them are dependent upon the stimulation of sense organs. To this class belong the pleasures of touch, of taste, of sound, of sight, of movement, as well as pleasurable states of more obscure origin involving the activity of the viscera. The pleasure of sex, in so far as it depends upon the stimulation of the sex-organs, belongs also in this class.

Among the sensory pleasures, those produced by the stimulation of the sense organs of the skin and of the muscles and tendons are of particular interest to us. The satisfaction which follows a warm bath and physical exercise, is due in large part to the stimulation of these sense organs. The effect of tickling, of scratching itching parts, of massaging and stroking, is at times comparable for its intensity and voluptuousness with the pleasures of sex. Massaging and stroking may induce widespread tensions similar to the general erethism of sexual excitement. Stretching also is, under certain circumstances, intensely pleasurable. Many years ago we reported a striking observation which may well be reproduced here. On rising in the morning, we had felt unwell; strange little shivers, not at all unpleasant, passed down the spine and along the legs and arms. They left in their wake sensations that invited to stretching, and every stretching of the arms, legs and torso, yielded a voluptuous pleasure[1]. This continued for a few hours and then gave place to general discomfort. At lunch time we had to go to bed, and for two weeks were kept indoors by a bad attack of the grippe.

---

[1] A sentiment of beatitude, also connected with the tension of muscles, has been observed in hysterical catalepsy. A patient of Charcot would become angry when recalled to the world and made to relax.—P. Janet, *Une Extatique*, pp. 229-30.

There was, perhaps, something similar in this experience of Mme Guyon : Once while at confession, she felt her head as if lifted up with so much violence that she thought her whole body was going to be raised above the earth. She enjoyed a delightful sensation " very pure nevertheless and spiritual." Afterwards, she suffered from great shivers and was unable to eat for the whole day.

There is another group of pleasurable states, never reaching the intense voluptuousness of the former, yet deeply enjoyable and satisfying. We allude to the affective consequence of the stimulation, no longer merely of sense organs, but of organized action-mechanisms (reflexes, instincts, innate tendencies, habits).

Happiness, as used both in common speech and in psychology, denotes a pleasurable condition dependent upon the attainment of what the individual considers of most importance to him, or a satisfactory progress towards that attainment. It implies a high degree of unification of tendencies and purposes. *Perfect* happiness results from the free, harmonious working of the whole being towards an inclusive purpose. Between the significance of happiness as here defined, and that of the pleasures of taste, of tickling, of muscle stretching, and the like, there is little similarity[1].

Now the mystic, in his search for divine love, has discovered that remarkable method of worship called the *Ascent of the Soul to God*. In it he finds a variety of sensory pleasures, those of relaxation, and at times of general erethism, of bright visions, of anæsthesias, and, eclipsing all these, pleasures and pains of sexual origin, delightful beyond anything else known to them. That is already much, yet he gets a great deal beyond that, things more directly to his purpose. For the mystic's purpose is far from being attained when he has secured the pleasures just named. During the moments that precede the extinction of consciousness in the trance, and afterwards as long as its influence lasts, he enjoys also happiness. It is a happiness due to the satisfaction of fundamental tendencies and needs. We know that before entering a holy life, our mystics were not content with existence as it was for them ; they felt needs that were not satisfied, and conceived ideals that could not be realized. Some of them were cruelly wounded in their self-esteem and, although married, were denied the spiritual as well as the physiological satisfaction of intimate companionship with a person admired, loved, and loving. In the mystical union they found a Presence that satiated the desires for self-esteem and self-affirmation, for affection and self-surrender, for intellectual harmony and moral perfection. They found or thought they had found the

---

[1] Reacting against the theory that would see in the enjoyment of ecstasy merely an expression of auto-erotism, P. Janet has emphasized the enjoyment that comes to his neurasthenic patients from a simplification and unification of the mental life. He has shown how, in many instances, with the disappearance of mental conflicts and the return of what he has called the " *sentiment du réel*," peace, self-confidence, and happiness have returned. But the share that sexual excitement assumes at the culmination of the beatific state of certain of his ecstatics must not be left out of consideration. On this point we have already said enough.

fulfilment of all their yearnings. And when they had returned to normal consciousness, they rejoiced in the momentous assurance of God's love and in the promise of his constant companionship[1].

---

[1] I find in the diary of a person whom I know the yearnings of a young man for pure love and tender companionship, expressed with an intensity of feeling so unusual, that I transcribe brief portions of it. When the mystic seeks the love of God, he is moved by the very same forces that find expression here. They are forces certainly not independent of the sex-impulse.

Sept. 23.—I often am filled with a passionate yearning for someone here to lavish my love upon and who would love me in return . . . Ah, that the days would come again when she (a sister) would pull my hair and run off with my things ! I wish she would prattle to me like so many children can. What would I not give for one gentle little fairy to come gliding into this old teacher's room [he is about 21 years old] after my day's work is done and stroke my face and talk to me about her little joys and troubles and draw me to sympathize with her, and play tricks on me, and kiss me ! But ah ! it cannot be—life's hard lines forbid it. However, I see only too clearly what I want. I want a powerful religion to absorb my whole nature and to make me thankful for what I have got and for what I do see of these dear little ones, and to make me love God in the highest, and work for Him.

Oct. 3.—[Mary, eleven years old, and Betty, together with grown ups, are at tea with him.] I ignored the presence of all but Mary. I suppose the others were well supplied. I know Mary was. I suppose the rest were in the room all the while, I know Mary was. The other may have talked, may have smiled, I know Mary did! In fact that tea-time may be summed up in one word, Mary.

Oct. 16.—I almost adore that child : no burden of care would be insupportable if she were near. I believe I could go cheerfully to death hand-in-hand with her ; but stop ! I must not talk like this.

Nov. 5.—What should I do without little girls around me ? I dare not think.

Dec. 18.—. . . But religion holds up to us a Friend who will never grow old or fade away. One whom you can love and live for without ceasing.

CHAPTER VI

THE METHODS OF CHRISTIAN MYSTICISM[1]

IN the preceding chapter we have considered the motivation of Christian mysticism. We must now examine its methods. Since the mystics are supposed to find contentment in union with God, our problem might be formulated as that of the means by which they establish contact with the Divine.

According to their theory and practice, the fundamental psychological condition of Union is *passivity*. It is only when the human will ceases to strive and surrenders to the divine Will that it becomes possible for God to communicate himself[2]. The biographical sketches contain evidence of the unanimity with which our mystics insist upon passivity as a condition of divine possession. They admonish the neophyte to renounce his will, to be still and listen ; then, and only then, he may expect to hear God's voice and feel God's power[3].

As a method subsidiary to passivity, the Christian mystics practise *asceticism*. God cannot be expected to bless man with his presence until man has done what he can to eliminate from his nature that which is displeasing to his Lord. And, since the flesh is the main source of the evil that is in him, his effort assumes chiefly the form of a battle against the bodily appetites : asceticism is a striving of the spirit to subjugate the flesh by starvation and suffering.

In its strenuous effort to curb the flesh and the pride of spirit, asceticism is in obvious opposition with the doctrine of passivity. For that doctrine in its radical form demands not only the silencing of evil propensities, but also the cessation of all efforts at self-betterment. The theory is found in that form in Tauler's writings : " So long as ye desire to fulfil the will of God and have any desire even after eternity and God, so long are ye not truly poor." Utterances to the same purpose may be found in practically all the great mystics. Nevertheless, and despite the implied contradiction,

[1] Comp. chap. XVII of Pratt's *Religious Consciousness*, and the corresponding chapters in Delacroix' *Etudes*.

[2] Murisier saw truly when he said that guidance by the idea of a divine person was the main characteristic of mysticism.—*Rev. Philos.*, 1898, pp. 469-72.

they have all more or less practised a self-willed asceticism. As a matter of fact, the more thoughtful of the mystics have noticed with surprise the unsatisfactory results of frontal attacks upon sin ; and, after a period of heroic but disappointing effort, they have altogether abandoned or greatly mitigated the severity of their ascetic effort.

Mere passivity, arrested bodily and mental activity, leads to sleep through drowsiness and somnolence. But when practised in order to attain union with God, it may culminate in an ecstatic trance with remarkable attendant phenomena. The Christian mystic looks forward not to mere sleep, not even simply to the blessed Nirvana of the Buddhist ; he goes to meet a personal God who loves him and whom he loves ; and he has in mind a more or less definite conception of what this meeting will mean to him. Thus, the mystical ecstasy is in part the outcome of the mystic's expectations, and, therefore, may be regarded as a product of auto-suggestion. But its frame-work, if one may speak so, is of another origin ; it is, as we shall see in another chapter, the direct product of physiological causes.

*   *   *

Now, this remarkable way of ascending to God—the mystical ecstasy—is not altogether an invention of the Christian mystics. It is the joint produce of chance discoveries and empirical gropings begun already in man's infancy. The more general of the desirable effects of relaxation and of passivity are too obvious to have long remained hidden. Some of their more special advantages were also discovered early. Long before the historical period opened, man had not only fallen in the habit of enjoying, in particular ceremonies, the bodily relaxation and the mental peace that come with the letting go of life's burdens, but he had learned to facilitate and complete self-surrender by the use of artificial methods—of narcotic drugs, for instance. These drugs not only bring about relaxation and somnolence, but the mental activity that persists seems alien to the subject's own will. Under the influence of these drugs he becomes passive, and yet he dreams dreams, sees visions, and enjoys an impression of delightful freedom and unlimited power. In the chapter on drug-ecstasy we have examined at some length the witchery of various narcotic drugs.

Later on drugs were replaced, in the production of sacred ecstasy, by other physical and by psychical means. The Yoga technique for entering Nirvana relies no longer on drugs. It makes the connecting link between the drug-intoxication of the savage and the psychical method of the Christian mystic.

The savage was almost entirely at the mercy of the direct physiological action of the drug; desires and expectations (auto-suggestion) added little to its effects. If he took mescal, he enjoyed as god-given the wonderful coloured lights and the feelings of detachment and power that it produced. It is otherwise in Christian mysticism. Whatever the topic of the meditation by which he may begin his devotions, the mystic never loses sight of the righteousness and of the love of the God he aspires to meet. As long as any consciousness remains, and long after the external world has disappeared, these thoughts, with the feelings and emotions which accompany them, remain present and exert a directing action.

The peculiar situation under which these remaining ideas find themselves in consciousness vastly increases their power; for the limitation of the mental activity, which is an essential feature of trance-states, constitutes a condition of increased suggestibility to whatever ideas may still be present. It is particularly important to recall that under the conditions of the Christian trance, love occupies the very centre of consciousness and remains there as long as any spark of consciousness lingers. We have seen that under these circumstances platonic love is fanned into a burning flame which involves the organs of sex. The love-energy thus mobilized and prevented from following its natural outlet, gives rise to a variety of remarkable phenomena.

The idea of God's righteousness also exerts on the entranced mystic its own particular effects. Some of them are monitory; they appear in the form of voices and visions. One may say that, in general, the mystic finds himself assuming the attitude of righteousness which he ascribes to God.

The condition of the entranced mystic is in certain respects, as we shall realize more and more clearly, similar to that of a hypnotized person under the sway of ideas that have been suggested to him; with the difference, however, that the mystic is his own hypnotizer; or, if one prefers to put it that way, that God (as present to his consciousness) is the hypnotizer. But this generalization will come with more power when we have seen how a series of trance-states issues from the practice of passivity.

I. Asceticism, its Causes and its Utility.

The forms assumed by Christian asceticism are sufficiently well-known to warrant passing immediately to the consideration of its causes and of its results. Rational causes can readily be found; yet, it would be a gross misunderstanding of human nature to suppose that Christian asceticism can be completely accounted for as an expression of rational purposes. The main rational causes of

Christian asceticism seem to us to be the following five[1]. They are of very unequal importance.

1. *Spiritualization.*—Whoever regards the "flesh" as the enemy of the "spirit" must look upon the pampering of the body as a fostering of evil; while the reduction of the bodily appetites or their elimination must appear as at least a step toward spiritualization. The influence of this belief is written large over every page of the history of Christian asceticism.

2. *Heroism.*—This motive fuses so readily with the preceding that its presence is not always recognized. It is strikingly exemplified in the following non-religious experience: "Often at night in my warm bed I would feel ashamed to depend so on the warmth, and whenever the thought would come over me, I would have to get up, no matter what time of night it was, and stand for a minute in the cold, just so as to prove my manhood[2]." Viewed in that light pains may be endured and sacrifices cheerfully made. This attitude of mind is known to most high-spirited men of fine moral fibre. It has usually a share in the fortitude of the ascetic.

3. *Self-sacrifice as a proof of devotion.*—To suffer pain for the sake of someone else is a way of demonstrating the extent of one's disinterested love. The earthly lover yearns for a chance to show that there is nothing he would not endure for the beloved. Divine lovers do not wait for the opportunity: they create it. Our mystics tell God that there is nothing they would not do for him and they make a beginning by inflicting upon themselves fearful torments.

4. *The meritoriousness of renunciation and suffering.*—There exists a widespread, if unformulated belief in the meritoriousness of self-inflicted suffering. It is felt to be a sort of currency available as payment for things desired. Young children occasionally show how natural is that idea. A lady relates how at the age of about five years, when her mother was dangerously ill and her recovery despaired of, it occurred to her that if she gave up a toy horse to which she was very much attached her mother would recover. Unable to make the entire sacrifice at once, she threw into the fire first the saddle and the bridle, and later the rest, after which the mother recovered[3]. Practices thus motivated are found in all religions.

It comes to pass also that a direct purifying effect is ascribed to suffering: it is supposed to have a cathartic action.

[1] Compare the six sources of asceticism mentioned by William James in the *Varieties of Religious Experience*, p. 296, ff.

[2] *Loc. cit.*, p. 300.

[3] Th. Flournoy, *Une Mystique Moderne, Archives de Psychol.*, 1915, vol. XV, p. 18.

5. *Imitation.*—The desire to be like Christ in all things, even in his suffering, is often present in Christian asceticism. It may not seem fair that we should escape suffering when Christ endured, even unto death, for our sake.

There is also the desire to establish a closer bond with Christ by making ourselves like him in this particular. After denying himself drink for several days, Suzo found comfort in this communication from his Master; " See, I also have suffered the anguish of death, and they gave me but a little vinegar and hyssop; and yet, all the cool springs of the earth were mine[1]." In addition to the present motive Suzo felt also in this instance the appeal to his manhood.

* * *

However considerable the influence of these several rational motives may be, they are supplemented by irrational ones. The following observations point to motives of that order. When self-infliction of bodily pain and subjugation of the body are regarded as conditions of admittance to divine favours, it would seem that asceticism would be practised most of all before the first ecstasy; and that it might be mitigated, if not abandoned, during periods of frequent divine visitations. But it is ordinarily otherwise: first comes the setting on fire by a passionate love-embrace and then begins the extravagant asceticism. Its height usually corresponds with the period of most frequent ecstasy, and both decline together. Mme Guyon notes, for instance, that during the years of God's withdrawal, self-mortification became difficult and that she shrank from pains formerly endured with pleasure. And yet it is certainly during the periods of God's absence that the main rational reasons for asceticism are the strongest. It is while Suzo enjoyed as many as two trances daily that his ascetic practices were so extravagant as to endanger his life.

The probability of an irrational causal connexion between the intensity of the tendency to asceticism and the love-ecstasies can hardly be denied by anyone familiar with the facts set forth in the section on the sex-motive. We saw there how Christian mystics are brought into a condition of unendurable pain by a sexual excitement without natural outlet. They writhe in an indescribably delightful anguish and cry out to God that it is enough, that he should let them alone for a while. The exasperation of the sex-impulse continues for a time after the ecstasy is over; and is renewed in weaker degrees between the ecstasies; for, the idea of the Great Lover and of his caresses is almost continuously present.

[1] *Leben*, chap. XVIII.

In a situation such as this, relief is frequently sought in violent, uncontrolled movements and even in self-inflicted pain[1]. A discharge of the pent-up energy is thus effected. Is not this what happens in great sorrow, when, under the shock and the pain of a disaster, one behaves like a raving maniac? No purposive action appropriate to the circumstances being at hand, the energy released by the distressing situation is spent in violent, irrational behaviour.

The connexion between sexual excitement and asceticism finds support in many a mystic's utterances: Sister Jeanne des Anges, Superior of the Ursulines of Loudon, wrote in her *Autobiography*: " These impurities and the fire of concupiscence which the evil spirit caused me to feel, beyond all that I can say, forced me to throw myself on to braziers of hot coal. . . . At other times, in the depth of winter, I have sometimes passed part of the night entirely naked in the snow or in tubs of icy water[2],"—all this to cool the fires of concupiscence.

But, if we express the opinion that sexual excitement urges to insane extravagances in asceticism, we are not to be understood as affirming that in no other way can such extravagances come to pass ; they may have other irrational motives. When St Marguerite Marie reports that she found a great delight in doing a thing most repulsive to her (licking sputum with her tongue), her statement may be understood in several ways : the *delices* mentioned may mean really only a keen sense of relief at having done an unpleasant action to which she was imperatively prompted. Or the supreme joy may have come with the demonstration of spiritual mastery over what she regarded as the resistance of the body. Or, yet, both explanations may be true at once.

The human being is so complex that there is no *à priori* difficulty in accepting a statement affirming that something very painful is also highly enjoyable. The pain may refer to one of the effects of the deed, and the delight to another. The man who makes a wry face when swallowing whiskey, finds it unpleasant to the taste, though it may be delightful to him in its more remote effects.

*　　　　*　　　　*

Concerning the very complex question of the utility of asceticism, we shall make two remarks only : Like frontal attacks in warfare, the effort to root out evil by facing it, keeps the enemy on the alert

---

[1] Much in sexual perversions is to be accounted for in this manner ; i.e., as the outcome of an irritation arising in an incomplete expression of the sex-impulse.

[2] As quoted by H. Ellis in his *Studies in the Psychology of Sex : Modesty*, etc., pp. 240-2.

and brings out resistance. It maintains in the field of attention the thought of the evils from which it would be desirable to withdraw attention. The damming of a strong current may be impossible when the digging of another bed may be feasible.

Our second remark is that the most influential among the practical mystics came to realize, more or less clearly, that asceticism at least in its extreme forms, is not an economical use of energy The more they progressed in their career, the less they relied upon hand to hand conflicts with the evil that was in them, and the more they trusted in passive contemplation of the perfections of God, in benevolent activities and in God's Holy Grace.

*　　　*　　　*

II. Passivity and the Stages of the Mystical Union.

Passivity, when practised under certain conditions, ends in ecstasy, the spectacular kernel of grand mysticism. It is in ecstasy that germinate the assurance of union with God, and the conviction of illumination and revelation. A special chapter will have to be devoted to a study of the nature of ecstasies, religious and otherwise, and to the explanation of the surprising beliefs connected with it. Here we propose merely to set forth the mystics' own conception and explanation of divine ecstasy. And, as they have ascribed much importance to an alleged succession of degrees or stages through which the soul ascends to ecstatic, divine possession, we shall begin with an exposition of these stages.

One of the first enumerations of the stages through which the soul is supposed to pass before complete identification with the Divine, is that of Hugo of St. Victor (1141). He recognized three degrees : *Cogitatio, Meditatio, Contemplatio*[1]. Although later mystics have introduced much more refined classifications, the essential meaning of this early generalization has not been contradicted by any of them. According to St. Victor, in Contemplation the soul leaves the world behind, withdraws into herself, and is simplified. At the end, she loses even the consciousness of her existence and is lost in God.

It would be very tedious and quite unprofitable to follow the many mystics who have attempted to describe the *Journey of the Soul*. When one recalls how difficult it is to observe correctly something so subtle and evanescent as mental states, and how lacking these observers were in mental training and even in the conception of scientific accuracy, one is not surprised to find that their

---

[1] Albert Stöckl, *Philos. des Mittelalters*, vol. I, pp. 353-4. The disciple of Hugo, Richard of St. Victor, makes six degrees instead of three. Nevertheless, their descriptions do not differ in any important respect.

descriptions agree only in their main lines. It will be sufficient for our purpose if we limit our examination to the formulations of the few among the great mystics who, because of conspicuous talent, overcame in a measure the difficulties of the task.

* * *

The ascending series of the mystical states according to Santa Theresa.—The art of Christian mystical worship is generally supposed to have found its culmination in the teaching of the great Spanish Saint (1515-82). None before or after, in the Roman Church, has surpassed her in fulness of experience and in talent of introspection. Her writings have become the standards in the description of this sort of experience[1]. Praise of Santa Theresa's talent should, however, not prevent us from realizing that she belonged to an ignorant and superstitious age. If the main lines of her pictures are consistent and definite enough, the rest is in part incoherent and at times contradictory. Neither should we lose sight of the fact that, however accurate she intended to be, she suffered the triple penalty of being a systematizer, of wishing to edify, and of desiring to make her experiences fit into the traditional dogmatic scheme of the Church of which she was a devout adherent.

In the *Autobiography*, the Ascent to God is divided into four stages or " states " : Meditation, Orison of Quiet (or, as others say, Contemplation) ; the Sleep of the Powers (or of the Mental Faculties) ; and Ecstasy, including Rapture. But in *Interior Castle*, these four stages are divided into six, and a new one is added. We shall see that there are sufficient reasons for rejecting this last degree as being the product of a confusion and for regarding the four stages of the *Life* as the more satisfactory division.

1. *Meditation* (Chapters XI-XIII)[2]. Meditation is man's work, " assisted by divine grace." As subject of the meditation one of the mysteries of the Passion may be chosen ; for example, our Lord on the cross. The aim of the soul must be to increase love and courage in the service of God. She may think of Jesus Christ as present to the senses, seek to fan her love for him into a bright flame, to keep in

---

[1] The main sources of information upon the mystical degrees and mystical life in general, are the *Autobiography* or *Life*, and the *Inner Castle or the Dwellings of the Soul*. Chaps. XI to XXII (written in 1562) of the *Life*, are consecrated to a description of the four stages by which the soul ascends to God. In *Inner Castle* she took up again, in 1577, i.e., fifteen years later, the description of the Ascent of the Soul.

All references to the *Life* are, here as previously, to the French translation by Marcel Bouix, Paris, 1857. The references to the *Book of Foundations* and to *Inner Castle* are respectively to the second and third volumes of the *Oeuvres Mystiques de Sainte Thérèse*, by the same translator, Paris, 1869.

[2] In the following descriptions, I have followed closely the phraseology of the Saint.

his company, speak to him, implore him, complain to him, and rejoice with Him.

Although it may at times be arduous to keep one's mind upon the subject of the meditation it is within man's power. But to endeavour to pass to the higher stages by one's own effort, would be " futile " and " presumptuous," for they imply a suspension of the activity of the understanding.

2. The *Orison*[1] *of Quiet* (XIV-XV) is a "foretaste of supernatural favours." It is God who elevates the soul to this union with him. Understanding and memory act only at intervals and in a peaceful manner. Their functions are reduced to assisting the will in the enjoyment of the blessedness offered it. At times, however, they disturb the intimate union of the will with God. The will, striving to maintain itself in union, " works in a marvellous way without the least effort in order to keep alive this small spark of divine love."

If, in Meditation, effort, sometimes irksome, dominates ; here it is enjoyment. The saint describes in glowing terms the delight of the Union of Quiet[2].

3. *The Sleep of the Powers*[3] (XVI-XVII). For a long time St Theresa did not know how to separate this state from the preceding. Both consist in an imperfect union with God and are fruits of his merciful grace ; and in both the activity of the mental functions is much reduced. Her efforts at distinction, enlightened though she is by the divine Master, are hardly satisfactory ; and one must admit the obvious fact, namely, that there is merely a difference of degree and not of kind. The most significant statements she makes regarding this stage are that " the powers of the soul are incapable of occupying themselves with any other object than God ; they are altogether taken up with the enjoyment of this excess of glory " ; the only task of the soul is to surrender entirely, to be ready to die if necessary. In order to paint this enjoyment she draws upon the most vivid hues of her rich palette : " it is a glorious delirium, a celestial madness " ; the soul feels herself dying to the world while reposing rapturously in the enjoyment of God. Compared with the second, this stage is characterized by a deeper degree of absorption in God and enjoyment of him.

[1] The word " orison " is used here, rather than " prayer," in order to reserve the latter for the more ordinary form of relation with God.

[2] Compare on this stage, *Interior Castle*, Fourth Dwelling.

[3] Compare on this stage, *Interior Castle*, Fifth Dwelling. In that book the name " Orison of Union " replaces " Sleep of the Powers."

The saint informs us that during the last five or six years she has often been favoured with this degree of union[1].

4. *Ecstasy, or Rapture*[2], *or Flight of the Soul*[3] (XVIII-XXI). In the two preceding states the soul belongs still sufficiently to herself "to be able to indicate, at least by signs, what she experiences "; but, in ecstasy, " the soul is absorbed in enjoyment, without understanding that which she enjoys. . . . The senses are all so completely occupied by that enjoyment that none of them can . . . pay attention to anything else. . . . The delights which overcome the soul are incomparably greater (than in the preceding stages), . . . and the soul and the body are equally incapable of communicating them." " The soul seems to leave the organs which she animates." " She falls into a sort of swoon. . . . It is only with the greatest effort that she can make the slightest movement with her hands. The eyes close of themselves ; and, if they are kept open, they see almost nothing. . . . If spoken to, the soul hears the sound of the voice but no distinct word."

The impression of levitation is frequent : " Often my body would become so light that it had no longer any weight ; at times I no longer felt my feet touching the ground." Ecstasy comes on more suddenly than the other states, and can with much less success be resisted : " When I wanted to resist," writes the Saint, " I felt under my feet astonishing forces which lifted me up." The suddenness and violence of these onslaughts are at times so great that she stands in fear of them.

---

[1] Semi-somnambulism (XVIII ; 185-6). I mention here this condition because it is taken up at this point in the saint's narrative. But it should be understood that nothing else in her writings would warrant the opinion that semi-somnambulism appears only after the third stage. As a matter of fact, she does not number it at all, and the name it bears here is of my own chosing.

If in the Orison of Quiet—and it seems to be the same in the Sleep of the Faculties—the soul keeps itself motionless for fear of losing contact with God ; in semi-somnambulism it " can lead at the same time both the life of contemplation and of action. While remaining united to God, it can attend to charitable objects, read, divert itself, etc. . . . it is like a person who conversing with another and hearing himself addressed by a third, gives to each a divided attention." Santa Theresa is not the only mystic who, at times, went about attending to ordinary business in this divided state of attention. Mme Guyon, St Marguerite Marie, and others, did likewise.

[2] Certain authors consider that Santa Theresa uses the term " rapture " (*ravissement*) to denote a particular kind of ecstasy. This does not seem to be the case. We know of no sufficient reason for setting aside this utterance of the Saint : " Rapture is called by diverse names, all of them expressing the same thing ; it is called elevation or flight of the spirit, transport, ecstasy." *Life*, XX, 215. See below for the distinction made by Poulain between Ecstasy and Rapture.

[3] Compare on Ecstasy, *Interior Castle*, Sixth Dwelling, especially IV-VII.

Santa Theresa is baffled by the mystery of a soul apparently unconscious and yet, as she thinks, aware that she loves and enjoys : " The will is doubtless occupied with loving, but it does not understand how it loves. As to the understanding, if it understands, it is by a mode of activity not understood by it ; and it can understand nothing of that which it hears. As to me, I do not think it understands, because, as I have said, it does not understand itself. For the rest, there is here a mystery in which I get lost[1]."

Here, as before, under the preconception that she is describing conditions sharply distinct, if genetically related, she strains to find absolute differences ; and, as before, she fails. Her final modest conclusion admits the failure : " In my view, Elevation of the Soul (Ecstasy) differs from Union " ; nevertheless, she concedes that they are " at bottom the same thing," only, in the Flight of the Soul, "God communicates to the soul a much greater indifference to, and detachment from the world. . . . Who does not see the difference between a small and a large fire ? Nevertheless, the one is as truly fire as the other."

Ecstasy is of very short duration. Here she speaks of half an hour ; elsewhere she is much less definite. As the powers return, it is the understanding and the memory that come to themselves first, while the will persists longer in union. At times, after a partial return to normal consciousness, the will is again caught up in Ecstasy[2].

*   *   *

A strong current of sensuous pleasure runs through the divine favours. St Theresa insists that one of the main concerns of the soul in Union and Ecstasy is to enjoy God. Many years later, when writing the *Book of Foundations*—Raptures had become very rare—she had perceived the danger lurking in our pleasure-loving nature : " The attraction which pleasure possesses for us is so keen that God has hardly given to the soul a taste of these spiritual delights that she entirely surrenders herself to them. She would remain as it were motionless in order not to disturb the sweet experience ; for nothing in the world she would want to lose it[3]." It is, however, only the Raptures lasting several hours that she condemns : " It would be better," she writes, " to use in the active service of God the long hours spent in this sort of intoxication. . . .

---

[1] Compare *Interior Castle*, Sixth Dwelling, IV, 431-4. The " mystery " will come up for elucidation in the chapter upon mystical revelation.

[2] The reader should compare Santa Theresa's description with that of the trance produced by drugs in chap. II of this book.

[3] *Book of Foundations*, p. 83.

I advise, therefore, the abbesses to eliminate these long trances[1]."
But if the delights are "spiritual" and from God, as she affirms in
this very passage, why not surrender to them and seek to enjoy them
as long as possible ? The Saint does not raise that puzzling question.
She is aware, in any case, that pleasure is not a sufficient justification
for the existence of mystical states. The gracious Lord grants them
as encouragement to holy living. One may well insist on this point,
for the mystics have not always been given the praise they deserve
for realizing that asceticism, on the one hand, and ecstasy, on the
other, are means to an ethical end. That which is to be attained
is humility and obedience ; and, above all else, the love of God and
man[2]. "Our rules in their entirety," writes the Saint, "are merely
means in order to attain more completely this end[3]."

Whatever the number of divisions made in the Journey of the
Soul and whatever variations in the names used to designate them,
later descriptions are in substantial agreement with that of Theresa.
We shall illustrate this agreement in the instances of the two Roman
Catholic Mystics who, after Santa Theresa, have observed with the
most care their trance-experiences, namely, St François de Sales and
Mme Guyon.

*   *   *

*The ascending series of the mystical States according to the
Traite de l'Amour de Dieu, of François de Sales.*—This treatise of the
famous Bishop of Geneva is a mystical classic. It owes its great
influence to the power of introspection of its author and a superior
literary talent. Although he knew some of the works of St Theresa,
there is no ground for doubting that his descriptions follow his own
experiences closely. His mind, better trained and not so easily
drawn out of its way or entangled by picturesque though
unimportant details, grasped more clearly than that of the Spanish
Saint the main outlines of the pictures he wanted to draw. Leaving
out a number of unimportant subdivisions, his description may be
summarized as follows.

(1) The starting-point is *Meditation*. The soul seeks "motives
of love," draws them to herself and delights in them. Then, she
choses that which she deems to be most favourable to her progress
and enters (2) *Contemplation* which differs from Meditation in that
" the latter considers in their details objects that may awaken love ;
while Contemplation is a unitary, total view of the loved object."

[1] *Book of Foundations*, p. 85.
[2] *Interior Castle*, Third Dwelling, II.
[3] *Ibid.*, First Dwelling, II.

It consists in an immobilization of thought upon certain ideas and images, chosen because of the tender feeling they evoke. "Although Meditation takes place almost always with difficulty and involves thought and critical consideration, the mind passing from one idea to another, seeking in different places the love of the Well-Beloved; Contemplation is always pleasurable because it presupposes that one has found God and His holy Love."

(3) At this point the soul is ready to pass into *Amorous Abstraction* (*Recueillement Amoureux*). But this cannot be accomplished by her own effort, the rôle of the human will is at an end; it is the work of God's holy grace. In that state, the soul enjoys a certain gentle sweetness (*douce suavité*) which testifies to the presence of God. Mental activity is reduced almost to nothing. The soul is conscious that God is near, and "makes a kind of effort to approach Him; she turns in the direction of her most lovable and beloved Bridegroom. An extreme reverence and a sweet fear sometimes fall upon the soul which is in that state." It happens also that "she remains as it were without life; she speaks and answers with difficulty, all the senses are benumbed," until the Bridegroom allows her to return to herself. When in Amorous Abstraction, the soul still possesses consciousness of the presence of the Bridegroom; she remains *en rapport* with him; she hears his voice, but can no longer answer him, or only with great effort.

The reader will have observed that Meditation, Contemplation and Amorous Abstraction correspond closely to the first three degrees of the classification set forth in Santa Theresa's *Life*.

(4) It sometimes happens that the trance deepens until there is a complete loss of consciousness; "the soul ceases even to hear the Well-beloved; she feels no longer any sign of His presence. Then, on awakening, she can say truly, ' I slept with my God and in the arms of the divine Presence and Providence, and I knew it not.' " The Bishop of Geneva describes with the pen of an artist the sensations of the soul as she feels herself gliding into the arms of the divine Lover and there falls asleep. The soul, says he, does not throw herself upon, or press herself against the Bridegroom, but passes gently as a liquid, flowing substance into the Divinity that she loves. This final condition is the *Liquéfaction of the Soul in God.*

*   *   *

The Ascending series of the mystical states according to the " Short and Easy Method of Orison " of Mme Guyon.—In this little book the descriptions are still terser than in the Treatise of St François de Sales. All accessory features are left aside and the main lines stand out with perfect clearness She also makes four degrees :

1. In *Meditation* " one must linger gently over some substantial thought, not reasoning about it, but merely fixing the mind . . . the subject should be selected with a view to fixing the mind."

2. " The principal exercise should be the presence of God." One must fix one's attention " by the affection rather than by the activity of the understanding. The soul rests, then, in a light amorous repose full of reverence and faith. . . . This should be an orison not of the thought, but of the heart."

3. " When the soul begins to perceive the odour of the divine perfumes . . . it is of great importance that she cease from all effort in order that God Himself may act. Remain quiet. It is necessary to breathe gently on the flame; so soon as it is lighted, cease blowing, for he who continues to blow will extinguish it."

4. Consciousness disappears. God has taken entire possession of the soul.

*   *   *

Santa Theresa, St François de Sales and Mme Guyon are agreed : the first step to take in the Ascent to God is to limit the range of the mental activity by choosing a subject of meditation, and then to concentrate the attention with as much completeness as possible upon the chosen theme. But the " concentration " here intended is not the activity of the thinker who seeks points of difference and similarity. In this technique, Contemplation means simplification ; all effort must cease in order to passivity. " Contemplation," says St François, " is a unitary, total view of the loved object " ; Mme Guyon writes of the same degree, " it should be an orison not of the thought, but of the heart " ; and Santa Theresa speaks of a " great reduction of the mental activity," and declares that the powers of the soul are unable to do anything except enjoy. Complete passivity brings with it a sense of absolute repose in God and a variable degree of warmth of enjoyment. It is followed in the completed instances by a moment of total unconsciousness.

It may be as Hocking says : in Meditation the mystic may recollect " those deepest principles of will, or preference, which the activities of living tend to obscure[1]." But in so far as it is the first step towards union with God, the function of Meditation is merely to lead up to passivity by arresting the activity of the mind. When, therefore, the mystic begins his Ascent with what he calls Meditation, he does not set aside the method of passivity. And his way of preparing himself, if not the best, is, in any case, effective. His utterances about what he means by Meditation and what he expects of it, leave no room for misunderstanding. The first step of the

[1] Hocking, *loc. cit.*, p. 376.

Christian mystical method is in substance the first step of the hypnotic method ; it begins with the fixation of attention upon some thought or external object in order to circumscribe mental activity.

* * *

The Buddhistic and the Islamic mystical trances and also hypnosis are essentially similar in their form to the Christian mystical trance.

The Mystical Trance in Buddhism.—The Blessed One spoke thus : " Through the subsidence of reasoning and reflection, and still retaining joy and happiness, the monk enters upon the second trance, which is an interior tranquilization and intentness of the thoughts, and is produced by concentration. But again through the paling of joy, indifferent, contemplative consciousness, he enters upon the third trance. But again through the disappearance of all antecedent gladness or grief, he enters upon the fourth trance, which has neither misery nor happiness, but is contemplation as refined by indifference. But again through having completely overpassed all perceptions of form, through the perishing of perceptions of inertia, and through ceasing to dwell on perceptions of diversity, he says to himself, ' Space is infinite,' and dwells in the realm of the infinity of space. But again through having completely overpassed the realm of the infinity of space, he says to himself, ' Consciousness is infinite,' and dwells in the realm of the infinity of consciousness. But again he says to himself, ' Nothing exists,' and dwells in the realm of nothingness. But again through having completely overpassed the realm of nothingness (the realm of ' neither perception nor yet non-perception '), he arrives at the cessation of perception and sensation[1]."

The Mystical Trance in Islamism.—By concentrating the mind upon some thought or by endless repetition of a word, the soufi empties his mind, loses the sense of the reality of the external world, and realizes a state of " psychic homogeneity " from which all distinctions have disappeared and in which nothing remains but a general awareness of existence : his own life and that of the universe seem merged together.

" The Mussulman ascetic (before reaching ecstasy) passes through three phases : preparation, perfection, expectation of ecstasy. In the preparatory phase the attention and the will are trained. The mystical ' apprentice' is directed to concentrate his mind upon some moral or philosophical topic. This in order to give him the habit of concentration, to avoid distraction, and to become accustomed to the use of symbols. He is to practise these exercises of concentration at

[1] Henry C. Warren, *Buddhism in Translations*, pp. 347-9, abbreviated.

first in the middle of the bustle of city life, in the public squares, in the bazaars. This is an obligatory test.

" In the second stage the ascetic lives solitary in the corner of the mosque or better in a cell of the *zaouia*, a room a few feet square, without ornaments, without furniture, almost without light. He practises fasting, vigils, silence, and the control of his thoughts. His aim is twofold : first, to curb his passions ; second, to isolate the object of meditation from its sensible qualities, to break his connexions with the phenomenal world. The mortification which he inflicts upon himself is to make him indifferent to pleasure and pain. Meditation upon metaphysical subjects more and more abstruse will convince the disciple of the non-reality of the external world.

" He is to train himself in the practice of the mental *dikr*, that is to say, of the meditation of a sentence of the *Koran*, of a formula, of a word. The verbal *dikr* or the repetition *ad nauseam* of the same words, is a degenerate form of the mental *dikr* ; it is a simple mechanical means employed by the Mussulman brotherhoods because a majority of the members have not the capacities required to become true soufis. The purpose of the mental *dikr* is to ' extract the divine essence from all the concepts of the understanding, out of all the ideas of the mind ' (Abd el Aben). The *dikr* causes the *soufi* to forget his family and business-affairs, his name, his own physiognomy, and his humanity. Thus by the successive elimination of all the accessory qualities of a thing or a concept, he approaches nearer and nearer to a homogeneous state.

" In the third stage, a state of peaceful expectancy is reached, very hard to describe. Personality has almost disappeared. The simplification and the narrowing of consciousness have reached their extreme limits.

" In complete ecstasy the *soufi* is lost as a wave in a sea of unity, and he has the intuition of being inseparable from it, he lives of the general life without sensible qualities, ' as an atom lost in the light of the sun[1].' "

The Hypnotic Trance.—The methods in common use to produce hypnosis include, as does the method to induce mystical ecstasy, the fixation of attention and directions (suggestions) intended to produce relaxation and mental passivity and, ultimately, sleep.

The first degrees of the hypnotic trance are similar to, and follow the same progressive order as the degrees of the mystical trances described in this book. Somnolence is the first indication of approaching trance ; the eyes close, the activity of the mind is greatly reduced.

[1] Probst-Biraben, *L'extase dans le Mysticisme Musulman, Rev. Philos.*, vol. LXII, 1906, pp. 490-8.

In a later phase, movements have become impossible. The subject may still hear and understand, but he is no longer able to answer, unless " suggestion " be used to restore his motor power. At that stage, hallucinations can be readily produced. There is no or little external perception to contradict the hallucinations, neither is there enough independent mental activity to cause their rejection.

If at that stage the subject be left to himself, he either wakes up or passes into what seems to be an ordinary, complete sleep. From that sleep he returns to consciousness in a normal way.

Further suggestions by the hypnotizer, or physiological causes may determine the appearance of artificial somnambulism—a condition in which the subject, without being responsive in a normal way to external stimuli, has nevertheless recovered the ability to move. He now acts out his dreams and the ideas put into his mind by the hypnotizer.

If the mystical trance stops at the " complete sleep of the powers," it is because, as the mystic grows somnolent and mental activity ceases, his idea of God fades out and he loses the stimulating and directing influence exerted by that idea. Therefore it is that, instead of passing into artificial somnambulism, the mystic falls into an ordinary sleep. Whereas the attention of the hypnotized is actively maintained upon the hypnotizer by the suggestions received from him.

The deepest hypnotic stage (somnambulism) may be reached at the first attempt, and so rapidly that the preceding stages can hardly be observed. Usually, however, it is otherwise ; and often no amount of perseverance brings complete success.

The only essential differences existing between the mystical and the hypnotic trance are due to the direct action of the hypnotizer upon the hypnotized, and to the differences between that which is expected of God by the mystic and of the hypnotizer by his subject.

* * *

III. The Confusion of the Degrees of Depth of the Trance with the Degrees of Moral Perfection.

The mystics affirm that the degrees of depth attained by the trance keep step with the moral progress of the individual. There is here a curious and far-reaching double error : the deepest stage of the mystical trance is regarded as being attainable only gradually ; and success in that respect is said to follow upon or correspond to the moral progress of the soul. The graver of these two errors is, obviously, the assimilation of increasing degrees of passivity in the mystical trance with progression of the soul towards perfection.

Complete " surrender to God " in a trance, and complete surrender of the selfish will in the affairs of daily life, are, as a matter of fact, very different things. That Santa Theresa should have identified things so different may well excite surprise. Yet it must be said in her behalf that, in this egregious confusion, the Spanish Saint was following an established tradition ; and was, in turn, followed by Roman Catholic theologians.

Let us observe first that, as a matter of fact, the attainment of the highest ecstatic stage need not be delayed. It is at times reached with the very first experience; in other instances, the ecstasy develops and reaches its final stage in the course of a few weeks, months, or years. If the reader will revert to the biographical documents, he will find that very early in their ascetic careers, Suzo and Catherine of Genoa enjoyed ecstasies apparently as complete as any experienced subsequently. They were not aware of the graded progression of which St Theresa and others make so much. Mme Guyon also found herself at the outset of her mystical career, at a single bound as it were, on the top round of the Ladder of Love. Of the orison with which she was favoured after the first interview with the Franciscan monk, she says, " it was altogether empty, without images ; nothing happened in my head ; it was an orison of enjoyment and of possession of the Will." During her first exaltation period, her orisons were " without acts," or " speech " ; without any " distinctions " ; movement was impossible, love alone remained. So far as ecstasy is concerned, there does not seem to have been any progress beyond that point—there was not room for any, for it had attained complete unconsciousness—and yet, she had a long journey to pursue before her whole being was regarded by herself as completely attuned to God's will. The first of the thirty-one trances of Mlle Vé was just as complete as the last. As to St Theresa herself, the account she gives of her trances is far from agreeing entirely with her theory.

The confusion we are discussing appears in its most shocking completeness in the systematization which, in her advanced years, the Spanish Saint had the misfortune to set forth under the title, *Inner Castle, or the Dwellings of the Soul*. That book was written in 1577, i.e., fifteen years after the part of the *Autobiography* containing her classification in four stages. It presents the Journey of the Soul as performed in seven stages. The first degree (Meditation) of the earlier classification is now subdivided into three. Thus, the four stages of the *Life* become six degrees or " dwellings." They are represented in her fanciful imagery as disposed about a new and central one, the seventh, which is God's abode and the goal of the Journey. The only important difference between this and the earlier description and classification is the addition of this new final stage, called " Spiritual Marriage or Deification."

Spiritual Marriage or Deification (II-IV). This name is intended to indicate the completeness and the permanence of the union that has now taken place. There is no longer any distinction or separation between the soul and God ; God and only God liveth in her. And the bride is no longer banished from the presence of the Bridegroom for periods of varying length ; she abides in the presence of her Lord.

The most surprising characteristic of this new condition is that it does not, as do the preceding stages, involve an obscuration of consciousness and a consequent abatement of activity. Contemplation has been left behind. Instead of wishing to die in order to enjoy more fully the bridegroom, the soul is now desirous of remaining on earth in order to serve the divine Master ; altogether steadfast, she is continuously absorbed in planning and performing good works. The great pains and the gnawing misery of dryness have vanished; "the soul is in a way freed from the inner disturbances which is endured in all the preceding dwellings." "That which surprises me most," declares the Saint, "is that when she has reached this condition the soul becomes almost a stranger to the impetuous raptures of which I have spoken ; even Ecstasy and the Flight of the Soul become very infrequent." The mysterious pains also have gone.

Realizing that the preceding picture of the Spiritual Marriage is to some extent idealized, the Saint adds a few corrective strokes. The soul is not absolutely sinless, she stumbles still, but never seriously ; and then, she quickly recovers, for the sight of her imperfection does not make her a prey to dejection. Neither is the body always free from pain ; but though it suffers, the soul remains serene and loses not the sense of God's sustaining presence.

The description is sufficient to make clear that this Spiritual Marriage does not belong to the series of brief, specific, trance states described under the names Meditation, Orison of Quiet, Sleep of the Powers, and Ecstasy. It is characterized by traits entirely incongruous with those belonging to that series. In Ecstasy, progress in the quiescence of mental activity, which marks the ascent from Meditation reaches its culminating point : the soul has become entirely unconscious of the world's existence and is altogether incapable of doing either God's will or her own. Whereas in Spiritual Marriage there is conscious activity of body and mind ; ecstasies, catalepsies, semi-somnambulism, and even visions have gone ; the soul is self-conscious, clear, and fulfilling God's will among men. What St Theresa has pictured under the name Spiritual Marriage or Deification is therefore not an additional and final stage of a trance-development—there is no stage beyond what she names Ecstasy—but her conception of the final condition of the purified soul, partly or entirely free from the accidents of rapture, ecstasy, dryness, etc., performing among men, in a steadfast way and without effort, the will of her divine Master.

Incredible as it may seem, this confusion of a fully conscious, unselfishly active, rational person, with the condition of someone entranced, i.e., deprived of his mental and bodily powers, runs throughout the writings of the great mystics. Two preconceptions made this confusion possible : (1) Ecstatic trances are divine favours given both as rewards for moral progress achieved and as encouragement or assistance in further effort. (2) Loss of sensory and of motor ability, and final total unconsciousness, mean divine possession. The tendency to confuse the passivity of unconsciousness with the universalization of the individual will is facilitated by the fact that the mystic enters the trance with his mind fixed on God, his attitude is for the moment that of the purified soul ; he feels only the generous promptings of the love-intoxicated[1].

It is well to recall that St Theresa never altogether lost sight of the belief that the trance states, capped by ecstasy, were special favours, occasional, extraordinary blessings, intended as means of perfecting the soul for the work to be performed for God on this earth. That, as she grew older, this truth became increasingly clear to her, cannot be contested. In *Inner Castle*, for instance, she is concerned much more with the condition and behaviour of the soul outside of the specific mystical states than with these states themselves.

*   *   *

[1] The honesty of purpose of Santa Theresa leads her here, as also in other connexions, into contradictions. In the very book in which she sets forth the unwarranted systematization we are criticising, she lets the following passages fall from her pen :
" There is an infinity of Dwellings ; the souls enter in them in a thousand ways " (I, II, 293). " One might suppose that in order to reach this Dwelling (the fourth, according to the classification of *Inner Castle*) it is necessary to have tarried long in the preceding ones." It is ordinarily so ; " there is, nevertheless, no fixed rule, because God distributes His favours when and how it pleases Him" (IV, I, 332). She goes so far as to recognize that final perfection may be attained without passing through any of the degrees she has described : " I would have you know, my daughters, that in order to . . . this union of pure conformity to the will of God (a state of active, perfection), it is not necessary that the powers of the soul be suspended. God, who is all powerful possesses a thousand different means for enriching souls and leading them to these Dwellings without making them pass by the short cut of which I have spoken, I mean without elevating them to that intimate union with Him" (V, III, 386).

At what period of her life does the Saint place the Spiritual Marriage ? No very definite answer can be given to that question. Delacroix says guardedly that she rose to that condition during the last ten years of her life[1]. Those who, with him, take her systematization perhaps too seriously, may be puzzled by the contradictions in which she has involved herself. Although from her own statements in the *Castle*, it seems that she reached Spiritual Marriage in 1572, she writes as late as 1579 as if she were yearning after the absent lover as during the barren periods of earlier years : " My heart is consumed with a desire to enjoy you and it cannot, captive as it is in this earthly prison. Thus, all stands in the way of my love. . . . But, alas, Lord of my Soul, how can I know with certainty that I am not parted from you[2]."

On the other hand several times much earlier she claimed to have reached Union, and to have been altogether happy in God's love. As early as the year following her entrance into monastic life, hardly on the threshold of the holy life, she lived " blamelessly " for a while. The most significant moment in the history of her moral progress, is probably the crisis in the year 1558, when, after twenty years of self-disapproval and unavailing struggle, she finally broke entirely with the World. God " changed entirely " her heart, and her resolution to give up everything for his sake " became unshakable." If one insists upon dating the Spiritual Marriage, it should be, it seems, from that year. The completeness of union was, nevertheless, temporary ; the natural man reaffirmed himself, and periods of depression and staleness, during which she lost the sense of God's love and of harmony with his will, made her again and again cry out as in despair for the return of her absent Lover.

There is no doubt that extraordinary favours became increasingly rare and finally disappeared entirely. As the end approached, her life moved at a more even pace. She ascribed this " progress " to the action of God, and thought that these divine instruments of sanctification were withdrawn because superfluous. One might, instead, regard their withdrawal as due to the natural effect of advanced age. According to her own account, she was at least fifty-seven years old, and perhaps sixty-six, when the stable, even tenor of the Spiritual Marriage began. At that time of life people love otherwise than at twenty ; transports and paroxysms are no longer within their means. In this connexion the rôle that we have had to assign to the sexual life in the production of the love-ecstasy must not be forgotten.

[1] See, regarding this point, Delacroix, *loc. cit.*, pp. 58-9.
[2] As quoted by Delacroix, *loc. cit.*, p. 59.

One might also take into consideration, as a cause of the disappearance of certain extraordinary favours, the cessation of inner moral conflicts. In so far as she was unified, remarkable automatisms in the form of monitory visions and auditions would cease, for they are products of inner conflicts. And, finally, one might add the important circumstance that, with the deadening of age and the attainment of a certain degree of moral unity, she entered upon a life of strenuous external activity. That fact was not without influence in bringing her to a more ordinary and healthier way of life.

*   *   *

The Ascending Series of the Mystical Degrees according to a Roman Catholic Theologian. Repeated attempts have been made by ecclesiastical writers, who do not claim direct knowledge of mystical phenomena, to systematize the many descriptions left us by practical mystics. Among the recent attempts approved by the Roman Church, the most thorough is probably that of A. Poulain[1] of the Society of Jesus. Sufficient interest attaches to the teaching of that Church and to the manner with which its scholars treat this problem to justify the following exposition.

In order to be accepted as true by the Roman Church, a mystical experience should " contain a knowledge of a kind that our own efforts and our own exertions could never succeed in producing." Any mysticism which cannot be made to bear out this " truth," is declared false mysticism by that Church[2]. Poulain's interpretations conform to this requirement.

Under the general head of " orison," he classifies both ordinary prayer and the mystical states, but he affirms an absolute separation between these two kinds of orison : the first can be performed whenever man wants ; the second cannot, it waits upon God's grace[3].

The four Degrees of Ordinary Prayer. There are four degrees of ordinary prayer : *Vocal Prayer*, which is recitation ; *Meditation*, also called Methodical or Discursive Prayer ; *Affective Prayer* ; and the *Prayer of Simple Regard or Simplicity*. The passage from one to the other of these is by insensible gradation. Affective Prayer is merely a prayer in which " the affections are numerous or occupy much more space than the considerations and the arguments[4]."

The highest degree of ordinary prayer, the Prayer of Simplicity is obtained when the simplification of the intellectual contents of consciousness and the diminution of the sense of self-activity, are carried sufficiently far and affect even the will, " which then becomes satisfied with very little variety in the affections[5]." In this state, the soul may be drawn " to content herself with thinking of God or of His presence in a confused and general manner. It is an

[1] *Des Grâces d'Oraison*, translated into English from the sixth French edition, under the title, *The Graces of Interior Prayer*, London, Kegan Paul, Trench, Trubner & Co., 1912, XXIII, 637.

Father Poulain is widely acquainted with Roman Catholic mystical literature. Santa Theresa is his most trusted guide. But although his respect for the utterances of orthodox mystics is prodigious he is nevertheless obliged, in order to make them agree with themselves, with each other, and with sound doctrine, to disregard many a definite statement. This delicate duty he accomplishes dexterously and discreetly.

[2] *Ibid.*, p. 3.

[3] Poulain, p. 1-2, the reasons for this interpretation are given in the sequel.

[4] *Ibid.*, pp. 7-12.

[5] *Ibid.*, p 8.

affectionate remembrance of God. If this be consoling, the soul feels a sacred flame which burns on gently within her and takes the place of reasonings[1]." The main difference between Meditation and the higher sorts of prayer is simple enough : " Either we reason, and then it is meditation ; or we do not reason, and then it is affective prayer or the prayer of simplicity[2]."

The four Degrees of Mystical Prayer . Sooner or later many persons arrive at the highest of the ordinary forms of prayer. It has even been held that every Christian ought to attain to it. But to pass from that prayer to the Prayer of Quiet—the lower degree of the mystical, i.e., supernatural forms of orison—is to cross an " abyss[3] " ; and none can do so unless by God's special favour. That which constitutes the alleged abysmal separation is explained thus : " There is a profound difference between thinking of a person and feeling him near us, and so when we feel that someone is near us, we say that we have an experimental knowledge of his presence[4]." " In the mystic state, God is not satisfied merely to help us to think of Him and to remind us of His presence. In a word, He makes us feel that we really enter into communication with Him[5]." The knowledge of God, gained in the mystic union, is not deduced from the nature of the experience or its content, it is an *immediate* knowledge. The soul *perceives* God, but not by the ordinary senses. God is made present to the soul without any material form. " That which constitutes the common basis of all the various degrees of the mystic union is that the spiritual impression by which God makes known His presence, manifests Him in the manner, as it were, of something interior which penetrates the soul ; it is a sensation of inhibition, of fusion, of immersion[6]." " Interior touch " is the term that seems to Poulain best to designate the particular nature of this knowledge.

From the above remarks, it would appear that the main, the substantial effect of the divine action in mystical orison is the realization by the ecstatic of a divine Presence, not of a merely " deduced " conviction, but an *immediate* experience of it. He perceives God by the feeling, by an " interior touch." In these and other words, Poulain strives to describe the characteristics of the particularly vivid and convincing impression of a divine Presence which is, as we also hold, the very centre of the Christian mystical experience.

There are only four degrees of mystical prayer. When any mystic seems to refer to some additional state, he merely uses other names for these same four degrees or for some particular aspects of them. Poulain's description of these states corresponds with that of the last four degrees in Santa Theresa's *Interior Castle*. In general he follows her as closely as consistency permits and even beyond.

(*a*) *Prayer of Quiet*. Divine action is not strong enough to hinder distractions ; the imagination still preserves its freedom.

(*b*) *Full Union*. The soul is *fully* occupied with the divine object ; it is not diverted by any other thought ; in a word, it has no distractions. On the other hand, the senses continue to act more or less ; so that it is possible, by speaking, walking, etc., to put ourselves into relation with the external world, and thus to bring the orison to an end.

(*c*) " In *Ecstasy* the divine action has considerable force, and all communications with the outside world by means of the senses are interrupted, or almost entirely so. Thus we are no longer capable of any voluntary movement nor are we able to come out of our prayer at will[7]."

[1] *Ibid.*, p. 13.

[2] *Ibid.*, p. 11.

[3] *Ibid.*, p. 65.

[4] *Loc. cit.*

[5] *Ibid.*, pp. 64-5.

[6] p. 90-1. See about this question the whole of chapter V, " God's Presence Felt," and of chapter VI, " The Spiritual Senses."

[7] *Ibid.*, p. 54. Where I do not quote, I have followed very closely Poulain's own wording.

These three stages differ, we are told, not in kind but in degree ; one passes from the first to the others by insensible gradation. None of them is of long duration. They may last but a few minutes and then may repeat themselves at brief intervals. They may develop slowly or appear abruptly. They may pass into a natural sleep[1] and may even, in Poulain's opinion, take the place of sleep. This last would explain how it is that some saints could without apparent fatigue spend a great part of their nights in prayer[2].

It is chiefly during ecstasy that visions and revelations are granted. The sense of the presence of God is at times so intense, God is so close, that it becomes a " spiritual embrace," characterized by very ardent delight[3].

When ecstasy makes a sudden, violent appearance, it is called " rapture." There may be violent suffering during the transport of ecstatic joy. The body continues in the position it occupied when the rapture came upon it. After a rapture there may be difficulty in resuming the ordinary occupations. The memory of what has been seen is retained ; but the soul does not usually know how to·express this exalted knowledge. As a rule it is felt that the under-standing has been amplified[4]. On this last point he insists in order, it seems, to separate divine ecstasy from trances that are symptoms of disease. The argument by means of which he supports his affirmation are no other than those offered by the mystics themselves ; he accepts them uncritically. The chief of these arguments is based upon alleged revelations—revelations too exalted to be understood[5].

(d) *Transforming Union*. Poulain prefers this term to Spiritual Marriage or Deification ; otherwise his description follows closely that of St Theresa. And, like her, he regards this final and stable condition of the perfected soul, seeking with full consciousness the advancement of God's Kingdom on earth, as completing the series of the brief, specific moments of limited or non-existent consciousness he has just described.

* * *

Poulain affirms the existence of a " chasm " between the last degree of ordinary or natural, and the first degree of mystical or supernatural orison : when the Prayer of Simplicity has been reached, man's work ceases ; or, rather, nothing more remains for him to do except the negative task of surrendering, of letting God have his way. Yet, in his description, the chasm is bridged ; he affirms God's action in the natural, and man's action in the supernatural stages. Of the Prayer of Simplicity (the last of the states of ordinary prayer) he says, " The persistence of one principal idea and the vivid impression that it produces, point as a rule to an increased action on God's part[6]." And, a little further on, " The prayer of simplicity, then, requires efforts at times, especially in order to curtail distraction, just as this is so with the Prayer of Quiet (the lower supernatural state) itself. Everything depends upon the force with which the wind of grace blows[7]."

* * *

[1] *Ibid.*, p. 227.

[2] *Ibid.*, p. 227-8.

[3] *Ibid.*, p. 228.

[4] *Ibid.*, pp. 244-5.

[5] " Magnificent sights, profound ideas present themselves to the mind. They are powerless to explain in detail what they have seen, however. This is not because the intelligence has been as it were asleep, but because it has been raised to truths which are beyond the strength of the human understanding. Ask a scholar to express the intricacies of the infinitesimal calculus in the vocabulary of a child or an agricultural labourer," p. 253. The problems raised here are discussed in chapters VIII, IX, and X of this book.

[6] *Ibid.*, p. 8.

[7] *Ibid.*, p. 14.

IV. The Distinguishing Traits of Supernatural Mysticism.

Individual mystics as well as the Roman Church have laboured to separate " true " from " false " mysticism. They have raised the question in this triple form : Is it a natural phenomenon ? Is it the work of the devil ? Is it the work of God ? The task of differentiation has proved most troublesome. General agreement seems, however, to have been reached by mystics and theologians of the Roman Catholic Church, upon the eight following characteristics[1] :

1. Divine communications, whether verbal or otherwise, possess greater distinctness and clearness than either human or diabolical communications.

2. They are expressed in us, but not by us : we listen, we are passive. They are often heard when we are not thinking of the subject to which they refer, and even when we are occupied with other thoughts.

3. Their meaning possesses a transcendental character, beyond human intelligence ; and is therefore usually incommunicable.

4. The meaning they convey seems, in a mysterious way, independent of the words used ; the same words may convey several meanings.

5. They come with power and authority, and produce a deeper and more lasting impression than natural words.

6. They produce peace in the soul. Worry, doubt, discouragement, etc., vanish, and are replaced by joy and happiness or by a pain free from any distressing implication.

7. They stimulate progress in the Christian virtues ; in particular, they incline to obedience, humility, and the praise of God ; and they increase faith in the teachings of the Church.

8. They have no bad physiological effects[2].

---

[1] Compare Poulain, *loc. cit.*, pp. 303-6 ; A. B. Sharpe, *Mysticism : its True Nature and Value*, London, Sands & Co., 1910, chap. IX, pp. 35-7, 159, ff. ; Josef Zahn, *Finführung in die Christliche Mystik*, vol. I, of the *Wissenchaftliche Handbibliothek*, Paderborn, 1908, § 36, p. 427, and § 38, p. 486.

[2] The reader may like to know Santa Theresa's opinion on this topic. It is in *Inner Castle* that her ripest judgment is found—a judgment enlightened by long years of reflection and by discussions with several theologians. In the third chapter of the Sixth Dwelling (pp. 426-8), she mentions five traits which differentiate " words " of divine origin from others. But, although she speaks with especial reference to divine manifestations in the form of verbal guidance, in her opinion the traits mentioned apply to all divine actions in man.

a. Divine auditions express meaning so clearly and impress themselves on the memory so deeply, that one cannot forget the slightest syllable ; whereas, those that come from our imagination are far from possessing that clearness. They resemble in a way, words heard in a dream.

b. They are often heard when we are not at all thinking about the subject to which they refer ; and, at times, even when we are conversing about other

It will be observed that these traits fall into two categories: some of them describe the experience itself, they are intrinsic to it ; others are its fruits. The intrinsic traits may be summed up in the words, suddenness, unexpectedness, passivity, illumination or revelation, and ineffability. We shall see in chapters IX and X that ecstasy regarded as "naturally" caused possesses also these five characteristics.

However interesting to the psychologist and significant to the experiencer himself the intrinsic characters may be, they are quite useless when an objective test is required. The director of souls, upon whom is thrust the awful task of recognizing the true nature of alleged mystical experiences, has always relied as a matter of fact either exclusively or mainly upon extrinsic traits, in particular, upon the moral test and revelation. When the ecstatic seems to make moral progress and is kept humble and submissive to the pronouncements of the Church, his experiences are likely to be classed as true mysticism. No revelàtion, no miracle, which causes moral or physical harm or which contradicts established Church truths, can be accounted divine[1].

In Protestant circles, the facts which are now most insisted upon as signs of the divine nature of mystical ecstasy are also those listed under items six and seven[2].

*   *   *

A Classification of Trances and Remarks regarding the Conditions of their Production.

The trances falling within the scope of this book may be classified under four rubrics : *simple trance, ecstatic trance, mystical trance,* and *ecstatic mystical trance.* It is with this as with any other classification,—there is no sharp line of demarcation between the several kinds of trances ; and, moreover, varying degrees of intensity of the several features of the trance produce great differences within each class.

1. *Simple trance :*—According to the dictionary, a trance is "a state in which the soul seems passive, or to have passed out of the body ; a state of insensibility to mundane things." In substantial agreement with this definition,

---

matters. Besides, they may have reference to ideas that merely flit through the mind, or to ideas that have passed, or to things of which we have never thought.

c. The soul merely listens to the words that come from God ; whereas it, itself, forms those that come from the imagination.

d. A single one of these divine utterances expresses in a few words that which our mind could express only in many.

e. Divine words possess (in a way which she finds impossible to describe) several meanings outside of the one they express by their sounds.—*Inner Castle,* VI, 3, pp. 426-8. Compare this division of the traits characteristic of true mystical ecstasy, with a division in three points, pp. 418-23.

[1] Compare Hugel, *loc. cit.,* II, p. 47, ff. ; Sharpe, *loc. cit.,* p. 160.

[2] Delacroix has interesting remarks on the theology and the psychology of Divine Grace in his section on Passivity, *loc. cit.,* p. 397.

we have used the term to designate a condition characterized by : (1) Partial
or total disappearance of the sensory and motor functions, which produces a
more or less complete loss of the awareness of the external world and of the
body ; (2) Reduction or total cessation of the higher mental functions.

A trance is said to be complete when every form of consciousness has ceased.
Were it not customary to use the word trance only when the state described
above is produced under unusual or abnormal conditions, ordinary drowsy
states and normal sleep would ,be called trances.

The trances considered in this book have usually been complicated by
ecstatic feeling and are, therefore, not simple trances. Had Tennyson been
ingenuous enough to take his experience at its immediate, crude value, instead
of transforming it by giving it a supernatural significance, the condition in which
he placed himself by repeating his own name would have been a simple trance.

2. *Ecstatic Trance :*—The common definition of ecstasy is " an exalted
state of feeling which engrosses the mind." A state of feeling so intense that
it absorbs the mind produces the two characteristics mentioned above as those
of trance. Every ecstasy is, therefore, to some extent a trance.

The trance-ecstasy may rise to amazing intensities of feeling and emotion
while the awareness of the external world decreases and, then, total unconsciousness may supervene more or less suddenly.

During certain phases of incomplete ecstatic trance, and together with the
wave of feeling and emotion, a considerable intellectual activity may go on,
as in the cases of Jean, of Rousseau, and in the instance related by Dostoievsky.
Under these circumstances, nevertheless, whenever it is possible to appraise
objectively the quality of that activity, it is found that it falls far below the
opinion of the ecstatic.

3. *Mystical Trance :*—Trances become mystical when they are regarded
as divine possession or as due to a divine intervention.

4. *Mystical Ecstatic Trance or, more simply, Mystical Ecstasy :*—A Mystical
trance which does not include ecstatic feelings, i.e., which is not an *ecstatic
mystical trance*—is little more than a theoretical possibility, for belief in a divine
Presence can hardly fail to arouse violent and engrossing emotions.

The preceding pages contain abundant illustrations of this class of trance.

* * *

There are ecstasies, mystical and otherwise, which are completely unprepared-for by the individual to whom they come ; his will counts for nothing
either in the time or in the form of the primary phenomenon. Such are ecstatic
prodromes of epilepsy, the cases (in chapter ix) of M.E., of St Paul, of
Symonds, and many instances among the great mystics,—for instance, the
ecstasy of St Catherine of Genoa when at confession.

But even in the completely unprepared-for instances, the trance may be, as
in the epileptic attack, anticipated by means of warning signs. The Great
Experience of Mlle Vé is preceded, several days in advance, by certain vague
impressions or symbolic pictures. Much more definite and reliable are prodromes
immediately preceding her ecstasies. They indicate " disturbances more
or less profound of circulation, respiration, muscular tonicity, sensibility,
and probably of all the other functions (if one could examine them)'."
These disturbances " correspond entirely to what may be observed in so
many mediums when they pass from the normal state to that of trance : the
blood withdraws from the extremities, they become cold ; at the same time
the face is congested ; there is shivering and trembling ; the limbs become
numb, " jerks " take place and are followed by contractions or paralyses;
touch sensibility is dulled ; they complain of buzzing in the ears or of the sound
of great waves ; it seems to them, as to Mlle Vé, that their spirit detaches itself
from matter, leaves the body behind, ascends, flies, etc.[1]

There are also trances which follow upon a preparation by the subject.
At times, this amounts merely to the production of conditions favourable to the
appearance of the trance. It is, then, merely facilitated, not completely
determined. Mlle Vé could not get her Great Experience exactly when she

[1] Flournoy, *loc. cit.*, pp. 177-8.

wanted it; but, by placing herself in a certain mental attitude, she could increase the chances of its appearance.

In certain persons trance can be brought about practically at will. They are induced, auto-suggestively, according to the method of the Hindoo Yogin, of the Mahommedan Sufis, of certain so-called spirit-mediums (Mrs. Piper, for instance).

In the lives of the Christian mystics there is the sudden, unexpected rapture and there is the ecstasy prepared-for and brought about by a fairly reliable technique. For persons in the physiological condition of our great mystics, already habituated to the mystical ecstasy, it is usually sufficient to conform to the directions set down by the mystical masters in order to determine the love-ecstasy characteristic of grand Christian mysticism.

There are, however, moments in the life of all mystics when nothing more than peaceful somnolence can be produced ; neither the organic love-factor nor any of the generators of brain-storms—whatever they may be—can be made to function. There are also periods when not even peaceful quiescence can be secured ; the soul remains distracted and restless.

The passage from self-conscious activity to that of entirely passive consciousness, and of the latter to total unconsciousness, can, however, never be exactly anticipated. There remains always, just as in the production of sleep, an undetermined, a surprise element. Sleep also follows usually upon the realization of well-determined conditions : a certain degree of fatigue, absence of disturbing sensations from the external world and from the body, quiescence of the mind. Nevertheless, it may be said of sleep also that it steals upon us with mysterious secrecy.

It may be added that the unprepared-for trances are often the more violent. Ecstasies following upon the practice of the mystical trance-technique, or of any other method, rarely find in the nervous system conditions ripe for violent nervous discharges. The trance is then limited to a delightful somnolence, bathed in love-feelings, or it may develop further and bring on the complete " Sleep of the Powers." When brain-storm factors are set off, the trance assumes the violence of sudden and unprepared-for raptures.

CHAPTER VII

THE MORAL DEVELOPMENT OF THE GREAT MYSTICS AND ITS RELATION TO THE OSCILLATIONS OF THEIR PSYCHO-PHYSIOLOGICAL LEVEL

THE moral history of the great mystics is commonly regarded as a progressive unfolding, culminating in a state of perfection ; and the various phases of depression and exaltation through which they pass are thought to belong and to contribute, each in its turn, to that progression. This is an inexact understanding of the facts. Like the course of most lives, theirs is, on the whole, undoubtedly in the nature of a development, but the oscillations of level do not constantly and of necessity bear to that development the instrumental relation which is attributed to them.

Where the documents were full enough we have been able to come to a definite conclusion regarding the relation of the progressive moral growth to the oscillations of affective and volitional level, and also regarding the degree of ethical perfection attained by the mystics. With regard to both these aspects we have been led to differ from the opinion common in the Church and also, in some respects, from that expressed by psychological students. These conclusions may now be summarily restated.

Factors of two orders—physiological and psychical—acting either separately or conjointly, determine the so-called periodicity of the lives of the mystics. Among the minor oscillations with a purely physiological cause we have noticed, for instance, a period of exaltation synchronous with a pregnancy, and we have learned that exaltation is not a very rare occurrence in pregnant women. To the states of " dryness " no moral cause can usually be ascribed, not even by the mystic himself.

Disconcerted and tormented by these irrational, unjustifiable moods, he comes to regard them as God's mysterious way of punishing and purifying.

When the oscillations of energy and affective tone remain within moderate limits, they are entirely commonplace and normal. The forces of life ebb and flow more or less irregularly. In certain individuals of the so-called artistic temperament these oscillations are better marked than in others. They may even so far surpass the ordinary as to remind one of a class of definite mental disorders called " periodic psychosis," " circular insanity," and the like.

In that class of disease, phases of exaltation and of depression succeed each other more or less regularly. In the great majority of instances it is not possible to refer the succession of states to psychical causes. And when any exist, they seem accessory to the physiological causes.

In so far as an alternation of states is not caused by psychical factors, it constitutes a problem for the physiologist and the medical man, and not for the psychologist. We may add that as there is in our mystics no discernible regularity in the succession of exaltations and depressions, the use of the term " periodicity " is here out of place. It is, however, theoretically possible that a real periodicity would come to light had we in the instance of any particular person an exact knowledge of the dates of the appearance of every oscillation. Unfortunately the biographical accounts left by the classical mystics are very far from fulfilling that condition. The record kept by Mlle Vé of her ecstasies is the only sufficiently complete and exact instance in our possession, and here reference is not to " dryness " periods, but to ecstasies.

The number of days which elapsed between each of her first sixteen ecstasies is respectively[1] : 5, 3, 11, 7, 8, 5, 8, 6, 7, 11, 5, 8, 9, 8, 7. If one supposes that unusual circumstances, physiological, psychical, or both, retarded by three days the second of the two ecstasies separated by eleven days, the last seven ecstasies would follow each other at almost perfectly regular intervals: 7, 8, 8, 8, 9, 8, 7.

This regularity may have been due to a connexion with sex functions, the ecstasy serving as a derivation or sublimation. We know that Mlle Vé was afflicted with attacks of nymphomania and that, in several instances, the connexion between sex and ecstasy forced itself upon her attention[2]. But we may also see in this periodicity nothing more than the expression of the general physiological antagonism between fatigue and recuperation. The trances left her in a state of great fatigue, and a certain interval between ecstasies was required for recovery[3]. In any case we are to remember that, in so far as our knowledge goes, the sex-function does not usually impose its rhythm on ecstasies.

[1] Flournoy, *Une Mystique Moderne, Archiv. de Psychol.*, vol. XV, 1915, pp. 174-6.

[2] See the case of Mlle Vé, chap. IX of this book.

[3] Flournoy, *Ibid.*, p. 125.

The irregularity of the earlier ecstasies might be referred to the same kinds of causes as those determining the irregularites observed at the beginning of the establishment of many periodic physiological functions—of menstruation, for instance. If, after the first sixteen, the ecstasies decreased greatly in frequency and became irregular, it is because of the appearance of psychical factors antagonistic to their production, in particular, growing doubts about their divineness.

Whatever periodic physiological basis there may be for the appearance of ecstasy, the periodicity may be destroyed by the influence of psychical factors. A chance event, making her feel her loneliness, would stir up in Mlle Vé passionate yearnings for divine companionship, and the coming of the Friend or of the great Experience would be hastened. The rôle played by desire and expectation in the production of her ecstasies seems to be indicated by the circumstances in which they decreased in frequency and finally ceased altogether[1].

The way in which accidental events, by stimulating psychical forces, effect alterations of the mental level, appeared with unusual definiteness and convincingness in our survey of the lives of Santa Theresa and Mme Guyon. In the latter, an outbreak of love for a Franciscan monk and, on another occasion, for Father la Combe, displaced a period of misery and pessimism and ushered in frequent ecstasies and glorious exaltation. In the case of St Theresa we saw how vividly chance occurrences brought home to her a neglected ideal, led her to new resolves, and thus for a while lifted her to new psychical levels. In Suzo, the gradual realization of the futility of excessive asceticism, assisted by various chance occurrences, finally reached a climax. With the throwing away of his instruments of torture, he passed from a long period of depressed introversion to one of buoyant practical activity.

The external and accidental factors that impinge upon the inner life of the mystics, providing as it were the occasions for crises and turning points, destroy any semblance to real periodicity that might appear, were the inner growth independent of the multitudinous, unpredictable, external impressions to which every individual is subject.

* * *

The systematizers among the mystics have fallen into the surprisingly coarse error of confusing degrees of ecstatic trance with degrees of moral perfection. The cause of the confusion is clear. If ecstasy is, as they think, union with God, then the more deep or

[1] See chap. IX of this book.

complete it is, the more perfect is that union : the depth of trance measures therefore the nearness to perfection, and complete trance-unconsciousness means complete union of the individual with the divine Will. We have shown that Santa Theresa slipped into a double error of fact when she set forth the moral development of the soul as proceeding parallel to the increasing depth of ecstasy : (1) Ecstatic trance does not usually develop according to the graded scheme set forth by her. It happens not infrequently that the very first trance-experience reaches an intensity of feeling, a rapturous quality, never to be surpassed and that it ends in a moment of complete unconsciousness. (2) The self-surrender of the Christian to God and his active life in unison with God (i.e., the perfect Christian life as the Church conceives of it) are not identical to the passivity and unconsciousness of the trance-experience or, in general, to states of automatism controlled by the thought of God.

The confusion involved in the theory of St Theresa has obscured not only the vision of theologians but even, to some extent, that of scientific students of mysticism. It has not, however, deeply affected the lives of the mystics. The final period (period of external activity in the service of God), when, according to their own opinion, they were closest to God, gives the lie to the theory of perfection in passivity. Far from being passive tools in God's hands, sheer automata, they were self-determined individuals, even though their purposes were regarded by them as conforming to the divine Will. Suzo on his apostolic visits, discoursing upon the love of God; Catherine of Genoa, managing her hospital as a Good Samaritan; Santa Theresa, engaged in her life-work as a founder of reformed monasteries, were perfectly self-conscious and self-determined. The wonders of trance and of drowsy abstraction had lost much of their initial glamour and, together with extreme asceticism, had receded to a subordinate place. Despite their theories, these mystics had come to realize very definitely that the perfect condition of the Christian is not one of inactive delight in God's sensuous favours, or of automatic, somnambulistic activity. They knew that his goal is not the kind of union with God and the kind of sinlessness character-istic of the passivity of trance, but rather the elimination of evil promptings or at least the ability always to overcome them, and a steadfast activity controlled by conscious purposes in agreement with God's Will. Ecstasy and other moments of passivity or automatism were, in their matured opinion, exceptional favours granted by God for encouragement and reward.

There is no true periodicity either in the course of the moral development or in the succession of the states of exaltation and depression which diversify the lives of the great mystics. And, although these states, and also the ecstasies, each exert their influence, it would be a mistake to regard them as having a fixed place in a systematic development. They usually happen at unpredictable moments as the result of a combination of internal and external forces; and it seems evident that the same goal would have been reached even if the number of these oscillations and their time-distribution had been entirely different.

* * *

The more significant junctures in the moral history of our mystics are, it seems to us, the decision to seek in a religious rather than in the social world the gratification of fundamental tendencies and desires; the exclusion, from the idea of the self, of the tendencies and desires regarded as evil; the decisions taken in important and definitely localized conflicts between the natural and the spiritual man; and the resolution to turn away from extreme asceticism and introversion to an active life devoted to social welfare.

The inner forces entering as an essential part into the production and the solution of these crises consist in various tendencies and desires, in the organization of some of these into ideals, in the strength and persistency of the impulses supporting these ideals, and in the influence of the general physiological condition of the individual upon energy and persistency in their pursuit. The influence of the religious atmosphere, which the mystics breathed, upon the formation of their ideal and upon their efforts to realize it, must not be exaggerated; for, the initial steps once taken, they moved on the whole in advance of the religious communities to which they belonged.

The periods of exaltation (including ecstasies) and of depression have in themselves no ethical significance. Neither enjoyment nor suffering bears a direct, definite connection with the formation of character. Each may have a negative or a positive influence upon ethical development. The beneficial influence of the trance-ecstasies due to drugs or of those that arise spontaneously is, when they are considered in themselves, limited at best to a relaxation of muscular strain and to a rest from the effort of adaptation to the demands of civilized life. It is only in so far as the mystical states are interpreted that they become factors in character formation. When the periods of exaltation and the ecstasies are taken as indications of the approval of a righteous and loving God, they result in a stimulation of the tendencies in harmony with the divine Will. And when the moments of " dryness " are regarded as punishments from Above and indications of a fall from divine favour, their influence may either bring discouragement and even despair, or incite to new efforts in order to regain the lost companionship. Whatever the degree of agreeableness or disagreeableness of what befalls the mystic, when he regards his fortunes as God's way of fulfilling a benevolent purpose, his various experiences are turned into instruments of moral achievement.

* * *

In so far as the mystical form of worship involves moments of restricted mental activity, i.e., trance-states of various degrees of depth, during which the mind is focussed upon the perfect Object, it possesses a particular efficacy, the explanation of which lies in the fact that a trance is a condition of increased suggestibility with regard to the tendencies, desires, and ideas that dominate it.

* * *

Did the great mystics obtain that which they set out to find when they embraced the religious life ? As in the case of every human being, their main demands were for self-affirmation, the esteem of others, self-esteem, and love. And they did find recognition, love, and moral guidance in their relations with God and with the religious community in which they lived.

The satisfaction of these fundamental human needs resulted in a substantial unification of personality. The latter parts of the careers of our mystics show them able to manifest the whole energy of synthesized beings in the fulfilment of tasks considered as assigned by God himself and achieved in close collaboration, or even in union, with him. Regarding themselves as divine instruments in the establishment of a new social order, the Kingdom of God upon earth, their life became one of joyful activity broken only by transports of surpassing love and peaceful rest. We make the above statements of fact without attempting to estimate the real social value of the mystics' achievements.

But if we were to ask whether the mystics realized in themselves the Christian ideal of moral perfection ; whether the divine, the socialized will altogether displaced in them the egoistic, "natural" man, our answer would have to be in the negative in so far at least as Mme Guyon, St Theresa and St Marguerite Marie are concerned. They fell far short of their ethical goal and approached it no nearer than did a host of inconspicuous Christians. For a justification of this opinion, we refer the reader to the biographical chapter. Francis of Assisi, Catherine of Genoa, and others appear to have travelled further along the road to Christian perfection ; but, concerning them and most Christian mystics, the available information is too scanty to permit an assured opinion.

We are to recall that if the establishment of God's Will in them, and of His Kingdom upon earth, came to occupy the first place in the concerns of our great mystics, it played a quite inconspicuous rôle in their determination to enter the religious life. Self-regarding motives, egoistic in character, were the main determinants of their decision to renounce the World for the companionship of God. And, regarding the nature and quality of the ideal which they came to pursue with much ardour, it must be said that these mystics were in no wise innovators; they found it in the Christianity of their time. It is by their radicalism in the pursuit of that ideal, and by the methods through which they chose to realize it, that they singled themselves out from other Christians.

Critical notes on Delacroix and Hocking.—Delacroix achieved a substantial progress over his predecessors in the understanding of the unfolding of the mystical life. We can say with him, " Ecstasy does not realize the aim of the mystic, he seeks beyond it. He aspires to a total transformation of the personality." " Thus the mystic has rejected that form of divine contemplation, the ecstasy, which was incompatible with life, because, if permanent, it would have destroyed life. He has passed beyond contemplation in order to reach action[1]."

But where, as in the following quotations, he describes the final condition of the mystic as characterized by passivity and the abolition of the feeling of self, we must disagree with him. He seems to us to have been in this respect influenced too much by the theory of the mystics and not enough by the facts which that theory is supposed to represent : " Deprived of self-consciousness (*conscience de soi*), plunged in a sort of essential felicity and continuous ecstasy, provided when necessary with precise ideas and moved to timely actions, the mystic has really fulfilled the conditions of deification." " The development of passivity, the abolition of the feeling of self, do away with that distinction and that alternation (depression and exaltation). In a kind of total automatism, they realize an impersonal and uniquely divine life[2]."

This description of the final condition of the mystic fits certain oriental and inferior Christian mystics, but not those we have studied, not, in general, the mystics recognized by the Church as great. Many of these, however, have passed through phases corresponding to that picture.

*   *   *

Reference should be made here to Hocking's *Principle of Alteration*. There are men who plunge into the detailed study of facts with a single-mindedness such that their creative imagination is endangered, and there are men who impatiently shake the dust of facts from their wings and soar gloriously. The first are called scientists, the second philosophers. In the *Meaning of God in Human Experience*, Hocking is primarily a philosopher and his Principle of Alternation (pp. 405ff), however enlightening it may be in other connexions, is of little use when one seeks to account for the specific oscillations observed in mystical life.

---

[1] *Etudes d'Histoire et de Psychologie du Mysticisme, la Systématisation,* pp. 417-8.

[2] *Ibid.,* pp. 417, 423.

CHAPTER VIII

THE GREAT MYSTICS, HYSTERIA AND NEURASTHENIA[1]

Much that has been reported in the biographical chapter points to the presence in our great mystics of nervous disorders, and perhaps of hysteria. Because that disease has long been supposed to be always connected with sexual and moral perversions, to convict a person of hysteria has been regarded as equivalent to a moral condemnation. As this opinion is no longer accepted in authoritative medical circles, a belief in the moral integrity of a person need no longer prevent the recognition of the presence in him of that disease.

We shall come to the conclusion that St Catherine of Genoa, Santa Theresa, Mme Guyon and St Marguerite Marie suffered from hysterical attacks. As to most of the other mystics mentioned in this book, our knowledge is too scanty to permit a reliable opinion. Whether or not our diagnosis be correct, we hold that the former separate themselves clearly from the insignificant and worthless individuals who, until recently, were regarded as the only possible sufferers from hysteria. It is with this disease as with epilepsy: most epileptics are degenerates, and generally inefficient persons; but a small number—a Napoleon, a Dostoievsky—have combined epilepsy with genius. We draw attention to this occasional co-existence without feeling called upon to account for it.

It should be borne in mind also that even though great mystics should be hysterical, it is obvious that the moderate mysticism, common in the rank and file of worshippers of almost every Christian sect, is entirely free from that disease.

As no structural alteration of the nervous system has been found, hysteria is spoken of as a functional, and not an organic, disease. And there are even people who include among its symptoms only what can be both produced and destroyed by suggestion[2]. In this view either the patient suggests to himself the disorders from

[1] The main ideas expressed in this chapter are to be foun d in our articles on the Christian Mystics published in the *Rev. Philos.* for 1902.

[2] See J. Babinski and J. Fromont, *Hysteria or Pithiatism, Military Medical Manual*, London, 1918, p. 311.

which he suffers, or they are suggested to him. But it must be recalled that a condition of excessive suggestibility points to an abnormal condition of the nervous system.

The most characteristic symptoms of hysteria are anæsthesia, hyperæsthesia, paralysis, and contracture. These involve a part or the whole of a limb, or one side of the body, or even the whole of it. They may appear and disappear without apparent reason and their duration varies from the briefest moment to several years. The anæsthesia may bear upon the feeling of hunger, and then the patient may refuse food and fast during incredibly long periods with relatively little observable inconvenience. If the patient eats, the food is ejected. To this intolerance there are curious exceptions, which point to the rôle played by auto-suggestion: everything except the consecrated wafer of the Eucharist may, for instance, be vomited. Spasms of the pharynx (*globus hystericus*) may make swallowing impossible.

The motor disturbances assume a great variety of forms. Although the limbs are not paralyzed, there may be an inability to perform some specific movement. The patient may, for instance, not be able to walk and yet may be able to dance. Not infrequently there are violent attacks resembling more or less closely an epileptic fit of *haut mal*, but without entire loss of consciousness.

In addition to anæsthesia and hyperæsthesia, other sensory disturbances are frequently observed—in particular hallucinations of colour, of smell, of taste, etc. Moments of mental vacuity, of semi-sleep, and sharp pain in the head, around the heart, or elsewhere, are not uncommon.

Hysteria develops usually upon the ground of a predisposing temperament; but there is little need of predisposition when the person is submitted to sufficiently strong or lasting influences, favourable to the production of the disease. Mental or physical exhaustion, or a great emotional shock, may be its immediate cause. It breaks out often in connection with the activity of the reproductive functions; it is, for instance, relatively frequent at puberty, in pregnancy, in diseases of the uterus, and at the climacteric change.

It will occur to the reader that potent predisposing causes of mental instability were probably innately present in our great mystics. " The quickly and intensely impressionable, nervous, and extremely tense and active physical and psychical organization[1]" characteristic of Catherine of Genoa were equally characteristic of Santa Theresa and of Mme Guyon.

[1] Hugel, *loc. cit.*, vol. I, pp. 97, 119.

The inaptitude of our mystics for ethical compromise is probably due in part to their hair-trigger, hypersensitive nervous organisation. It is to that trait that they owe much of their remarkable absolutism in matters of conscience and of love. In tougher persons, moral considerations and scruples are more evanescent and physical love is not so easily discouraged. In them, the wear and tear of contradiction, the chafing of opposed tendencies, is not great enough to be unbearable. Not so with our mystics : mental conflicts are to them unendurable ; they must be solved. But why are they not content to solve them by letting themselves down to the level of the " natural " man, instead of tenaciously insisting that they must end with its subjugation and the victory of the " spiritual " man ? This trait, the importance of which we have already sufficiently indicated, is one of the traits which singles them out as belonging to a class other than that of the ordinary hysterical sufferers.

Already predisposed by their temperament to certain nervous disorders, these great mystics were almost unavoidably condemned to them by the circumstances of their lives. It has become more and more recognized that a prolific, if not the most prolific, source of psycho-neurosis is an abnormal sexual life. None of our great mystics enjoyed a normal sex-life ; either they lived unmarried and under an exciting love-influence—the women in contemplation of the Heavenly Bridegroom, the men of the Holy Virgin ; or, they were married without finding in that relation the physiological and the moral satisfaction which it should give. The section of this book treating of the sex-motive in mysticism offers undeniable evidence of recurrent attacks of erotomania in connexion with love-ecstasies.

To that potent inciting cause of nervous disorders was added the exhaustion systematically induced in ascetic struggles against the flesh—struggles lasting for years and associated with periods of depression and general moral misery, sufficiently long, frequent, and intense to reduce vitality to a dangerously low level. Who, knowing these facts, would be much astonished at hysterical outbreaks ?

But we must turn from the consideration of probable causes to that of actual symptoms which, in our opinion, justify the diagnosis of hysteria. Every one of the symptoms mentioned above appears repeatedly in St Catherine of Genoa, St Theresa, Mme Guyon, and most of them also in St Marguerite Marie. We shall briefly set them forth in the case of the first two of these prominent mystics. As to the others, the reader may refer to the biographical chapter and, for fuller information, to the original documents.

Hysterical symptoms in St Catherine of Genoa.—Our information regarding this Saint is drawn from the *Vita*, as presented by her admiring biographer, Friederich von Hugel. Phenomena symptomatic of hysteria, or related to it, were observed at various periods of her life, but it is during her last four years that attacks of the character now to be described became frequent. She would experience sensations of extreme heat and cold, not related to the external temperature, and also an excessive sensibility or insensibility to touch : " One day she suffered great cold in her right arm, followed by acute pain." " At times she would be sensitive to such a degree that it was impossible to touch her sheets or a hair of her head ; she would, if this were done, cry out as though she had been grievously wounded." Again, at another time, " she had another attack (*assalto*), when all her body trembled, especially her right shoulder. It was impossible to move her from her bed ; she did not eat, drank next to nothing, and did not sleep." On another day, " she had another attack, a spasm in the throat and mouth, so that she could not speak, nor open her eyes, nor keep her breath except with extreme difficulty." " In her flesh were certain concavities, as though it were dough, and the thumb had been pressed into it." On another day " her pains made her call out as loudly as she could, and she dragged herself about on her bed. And those that stood by were dumbfounded at seeing a body, which appeared to be healthy, in such a tormented state. And then she would laugh, speak as one in health, and say to the others not to be sorrowful on her account, since she was very contented. And this lasted four days ; she then had a little rest ; and, after this those attacks returned as before." Recovery from excruciating painful attacks was frequently as sudden as the onslaught of the disease itself. This is a well-known feature of hysteria.

On August 22nd or 23rd, she had an attack and " remained maimed (paralyzed) in her right hand and in one finger of the left hand. And then she remained as though dead for about sixteen hours." " She would, at times, be so thirsty as to feel capable of drinking all the water of the sea, and yet she could not, as a matter of fact, manage to swallow even one little drop of water[1]." Her biographers report that, nevertheless, she continued to receive the Holy Communion with ease and safety—and in this, they will be readily believed by those who are familiar with hysterical phenomena : the symptoms are determined to a very great extent—altogether, say some authorities—by the mental attitude and expectations (auto-suggestion) of the person.

[1] The preceding quotations from the *Vita* are drawn from Hugel's *The Mystical Element of Religion*, ·vol. I, pp. 197-209. See also vol. II, pp. 14-27.

The frequent and prolonged fasts which Catherine inflicted upon herself, with no evil effect apparent to those about her, were the object of their admiration and are still regarded to-day by writers on mysticism as proof of miraculous intervention. If one may trust the exactness of her biographers, she went during perhaps twenty years, "for some thirty days in Advent and some forty in Lent, with all but no food; and was, during these fasts, at least as vigorous and active as when her nutrition was normal." Hugel offers this naturalistic explanation of the miracle : "These fruitful fasts were accompanied, and no doubt rendered possible, by the second great psychical peculiarity of these middle years, her ecstasies." These two peculiarities, as he calls them, "arise, persist, and then fade out of her life together." Now, if one bears in mind that Catherine was "often in a more or less ecstatic trance from two to eight hours" (every day, he seems to mean) ; that, in this condition, "the respiration, the circulation, and the other physical functions are all slackened and simplified " ; and, finally, that the mind is then "occupied with fewer, simpler ideas . . . and that the emotions and the will are, for the time, saved the conflict and confusion, the stress and the strain, of the fully waking moments[1]," it will seem natural enough that during the shortened time of full wakefulness Catherine enjoyed what seemed to casual observers a normal strength and activity. That this behaviour, continued during twenty years, was, nevertheless, together with her abnormal sexual life, the probable main cause of her ultimate breakdown, is a likely conjecture. The moment came when she had to give up these extravagant fasts and would find it necessary "owing to her great bodily weakness . . . even after Communion, to take some food[2]." At this stage, even when she realized her need of food, she no longer could digest what would have been necessary to a healthy life.

The remarks offered by Hugel in explanation of Catherine's fasts are supported in a striking way by the observations of P. Janet and Ch. Richet upon the ecstatic Madeline. During the periods of frequent ecstasies, she, like other ecstatics, did with an amount of food which would have been " quite insufficient to others, without, however, suffering a reduction in weight[3]."

The voluntary and prolonged fasts met with in great mystics should be considered in connexion with "hysterical anorexy," a disorder consisting chiefly in the systematic refusal of food, in

[1] Hugel, *loc. cit.*, vol. II, pp. 33-4.
[2] *Ibid.*, p. 148.
[3] *Une Extatique, loc. cit.*, p. 227.

certain digestive disturbances, and in consequent inanition. In *Major Symptoms of Hysteria*,[1] Janet describes, and considers theoretically, that interesting disorder. The following information is drawn almost verbatim from that book.

Anorexy constitutes very often an early manifestation of hysteria. It is never of brief duration and often continues for many years. When it does, it does not involve a constant refusal of all food. Even when the fast has lasted for years and has been fairly rigorous, the person may seem to be in good health; he may even show "a greatly exaggerated physical and moral activity[2]." Sooner or later, however, comes the period of inanition, the bodily weight, so far relatively well maintained, now falls rapidly. The patient remains in bed in a semi-delirious, semi-comatose condition.

Janet distinguishes between a refusal of food due to a fixed idea and true anorexy; the latter involves the disappearance of hunger, probably because of an anæsthesia of the stomach. The first is found in the psychasthenic neuroses while the latter is an occasional symptom of hysteria.

With these crumbs of knowledge regarding anorexy, and with the incomplete information given us about St Catherine by Hugel, we may not be able to determine with assurance whether the "fasts" of that Saint were really manifestations of anorexy, but we have at least seen that the maintenance of weight and of strength during surprisingly long fasts, even in persons who do not spend much of their time in ecstasy, is a fact susceptible of explanation. We have understood also that these fasts, despite their apparent harmlessness, were probably the main cause of the final break-down of that unfortunate woman.

A final word must be said regarding moments of mental vacuity met with among patients suffering from hysteria and related disorders. Instances are to be found in the *Vita*, but fuller descriptions are given by St Theresa and by Mme Guyon. During a certain period of her life, the latter would fall into a somnolence in which impressions from without were perceived either vaguely or not at all. This would come upon her at any hour, wherever she happened to be and whatever she might be doing. One day, when her sick husband inquired about the condition of the garden, she went to it, at his repeated request, "more than ten times without seeing anything[3]"!

---

[1] *Major Symptoms of Hysteria*, Macmillan, New York, 1907, p. 228.

[2] *Loc. cit.*, p. 231. For an explanation of this fact, see the following pages.

[3] Instances of this mental vacuity will be found in P. Sollier, *Genèse et Nature de l'Hystérie*, vol. I, pp. 266, 267. The remarks under *Troubles de l'Attention*, and *Rêverie*, in Janet's *Les Obsessions et la Psychasthénie*, vol. I, pp. 362-9, are instructive in this connexion.

Hysterical symptoms in Santa Theresa.—In the *Revue des Questions Scientifiques* for 1883, there appeared a paper by a Jesuit, G. Hann, on *Hysterical Phenomena and the Revelations of Santa Theresa*[1]. This essay, crowned at a competition at Salamanca, was subsequently put on the Index. In that paper the author, who had studied under Charcot and other physiologists, drew a very faithful picture of the Saint's ailments and concluded thus : "We are in the presence of an instance of organic hysteria as characteristic as possible ; the disease reaches in truth its highest limit. . . . It is the *Grande Hystérie* with its prodromes, its contractures, and its attacks which recall closely the frightful fits of epilepsy." At the same time, Hahn indicated features which separate the Saint from the great majority of hysterical patients, and he offered reasons for his belief that her " revelations," or at least some of them are not of a purely natural origin.

It will be convenient to follow this Roman Catholic author in his demonstration of hysteria. It consists essentially of quotations from Theresa's *Autobiography* and of corresponding citations descriptive of hysterical symptoms—these latter quotations we shall place in parenthesis.

Theresa's nervous affection broke out violently during her novitiate and was for three years the cause of almost constant suffering. She relates that, in entering upon the holy life, she had reached the satisfaction of her highest wishes, but she adds, " in spite of so much happiness, my health did not resist the change of life and of food. My weakness (*défaillances*) increased, and I suffered from nausea so acutely that it frightened me. To this was added a complication of other ills. . . . My disease became so serious that I was nearly always on the point of fainting. Often I even lost consciousness altogether[2]."

She journeyed to a small town in quest of medical assistance but without success : " The disease of which I hoped to be cured had only become worse ; the pains about the heart were so acute that it seemed at times as if it was being torn to pieces by sharp teeth. (" Cardiac palpitations have a large place in the prodromal stage of the attack of hystero-epilepsy. All the patients complain of them."— Richer, *Etudes Cliniques*, p. 19). . . . My weakness was extreme ; an excessive disgust for food did not allow me to take

---

[1] G. Hahn, *Les Phénomènes Hystériques et les Révélations de Sainte Thérèse*. S.J., *Rev. des Questions Scientifiques*, Bruxelles, 1883, vol. XIII, XIV, in three parts. The hysteria described by Hahn is the one known to the School of Charcot.

[2] This and the following quotations are taken by Hahn from the French edition of Santa Theresa's *Life*, published by P. Bouix, Paris, 1852.

any food except liquids. ("Digestive disturbances seem constant. The patient has no appetite, or taste is perverted. Frequently, the patient vomits almost immediately what he has absorbed. Between the meals, nausea may appear as the result of spasmodic contractions of the diaphragm and of the œsophagus."—*Ibid*, p. 16). . . . I felt as if burned by an internal fire. My nerves contracted, with pain so intolerable that I had neither day nor night a moment of rest. To this was added a deep sadness. That is what I gained by the journey."

"Four days of frightful attacks" stood out conspicuously in her memory : "My tongue was torn to pieces from having been bitten. ("The mouth opens wide, the tongue sometimes is projected outwardly and moves from right to left."—*Ibid*, p. 46. If during the spasmodic movements the mouth closes, the tongue may be bitten. This occasionally happens during the seizures.) As I had eaten nothing during this interval, and as I was so weak that I could hardly breathe, my throat was so dry that it would not admit even a drop of water. (Hahn tells us that a more exact rendering of the original Spanish would be : " I felt *stifled* at the throat, so that I could not even swallow a drop of water." This would indicate, unmistakably, he thinks, the presence of the "*globus hystericus*.") My body felt as if dislocated, and I suffered from dizziness in my head. My nerves were so contracted that I was gathered together as in a ball. I could not without help move either arms, or feet, or hands, or head ; I was as motionless as if death had stiffened my limbs ; I had merely the strength to move one finger of the right hand. People hardly dared approach me ; my whole body was sadly bruised, I could not stand the contact of any hand ; I had to be moved with the help of a sheet which two persons held at each end. ("The frigidity of the limbs is such that the patient may be displaced, put on the stomach or on the side, without changing his attitude." "The general contraction may be so painful as to force dreadful cries from the patient."—*Ibid*, pp. 74, 141.) . . . During nearly three years I remained paralyzed. Nevertheless, I grew slowly better, and when, with the help of my hands, I began to drag myself a little upon the ground, I returned thanks to God."

Ultimately, with the help of St Joseph, she recovered entirely from her paralysis, but various other symptoms returned as late as the writing of the *Autobiography* and of *Inner Castle*. One reads in the latter, " As I write these lines, I pay attention to what goes on in my head, that is to say to that great noise of which I spoke at the beginning, the noise which has almost made it impossible for me to do this writing asked for by my superiors. It seems like the noise of many large rivers, of an infinite number of birds singing, and of sharp whistles ; I don't hear these noises in my ears, but I feel them at the top of my head." (" Nearly all the patients hear whistling in the ears, always more intensely on the side of the hemianæsthesia. They hear as the rolling of wagons, the ringing of bells, the sound of brass bands. L. hears birds singing in his head."—*Ibid*, p. 21.)

Many if not all the symptoms mentioned above are now regarded as indicative of the high degree of suggestibility characteristic of the hysterical condition. Mme Guyon has provided us with striking instances of suggestibility. We recall in particular how, having fallen from her horse and resumed her journey, she felt impelled as by an external force to fall on the same side ; and she had to resist by throwing herself with all her might in the opposite direction. We reported also that during a severe illness marked by paralyses, contractures, hyperæsthesias, etc., she returned to "the state of the child." The amazed Father la Combe would say to her, " It is not you, but a little child that I see." Similar instances, altogether disconnected from the religious life, are recorded in works on psychasthenia and hysteria. Janet speaks of persons who "play a sort of comedy ; they make themselves small, naïve, wheedling ; they pretend ignorance and like to be regarded as ' a little stupid.' This is because they want to be guided, . . . They want to be amused, played with ; in a word, they want to be treated like children[1]." " Qi., a woman thirty-five years old, is haunted by the desire to skip a rope, to clip her hair short, to let it down. There is here clearly an obsession." She explains her underlying feelings thus : " I would so much like to be small, to have a father and mother to hold me on their laps, to pat my head. . . . But, no, I am Madame, mother, housekeeper ; I must be serious, think out alone my problems. O, what a life[2] ! " The idea of the child Jesus, the object of her love, haunted Mme Guyon. In her suggestible condition her yearning worked itself out into the mimicry of a child.

*　　　*　　　*

The facts and considerations contained in the preceding pages lead inevitably, it seems, to the conclusion that our great mystics have suffered at various moments from symptoms characteristic of hysteria. Equally unavoidable, however, is the conviction that the hysterical sufferers ordinarily described by the psychiatrist do not match these mystics point by point. It cannot truly be said of the latter, as it can of the former, that they are purposeless weathercocks,

---

[1] Janet, *Les Obsessions et la Psychasthénie*, Paris, 1903, vol. I, p. 391.

[2] *Ibid.*, p. 392.

incapable of energetic, sustained, and intelligent effort for the realization of rational purposes.

It is with the symptoms of hysteria as with those of epilepsy : they appear in persons of widely different types. Sufferers from these disorders may be compared to machines with the same defect or group of defects. These may coexist with great differences in power, in quality of the material, in finish, and even in structure. Once let the defect be corrected, the several machines will prove themselves efficient in widely different degrees. As the human organism is infinitely more complicated than any man-made machine, the possible differences between persons afflicted by the same symptoms are far more numerous than in machines.

If sufficiently abused, the human body, like any machine, will break down at some particular point. Our great mystics were submitted to conditions of life so severely and persistently adverse to health that even the stoutest nervous system might have been expected to yield to the strain. This is particularly true of St Catherine of Genoa and of Mme Guyon, in whom the sex-needs, in their physiological and psychical aspects, as well as other fundamental needs and desires, were baulked and repressed in year-long conflicts. Suzo's and St Theresa's lots were less unfortunate. Yet they also had to live a life of continence and they were for years divided souls with regard to the things which most matter to man. Because of the ideal they had formed and of the method of life they had chosen, their deepest instincts and desires could not be gratified in the ordinary way. And they aggravated repressions and conflicts, in themselves sufficient to cause a variety of psychoses, by excessive and persistent ascetic practices, and thus exhausted themselves to the point of inanition. How many persons about us who successfully live a normal life would have withstood the ordeals to which these people have been subjected ?

The great mystics and neurasthenia.—Janet has given us a minute and masterly analysis of the characteristics of non-hysterical psychopaths[1], whom he classes together as manifesting a general psycho-physiological insufficiency. They suffer from an abnormal scrupulosity ; they hesitate, deliberate endlessly, are afraid to conclude and to act ; and this not only when commonsense would dictate extreme caution, but concerning insignificant matters or problems which normal minds would simply set aside as insoluble. Moreover, they are fickle and without constancy of purpose. They

---

[1] In *Médications Psychologiques* and in earlier books. It is unnecessary for our purpose to attempt to draw any distinction between " neuropathy " and " psychopathy."

are in general abnormally dependent upon external sources of strength and in particular upon affection and love.

As life is usually too complicated for them to cope with it successfully, they seek consciously or unconsciously to simplify it; they may cut themselves off entirely from society and live in seclusion. They are given to day-dreaming and to moments of mental vacuity during which they appear almost bereft of their senses. Feelings of dissatisfaction with themselves, of ennui, and of "incompleteness" are common. They exhibit at times a shocking callousness.

The connexion existing between these various traits is obvious. A silly scrupulosity, a diffidence and inability to act, a desire to simplify one's life, an inordinate craving for the support of authority and affection, mental vacuity, obsession, and monoideism—are all traits which may easily be conceived as proceeding from one and the same root, namely, a general psycho-physiological insufficiency.

Our great mystics manifest many or even all of these symptoms, but a careful observation of their behaviour reveals that (except perhaps during the brief moments when the intensity of their inner conflicts and the severity of their asceticism have temporarily disabled them) they do not have the same significance as in the ordinary patients of the psychiatrist.

The withdrawal of the mystics to religious communities has not the same meaning as the isolation of the psychopathic patient whose energy and mental resources are insufficient to meet the complexities of ordinary social life. If these mystics refused to accept life as it presented itself to them before they embraced the holy life, it was not primarily because of its complications but because it lacked qualities without which life was for them not worth living. They withdrew to the comparative seclusion of convents with the purpose of finding a new life which would gratify their fundamental cravings. And it was not without an impressive display of perseverance that most of them achieved their separation from the World. The obstacles which they overcame would have been effective bars for ordinary persons. And when, long after her novitiate, St Theresa felt that she ought to give up the few worldly relations she had kept, it was not in order to reduce her life to a manageable point. As a matter of fact she desired and enjoyed company; but, as it kept awake pride and vanity, she felt that it was to be renounced.

When these mystics struggle with their conscience about going out in décolleté, receiving a friendly visitor, eating a dainty morsel, or otherwise gratifying their senses, they are not displaying the scrupulosity of the asylum patient who refuses to eat certain dishes, is in dread of becoming too lean or too fat, must have his bed made in a particular way, does not dare utter certain words, etc. When self-indulgence is regarded as a cardinal sin (as it was in their religious world) to undertake a war to the death against fleshly inclinations is not necessarily a sign of insane scrupulosity. Their conduct in this connexion was logically determined by a theory widely accepted in the Christian Church, and their practice differed from that of the ordinary Christian in no other way than in being radical : they sought to achieve completely that which others were satisfied to get partially. The remorse they felt at their failures proceeded from the consciousness of the failure of the spirit to be master in its tenement of clay. The persistency with which they sought to use their suffering, whether self-inflicted or otherwise, for the furtherance of this great purpose, is one of the striking aspects of their lives. There is nothing which they do not venture to construe so as to make it grist to their mill. To what extravagant length they have gone in that direction is well illustrated by St Catherine when she was suffering from hysterical attacks.

The great mystics aimed not at simplification as such, but rather at a unification which would give the mastery to the impulses and desires regarded as of God. The ordinary psychopath has no such purpose : he seeks the elimination of the *more difficult* social relations, i.e., a descent to an easier level of life.

As to their alleged aboulia and need of external support, no one aware of the relation which existed between them and their religious directors will be inclined to deny that the latter were, on the whole, directors in name only, and that, at times, they were reduced to the rank of servants. Their lives once reorganized, unified on a higher level, the great mystics sallied forth into the World and proved themselves men and women of action of no mean ability. In this connexion we need only recall St Catherine's management of a large hospital, St Theresa's operations as foundress of monasteries, and Mme Guyon's and Suzo's apostolic activities. Mlle Vé was the successful director of an educational institution.

Without making light of the abnormal nature of periods of deep depression, of certain extravagances of behaviour, and of ecstatic trances conspicuous in the great mystics, and without forgetting that in them accidental causes of psychasthenia and hysteria acted upon temperamental predispositions to nervous instability and to dissociation, one may nevertheless reject the opinion according to which these symptoms of nervous disorder identify them with ordinary psychopaths and are necessarily indicative of a general mental and moral worthlessness. Identity of symptom does not mean identity of person. Deep oscillations of emotional tone, ecstasies, and even hysterical attacks do not necessarily imply the intellectual and moral insufficiency characteristic of Madeleine and her class. They may on the contrary be allied with traits which make the genius.

CHAPTER IX

ECSTASY, RELIGIOUS AND OTHERWISE : A COMPARATIVE STUDY

I. Spontaneous Ecstasies.

In the course of the preceding descriptions of Christian mysticism, many problems have been raised and a few have been answered. But the psychological investigation of the mystical ecstasy and of its several constituent or attendant phenomena is a task that remains before us. For the accomplishment of that task the ground has been prepared by introducing at the beginning of this book a study of the older and simpler forms of mystical ecstasy—those known to savages and to Hindoo civilization. Thus, genetic connexions between the present and the earlier forms of trance-worship have been provided.

In order to reach full fruition our investigation must add to the use of the genetic that of the comparative method of research. Outside of religious mysticism there are numerous instances of raptures possessing many of the traits commonly regarded as characteristic of the divine Union. These non-religious instances of ecstasy must be compared with those that have thus far occupied our attention. It is a misfortune (and the main cause of their little success) that the students of mysticism have usually kept their survey within the boundaries of religious and even of Christian mysticism. To attempt a solution of the problems of mystical ecstasy on that basis is just as hopeless as it would be to undertake the study of English philology while disregarding the related languages. We shall, therefore, seek whatever light may come from a survey of several classes of experiences which common opinion relates to mysticism.

*　　　　*　　　　*

Among the dread diseases that afflict humanity there is one that interests us quite particularly ; that disease is epilepsy. Its main manifestation is often preceded by curious signs, varying greatly from person to person, but fairly constant in the same person. In some instances, the " aura," as these premonitory symptoms are called, is in the nature of an ecstasy. In *Modern Medicine*, Dr Spratling reports the case of a priest under his care whose epileptic attacks were preceded by a rapturous moment. Walking along the streets, for instance, he would suddenly feel, as it were, " transported to heaven." This state of marvellous enjoyment would soon pass, and, a little later on, he would find himself seated on the curb of the side-walk aware that he had suffered an epileptic attack[1]. The same author mentions elsewhere two other epileptic patients, " teachers of noted ability," who speak of their auræ as " the most overwhelming ecstatic state it is possible for the human to conceive of[2]."

Similarly, the Russian novelist, Dostoievsky, himself an epileptic, describes in his novel *The Idiot* an ecstatic aura : " I remember among other things a phenomenon which used to precede his epileptic attacks when they came in the waking state. In the midst of the dejection, the mental marasmus, the anxiety which he experienced, there were moments in which all of a sudden the brain became inflamed and all his vital forces suddenly rose to a prodigious degree of intensity. The sensation of life, of conscious existence, was multiplied tenfold in these swiftly passing moments. A strange light illumined his heart and mind. All agitation was calmed, all doubt and perplexity resolved themselves into a superior harmony ; but these radiant moments were only a prelude to the last instant— that immediately preceding the attack. That instant, in truth, was ineffable[3]."

The following information regarding the several forms which the aura may take bears directly upon our problems. " The most common psychic aura is a sudden acceleration of the imagination, a quick overflowing of the process of thought in which the train of imagery is urged ahead with trembling, excited haste until the thread is snapped and unconsciousness occurs." Sudden temporary blind-ness, may constitute its most substantial part. " Auditory aura usually partakes of the character of roaring and voices, the sound of waves, etc. Such auræ occur in from two to three per cent. of all cases[4]." Hallucinations of taste and smell also occur. The re-appearance of normal consciousness is frequently marked by temporary mental confusion, during which phase automatisms may take place.

The preceding instances of epileptic auræ show the following features. (1) There is a total absence of causal, conscious factors. (2) They bear a specific relation to a physiological disorder. The

---

[1] Wm. P. Spratling, in article " *Epilepsy,*" in Osler's *Modern Medicine,* vol. 7.

[2] *Epilepsy and its Treatment,* p. 466.

[3] *The Idiot,* vol. 1, p. 296. Quoted from Spratling. There is a similar description in *The Possessed (Besi),* tr. Garnett, New York, Macmillan, p. 554.

[4] *Three Lectures on Epilepsy,* by W. A. Turner, Edinburgh, 1910, p. 6.

ecstasy is, therefore, in these cases, assigned to a purely physiological cause. (3) The aura comes suddenly and unexpectedly. The subject's rôle is entirely passive; it is as if an external power had taken possession of him. (4) The ecstasy may bring with it a sense of initiation, illumination, or revelation. (5) The experience is so wonderful that the most extravagant descriptive terms and comparisons seem to fall short of the reality; it is an *ineffable* experience.

These traits might naturally enough suggest superhuman causation, yet no metaphysical significance is ascribed to them. The priest did not think himself actually transported to heaven; neither did he believe that he had communed with God. Both the priest and Dostoievsky accept the scientific view: these raptures are the expression of a particular disease, and so, they say, " it is not a higher life, but on the contrary, one of lower order[1]."

In the works of Pierre Janet may be found instances in several respects similar to the preceding, although apparently not connected with epilepsy. In them, some conscious activity, sometimes regarded by the experiencer as its sufficient cause, precedes the ecstasy. But the conscious activity plays rather the rôle of an occasion; it is like a spark that explodes a train of powder.

Fy, while walking in the country, is intoxicated by the open air, " everything seems delightful "; she is going " to burst from happiness." " I have," she declares, " never before experienced that; the day passes like a dream (five times more swiftly than in Paris); I feel a better person, and it seems to me that there are no bad people, every face is sympathetic and it seems to me that I live in the Golden Age[2]."

Gs, contemplating Paris from the top of the Trocadero, is roused to intense admiration and for a moment he forgets his suffering. " It seems to me," says he, " that it is too beautiful, too grand, that I am lifted up above myself. At the time, it gives me an enormous pleasure; but it exhausts me; my legs shake, and it seems to me that, unable to stand that happiness, I am going to swoon[3]."

But, however vivifying and inspiring a beautiful day in the country or Paris from the Trocadero may be, these sights do not usually liberate storms of feeling such as are described by these two persons. The country and Paris acted upon them like a last drop that starts an overflow. Quite similar is the following instance taken from my own collection of documents. It belongs to a perfectly normal person.

[1] *The Idiot.*
[2] P. Janet, *Les Obsessions et la Psychasthénie*, Paris, 1903, vol. 1, pp. 380-1.
[3] *Loc. cit.*, 380.

" Once when walking in the wild woods and in the country, in the morning under the blue sky, the sun before me, the breeze blowing from the sea, the birds and flowers around me, an exhilaration came to me that was heavenly—a raising of the spirit within me through perfect joy. Only once in my life have I had such an experience of heaven[1]."

The case of Nadia is not essentially different. For, although two powerful emotional stimuli, love and music, provide rational causes, common sense cannot regard them as causes commensurate with the intensity of the storm they let loose. The love itself has hardly any rational basis ; Nadia has never spoken to the object of her passion and has seen him but a few times. She wrote to Pierre Janet, her physician, " The concerts given by X have been for me a revelation ; they have awakened such an enthusiasm in me that I have never recovered from it. I cannot explain its effect. When I left the hall after the first concert, my legs and whole body shook so that I could not walk, and I spent the night in tears. . . . But it was not painful, far otherwise ; it was as if I was coming out of a dream which filled my past life. I understood things more as they really are. I was in a veritable heaven of happiness. My only hope during many years has been to hear him again and to experience the same feelings. I believe that, as people said, I had a passion for him, but it was not an ordinary passion ; of that I am sure. He seemed to possess a supernatural influence over me[2]."

Nadia reminds one of love at first sight. Is not the *coup de foudre de l'amour*, as the French say, a phenomenon in several respects similar to the one we are discussing ? The passive rôle of the subject, the suddenness of the emotional onslaught, the ineffable happiness, the sense of discovery, establish a more than superficial resemblance. Unfortunately, there is no time to insist upon this parallel. Here is a final instance :

Jean occasionally experiences what he calls " *sensations sublimes et solennelles.*" This happens, for instance, when he thinks of himself as a representative in the Chamber of Deputies, where, before well filled galleries, he pronounces a great political speech. A slight shudder runs through his body—not an unpleasant shudder—his heart is calm and beats slowly . . .; instead of his habitual

---

[1] No. 40. " Sometimes, when I am away on the hills or in the woods alone, God seems very near. . . . It is then that my soul goes out to Him most fully, and that I am nearest to freedom from the limitations of time and space and matter, nearest to gaining a true sense of relative values. I do not then arrive at conclusions through any process of reasoning—I simply *know* for the time." From one of Pratt's correspondents, as quoted by him in *The Religious Consciousness*, p.358.

[2] P. Janet, *loc. cit.*, p. 387.

humble tread, with head down, he straightens up and strides along with an important air. His intelligence is exalted and keen, and he thirsts for knowledge ; above all, he enjoys a sense of happiness never otherwise felt. " These are," he says, " divine impressions that prove to me the existence of a soul in the body[1]."

The appellation " divine " applied by Jean to his emotion, and the illogical sequence of ideas by which he comes to a belief in the existence of a soul in the body, are well worth noticing. The same sort of reasoning is common enough among persons cherishing high intellectual pretensions : Jean, like Mlle Vé and the theologians of " inner experience," passes from a sense of exaltation and vivification to the idea of God as its cause.

Few, if any, persons will fail to recognize in their own history moments of exaltation comparable to the above, both in their quality and in their occasion. We are in the habit of regarding these moments as determined by some mental content but the noteworthy thing is that many of them are, in principle, no more rationally caused than Jean's ecstasy, or the raptures of No. 40. Did Jean actually pronounce mentally a noble discourse ? Did he develop with powerful logic a succession of great thoughts supported by vast erudition ? Certainly not. He did not actually say anything, or what he said mentally was mere shadowy fragments of commonplace, stump-speech oratory. But he pictured himself speaking in the impressive setting of the Chamber of Deputies ; he heard the applause of the galleries ; shivers coursed down his spine ; he straightened up, and thought himself convincing and witty ! Illusions of this sort are as common as they are psychologically interesting. To them hasheesh, mescal, alcohol and other narcotic drugs owe much of their charm ; and to them also is due in part the belief in the divine nature of the condition produced by these drugs.

All these non-religious raptures, both the epileptic and the others, happen suddenly and unexpectedly. The subjects feel as if in the hands of external agents. They are carried away by a wave of sensations and emotions, indescribably delightful. Moreover, they are under the impression that they have entered a new world, and so they speak of illumination, of revelation. We recall that these traits —*suddenness, unexpectedness, passivity, ineffability* and *illumination or revelation*—are the very traits which, together with beneficial moral consequences, are regarded by the Christian mystics as characteristic of true religious ecstasy.

The trait most insisted upon—a trait without which, according to the Roman Catholic Church, no ecstasy is a true religious ecstasy

[1] *Loc. cit.*, p. 381.

—is the revelatory, or, as the philosophers say, the noetic quality. A careful examination reveals the presence of that trait in every one of the preceding instances. Nadia alone, it is true, uses the word "revelation," but all these persons convey in unmistakable terms the unique, wonderful quality of their experiences. Both Nadia and Jean speak of a new understanding of things, and Dostoievsky, struggling to describe the indescribable, notes two aspects of revelation upon which the Christian mystics usually lay stress, its clearness and its certitude.

It might be said, by way of objection, that what we refer to in these instances as " revelation," is too lacking in conceptual clearness to deserve that name. But is it not well known that lack of conceptual definiteness has never been regarded by the mystics or their apologists as a sufficient reason for disbelieving in the revelatory quality of the mystical experience ? On the contrary, they have one and all insisted upon its inexpressibility.

*   *   *

We pass now to an instance of ecstasy regarded as religious both by the experiencer and by the World in general.

M.E. is a man of superior education and of great moral earnestness. Throughout his life he has wrestled with philosophico-religious problems. He is wont to see in life, or at least in its more dramatic events, the hand of Providence. It will be observed that the ecstasy fell upon him with startling unexpectedness. So far as he knew, nothing whatsoever, whether in his physical or psychical condition, could have foreshadowed its appearance. In this respect, this ecstasy does not differentiate itself from the rapturous epileptic aura. We shall have to ask ourselves whether it differentiates itself from it in any way except in the interpretation placed upon it by the subject and in the consequences of that interpretation.

" As to ecstasies, I have experienced one, among others, which I remember perfectly. I will try to tell you when and how it happened and what it was like. I was thirty-six years old. I was climbing with some young fellows from Forclaz to the Croix de Bovine in order to reach Champex. We were following a road bordered by blooming oleanders and looking down over a stretch of country dotted here and there with clumps of firs. The wind scattered the clouds above and below us, sending them down or driving them up in whirling eddies. Now and then, one escaped and floated over the valley of the Rhone. I was in perfect health ; we were on our sixth day of tramping, and in good training. We had come the day before from Sixt to Trent by Buet. I felt neither fatigue, hunger, nor thirst, and my state of mind was equally healthy. I had had at

Forclaz good news from home ; I was subject to no anxiety, either near or remote, for we had a good guide, and there was not a shadow of uncertainty about the road we should follow. I can best describe the condition in which I was by calling it a state of equilibrium. When, all at once, I experienced a feeling of being raised above myself, I felt the presence of God—I tell of the thing just as I was conscious of it—as if His goodness and power were penetrating me altogether. The throb of emotion was so violent that I could barely tell the boys to pass on and not wait for me. I then sat down on a stone, unable to stand any longer, and my eyes overflowed with tears. I thanked God that in the course of my life He had taught me to know Him, that He sustained my life and took pity both on the insignificant creature and on the sinner that I was. I begged Him ardently that my life might be consecrated to the doing of His will. I felt His reply, which was that I should do His will from day to day, in humility and poverty, leaving Him, the Almighty God, to be judge of whether I should some time be called to bear witness more conspicuously. Then, slowly, the ecstasy left my heart ; that is, I felt that God had withdrawn the communion which He had granted, and I was able to walk on, but very slowly, so strongly was I still possessed by the emotion. Besides, I had wept uninterruptedly for several minutes, my eyes were swollen, and I did not wish my companions to see me. The state of ecstasy may have lasted four or five minutes, although it seemed at the time to last much longer. My comrades waited for me ten minutes at the cross of Bovine, but I took about twenty-five or thirty minutes to join them ; for, as well as I can remember, they said that I had kept them back for about half an hour. The impression had been so profound that in climbing slowly the slope, I asked myself if it were possible that Moses on Sinai could have had a more intimate communication with God. But the more I seek words to express this intimate inter-course, the more I feel the impossibility of describing the thing by any of our usual images. At bottom the expression most apt to render what I felt is this : God was present, though invisible ; He fell under no one of my senses, yet my consciousness perceived Him[1]."

No wonder that this exquisite experience aroused in M.E. thankfulness towards the Giver of it, and a wish to know what he could do in order to show himself deserving of the blessing. He " felt " that he " should do His (God's) Will from day to day." This thought, so obvious that it might have appeared in any mind with

[1] Th. Flournoy, *Observations de Psychologie Religieuse, Archives de Psychol. de la Suisse Romande*, vol. II, 1903, V, pp. 351-7 (abbreviated). The translation is by Wm. James in *The Varieties*, pp. 67-8.

similar religious preconceptions, is taken as God's reply. This is the only revelation conveyed in a conceptual form. No one would insist upon its evidential value. But, in the opinion of M.E., the power, the goodness, and probably other qualities of God, and ineffable aspects of the meaning of life, were also revealed; he " felt " them.

During a mountain journey, and apparently in the absence of any natural cause, whether physical or psychical, M.E., is suddenly thrown into a rapture, the basal features of which are quite similar to those of the ecstasy of the epileptic priest. Was it, perhaps, an epileptic attack ? We do not know, and it matters little to us whether it was or not. What matters in this connexion is the observation that the seizure had no conscious cause. It was not brought about by a train of thought and emotion ; it appears to have been caused altogether by organic processes.

In his second letter to the Corinthians, St Paul has recorded a wonderful experience. When he comes to the subject of "vision and revelations of the Lord," the great Apostle relates how fourteen years before—whether in the body or out of the body, he does not know—he was "caught up to the third heaven," and "heard unspeakable words which it is not possible for man to utter[1]." This experience possesses the essential traits of the preceding ecstasies suddenness, passivity, illumination, ineffability. Did St Paul, as some affirm, suffer from epileptic attacks ? Here again the answer matters little. That which interests us is that, as in the case of M.E. and of the epileptic auræ, there were no conscious antecedents which might be regarded as the cause of the event.

How is a person experiencing an adventure of this kind going to account for it ? That will depend upon his beliefs, his knowledge of physiology and of psychology, and upon attendant circumstances. If he knows that the experience is a prodromal stage of epilepsy, he will not be tempted to see in it the work of a divine Being. The great Apostle, just as M.E., regarded his rapture as a divine intervention. Ignorant as he was of modern science, a sharer in the beliefs current about him in divine and diabolical possession, and a passionate disciple of the Lord Jesus Christ, risen from the dead and seen on the way to Damascus, how could St Paul have interpreted the storm of feelings and emotions that suddenly assailed him, otherwise than as he did[2] ?

[1] 1. Chap. XII, 1-4.

[2] One may quite legitimately ask whether the interpretation of his rapture given by M.E., would not have undergone the same change as the initial interpretation given by Mlle Ve, if his opportunity for observation had been equal to hers.

The description of a curious trance with which John A. Symonds, the poet and essayist, was afflicted may be introduced here. It will show us how an experience similar to the foregoing may be differently interpreted by a person highly cultivated and free from the beliefs traditional in mystical circles.

" Suddenly," writes Symonds, " at church, or in company, or when I was reading, and always, I think, when my muscles were at rest, I felt the approach of the mood. Irresistibly it took possession of my mind and will, lasted what seemed an eternity, and disappeared in a series of rapid sensations which resembled the awakening from anæsthetic influence. One reason why I disliked this kind of trance was that I could not describe it to myself. I cannot even now find words to render it intelligible. It consisted in a gradual but swiftly progressive obliteration of space, time, sensation, and the multitudinous factors of experience which seem to qualify what we are pleased to call our Self. In proportion as these conditions of ordinary consciousness were subtracted, the sense of an underlying or essential consciousness acquired intensity. At last nothing remained but a pure, absolute, abstract Self. The universe became without form and void of content. But Self persisted, formidable in its vivid keenness, feeling the most poignant doubt about reality, ready, as it seems to find existence break as breaks a bubble round about it. And what then ? The apprehension of a coming dissolution, the grim conviction that this state was the last state of the conscious Self, the sense that I had followed the last thread of being to the verge of the abyss, and had arrived at the demonstration of eternal Maya or illusion, stirred or seemed to stir me up again. The return to ordinary conditions of sentient existence began by my first recovering the power of touch, and then the gradual though rapid influx of familiar impressions and diurnal interests. At last I felt myself once more a human being ; and though the riddle of what is meant by life remained unsolved, I was thankful for this return from the abyss—this deliverance from so awful an initiation into the mysteries of scepticism[1]."

[1] J. A. Symonds, *A Biography*, London, 1895, pp. 29-31, abridged, quoted by Wm. James in the *Varieties of Religious Experience*, p. 385.

It is not unusual for fear to be felt when trance approaches unconsciousness. A trance, similar to that of Symonds, occuring in four persons closely related by blood is reported by Sir Crichton-Browne in his *Cavendish Lecture* on " Dreamy Mental States." " The youth who gave the fullest account said that suddenly he lost his hold of the universe and ceased to know who he was. Everything seemed changed in a twinkling, and he lost his relations to time and space. He felt intense terror while the attack lasted, lest he should never become himself again . . . . He was never unconscious during attacks that lasted ten or twelve seconds at the most . . . . At one time he could bring them (these feelings) on by gazing intently at his own face in a looking

The child who playfully throws himself from a height into the extended arms of his father suffers a shudder of anxiety, followed by a delightful sense of utter safety when in the embrace of the fond father. So does at times the mystic when, as he thinks, he yields up his personality to the divine Father. St Theresa and others report an instant of terror and a tendency to stop themselves on the brink of the abyss, and then the peace and the delight of divine embrace. Symonds, who in this connexion thought neither of the Heavenly Father nor of Christ, felt only the dread of approaching dissolution. He, no more than religiously inclined persons, could resist the prompting to interpret the primary data of his consciousness. But as his preconceptions were different, so also was his interpretation. It seemed to him that, together with his self-consciousness, the Universe would come to an end ; that both himself and the world were mere illusions.

There is no evidence that the primary conscious facts in the experiences of M.E., of St Paul, and of Symonds differed in any essential way from those of the unusual epileptic auræ reported above. But *they were differently interpreted.* M.E. and St Paul regarded their ecstasy as the work of God. That interpretation transfigured the primary experience and made of it a religious ecstasy.

It is advisable to insist upon the effect of the interpretation put upon the primary data. However delightful in itself, the epileptic

---

glass or . . . . becoming ' abstract and metaphysical,' as he termed it . . . . As they wore off in adult life, the last vestiges of them were experienced while he was drowsy and just falling to sleep."—*Lancet*, June 6th, 1895.

Mary Reynolds, who exhibited two " personalities," experienced during the transition from one to the other, a fright which she describes by saying that it was " as if I were never to return into this world."—S. Weir Mitchell, *Mary Reynolds, a case of Double Consciousness,* Trans. of the College of Physicians, Phila., April 4th, 1888, as quoted by P. Janet, *Major Symptoms of Hysteria,* p. 76.

In his experimental investigation of the subconscious, Abramowski mentions, in connexion with the disappearance of memories as one goes to sleep, " a condition of disquiet, something like fear." Two of his subjects report fear under similar conditions. " I felt fear," says one of them, " I had a moment of anxiety so marked that I wanted to interrupt the experiment and go out."— E. Abramowski, *Le Subconscient Normal,* Paris, 1914, pp. 201, 330.

In one of our own experiments with ether, one of the subjects was aware of fear as consciousness was on the point of vanishing. It was soon replaced by peace and happiness.

Mlle Vé speaks of a resistance to the progress of trance as being customary with her and almost involuntary. In her case the surrender comes with " a voluptuous and deep enjoyment." She tells us that she has often " compared that struggle and that surrender to the passionate struggle of a woman who loves but contends and resists before surrendering."—Th. Flournoy, *Une Mystique Moderne,* pp. 81, 83, 100.

ecstasy can have, for those who know its relation to disease, only a depressing effect. What a sardonic mockery this introduction of an epileptic attack by a moment of delirious happiness ! But if, like St Paul, M.E., and others, one refers the experience to a loving, divine Agent, it is no longer merely delightful, it becomes " divine " : the rapture is enriched by all the values and the glory which, in the mind of the subject, belong to God. Something similar happens to the possessor of a beautiful flower when he learns that it comes from the beloved. It is no longer simply an admirable flower, it is a talisman that miraculously kindles the inner life of the lover.

If sudden inexpressible delights are taken as a sign of God's presence, one should not be surprised if feelings of an opposite quality are construed as a sign of his absence. We have in mind neither the periods of "dryness" of the Christian mystics, nor Bunyan's sense of unpardonable guilt, but a particularly instructive instance of a person of high culture and intellectual power interpreting distress arising from the digestive functions as the absence of God. The following entry is found, under date March the 31st, 1873, in the *Diary* of no less a man than the Genevese philosopher Amiel[1].

" For an hour past I have been the prey of a vague anxiety ; I recognize my old enemy. . . . It is a sense of void and anguish, a sense of something lacking. What ? Love, peace—God perhaps. The feeling is one of pure want unmixed with hope, and there is anguish in it because I can clearly distinguish neither the evil nor the remedy. Of all hours of the day, in fine weather, the afternoon about three o'clock, is the time which to me is most difficult to bear, I never feel more strongly than I do then ' le vide effrayant de la vie '."

Now, physiologists say that the middle hours of the afternoon are hours of low vitality. And, as we might expect, dyspeptic persons—Amiel was one of them—suffer most during that period of the day.

That a man of the mental acuity of Amiel should have been ready to see in these feelings of want and anxiety the absence of God, may induce the reader to tolerate the surmise that Tennyson (a mystic), after eating a certain mutton chop, might have rhapsodized about a divine visitation had he not known that he had eaten the chop. Here is the incident as related by the poet himself. After having been for ten weeks the guest of a vegetarian friend, Tennyson complained that his blood had lost its warmth. Subsequently, probably as soon as he was delivered from his friend, he ate a mutton chop. He said of that feast, that it was " one of the most wonderful " experiences he had ever had. " I shall never forget the sensation.

[1] Amiel's *Journal* was put into English by Mrs. Humphrey Ward.

I never felt such joy in my blood[1]." Our surmise is that, had the poet been ignorant of its cause, he would have classed this surpassingly delightful and vitalizing experience with his religious, mystical illuminations. The high probability of this supposition will appear more fully presently, when we look into his mystical experiences.

*   *   *

Were one to judge by the instances I have given, one might think that the prodromal stage of epilepsy is always an ecstasy; and yet that is but seldom the case. The auræ may consist of the most varied experiences. There are instances when the aura is terrifying; the face of the subject expresses the most horrible fear. I chose only ecstatic cases because they are the only ones that interest us. It should be known, further, that a sense of joy and of abundant life is present in morbid conditions other than epilepsy[2]. In a phase of general progressive paralysis, the poor patient, reduced to a bestial condition, beams his enjoyment as he endeavours to answer one's questions about his health.

The same remark may be made with reference to the other psychical storms we have described. All those given here are rapturous in quality; yet there exist varieties with very different affective tones. There are, for instance, pathological fits of anxiety, of fear, of anger. These appear either in the complete absence of psychical cause, or at the slightest provocation. Everyone knows persons constitutionally disposed to wrathfulness and also their opposites, the ever placid and sweet. Pathological anxiety is not uncommon; here is an instance of it. A woman of forty-six years suffered at times from " a feeling of extreme nervousness and agitation, great restless anxiety, with a sense of uncontrollable dread of some unknown impending terror. Physically, the attack was characterized by violent trembling of the whole body, hurried breathing, irregular heart's action, and profuse cold sweating[3]." In his Study of Anger, Stanley Hall reports several instances of abnormal rage, in particular the case of a girl who had, about once a month, violent fits of rage[4].

*   *   *

[1] *The Works of Tennyson*, ed. by Hallam, Lord Tennyson, London, 1908, vol. 6th, p. 394.

[2] See, for instances of a state of pleasure in disease, Dr M. Mignard, *La Joie Passive, Jr. de Psychol. Normale et Pathologique*, vol. VI, 1909, pp. 97-123.

[3] "The Pathology of Morbid Anxiety," Ernest Jones, *Jr. of Abnormal Psychol.*, vol. VI, 1911-2, p. 102.

[4] *Amer. Jr. of Psychol.*, vol. X, 1898-9, p. 541.

In *A Study of Fears*, by the same author, are to be found striking instances of sudden, abnormal fears. *Ibid.*, vol. VIII.

Janet reports a good instance of recurrent violent anger in *Médications Psychologiques*, vol. II, p. 149.

The facts related in the present chapter warrant the following conclusions :—

(1) Whether they belong to the religious life or not, these raptures, or psychical storms, break out suddenly and overcome the subject. He feels as if in the hands of an external power, and he interprets what happens to him, in accordance with the custom of the time and his own private knowledge. These wonderful experiences include indescribable impressions, designated by the term illumination or revelation. Their traits—suddenness, unexpectedness, passivity, illumination, ineffability—therefore, are not characteristic of religious life alone.

(2) In many cases these psychical storms have no conscious cause. Neither perception, nor idea, nor emotion brings them about. They break out suddenly, as of themselves. In other instances, a beautiful landscape, the idea of a speech, music, etc., are the occasions of the discharge. I say the occasions, because there is evidently no exact correspondence between the conscious antecedents of the storm and the intensity and the quality of the rapture. We must, therefore, conclude that these phenomena have unconscious causes which may be sufficient in themselves or which may need supplementing. The facts seem to warrant the further conclusion that the unconscious causes are organic[1].

Not only rapture, but every phenomena of an emotional nature may be included in this last generalization. To say that our emotions are not entirely determined, either in their quality or in their intensity, by the facts which are commonly said to be their causes, is to utter a truism. The same so-called causes produce in the same person, in different circumstances, enormously different effects. I need only recall the domestic scenes with which too many families are acquainted. The assigned causes of these scenes, as a matter of fact, usually are merely insignificant occasions for the outbreak. Paris seen from the Trocadero, a sunny, peaceful landscape, a concert, an imaginary discourse, played, in the instances reviewed above, the rôle of the spark that ignites the powder. Pent-up nervous energy seemed merely to be waiting for a last addition, in itself unimportant, before setting into motion a complex series of physiological processes : trembling, lowering of the temperature, weeping, etc., and states of consciousness remarkable by their

---

[1] Referring to the mystical trances of Mlle Vé, soon to be considered, Flournoy writes, " On the whole, the divine experience of Mlle Vé may be compared to a periodic nervous storm, which each time gathers strength slowly, then breaks out suddenly, and disappears leaving behind more or less intense moral effects."—*Archives de Psychol. de la Suisse Romande*, vol. XV, 1915, p. 176.

intensity and quality. In the epileptic aura not even a spark from the outside is necessary: the discharge is altogether spontaneous.

(3) A third and last conclusion from our analyses refers to the extensive and profound transformation suffered by the primary phenomenon when it is interpreted and elaborated under the influence of desires and beliefs. In the instance of M.E., consciousness had no share in the production of the primary, the immediate, experience; Christian beliefs intervened only after its appearance. But they transfigured it by putting into it a divine meaning. In this ethically-minded person, the rapture became a powerful source of moral energy.

Some reference to the functioning of the nervous system in epilepsy may give some definiteness to our conception of the mechanism underlying psychic storms, of which epilepsy and ecstatic raptures are varieties.

In so far as we are concerned in the phenomenon, the essential fact in epilepsy is a sudden discharge of nervous energy, with a great variety in the routes followed by the liberated energy. The cause (or causes) of the disease does not interest us beyond the knowledge that it is purely organic. The almost endlessly varied forms assumed by psychic storms are due to differences in the distribution of the nervous energy. In *Grand Mal*, it is intense and general. The marked motor disturbances and the loss of consciousness indicate that the discharge has invaded the motor area as well as other portions of the brain. In " psychic epilepsy," on the contrary, only those parts of the nervous system correlated with sensory and ideational functions are affected ; consequently the symptoms are chiefly sensory. The type of hallucination will be visual, or auditory, or otherwise, according to whether the discharge affects the visual, the auditory, or other sensory regions of the brain. When tender or voluptuous emotions are produced, we must conclude that the nervous discharge has reached those parts of the nervous system, and perhaps those organs that are connected with these emotions. We may think of the degree of mental confusion and of unconsciousness as depending mainly upon the extension and the intensity of the discharge into the so-called association areas.

*   *   *

II. Ecstasies Connected with the Solution of Moral Conflicts.

In the preceding instances, ecstasy, whether religious or not, appeared or seemed to appear quite independently of any previous mental activity of the subject. Not only was it sudden and unexpected, but there was no obvious evidence that any antecedent desire or train of thought had prepared it. We came to the conclusion that organic causes could of themselves determine mystical raptures.

It would, however, be a gross error to think that the subject's desire and his mental activity in general never count for anything in the production of these remarkable phenomena. The previously considered ecstasies of the Christian mystics, although in a sense unexpected, were in most cases not only desired but prepared-for, often, by a systematic procedure.

The first two of the following instances (Mrs Pa. and Mme D.) do not involve a complete ecstatic trance. They are nevertheless placed here because they yield an impression of illumination or revelation, which is, as we have learned, a characteristic trait of mystical ecstasy.

Mrs P.—" I had gone on a visit to my brother after my husband's death, because I could not settle down or care to take up my life again on account of its utter absence of interest and the futility of all things. One morning I woke and lay watching the trees waving about outside my window, remembering a book by Henry Drummond I had read years before, but of which the only thing I seemed to remember was the part that speaks of God's life being in the trees. Suddenly (and I have always wondered why it had not occurred to me before) the thought came : but, then, the same life must be in the animals and also in man ; and, since man is recognized as being eternal, why, then, he must be part of God Himself. Then the realization came that there is only one Life anywhere, that there is only one God everywhere, in whom all, *as a matter of fact,* ' live and move and have their being,' out of whom even what we call evil must in some wonderful way have come as well as what we call good. Then, the feeling of exultation that nothing could hurt me, ever any more, not even death itself, for if in me is God's life, death has no power over it. . . . If I am of God and He in me, even so must He be in the body of every mortal man without distinction. So we are all ' sons and daughters of the Lord Almighty ' and all brothers and sisters in actual truth. The world suddenly seemed like one big family, taking away somewhat one's loneliness.

"Now, all this may not seem much to you, *but to me this realization was such a wonderful thing that for days I went in awe of the knowledge, wondering if the clergy whom I met knew about these things and, if so, why they did not tell the people*[1]."

The appearance in Mrs Pa's mind of the ideas expressed in this letter need not surprise us ; but we may well wonder at their effect. Hundreds of times those or similar ideas have passed through the minds of other persons to be dismissed speedily as inadequate or to remain without making any deep impression. The magnitude of the effect they produced in this instance must have been due to the psycho-physiological condition of Mrs Pa. She had moved from the United States, where she had lived with her husband, to new surroundings in Australia. Here she found kind people and new interests. She was still young ; life, love,—the libido, the Freudians would say,—could not be kept down endlessly by sorrow. One morning she awoke, rested and peaceful. The trees were gently swaying in the sunlight. A vague thought from Henry Drummond,

[1] From a letter written to the author in 1914.

that persuasive propagandist of the God of Love, flitted into her mind, and the world was transformed!

There are reasons in the circumstances recited above for thinking that Mrs Pa. was on the verge of one of those organically caused feeling-storms described in preceding pages and that the recall of Drummond's idea about God's life being in the trees acted as the additional charge needed to produce the spark.

But why did the elation continue far beyond the ordinary duration of an organic brain-storm? Let it be said first that it would be a mistake to suppose that its intensity was sustained without diminution beyond a brief space of time. Soon Mrs Pa. found a relatively stable level, considerably above her preceding condition it is true, but still far below that of the ecstatic crisis. The problem is therefore the persistency of this diminished state of heightened optimism and efficiency. Its solution is to be found, I think, in the following considerations :—(1) Time brought assuagement to her grief. (2) The absence of concentration of her potential affection upon one individual and the absence of sex gratification favoured the irradiation or sublimation of an apparently strong love-disposition. (3) The idea of a pantheistic God of love put into her head by Drummond, was just the kind of idea which her affective and intellectual equipment prepared her to accept. In a frigid and less intelligent person, the impression produced by that conception would have been probably less intense and more evanescent.

Madame D.—For many years Madame D., a woman of average education, mother of several children, had struggled with the problem of evil in the form which it assumes for those who believe in a God both omnipotent and benevolent. When, to her observations of the moral indifference of nature and the unspeakable cruelty of men, were added terrible events in her own family, her religious faith in the omnipotent Providence met shipwreck. She realized that an omnipotent God who should consent to what happens in the world would be a monster. But she had formed with the Christian God too many bonds, of too long duration, to be able easily to give him up. For years she wrestled with the dilemma : either a monster-God or no God at all. Neither horn of that dilemma was acceptable to her. Then, suddenly, came another solution. "In a struggle more violent and overwhelming than the others," she saw that she must give up the idea of a God-Providence. At the same time (I quote) "there came into my mind as clear as day the idea that the contradiction between an all-good, all-powerful God and that which happens in the world is simply due to the fact that God is absent from the world." He is really the great Creator and the loving Father of humanity; it is He who has given us all the good things we enjoy; but He is not responsible for what now happens in the world, for He has withdrawn from it. "God absent from the world. What an enlightening and helpful explanation! It was on a Thursday between four and five o'clock in the afternoon (she names the street and the exact spot on the sidewalk) when I was coming home from a visit to my friends X, that this light came to me suddenly out of my darkened sky. O God, how happy I was to find you in heaven after I had lost you on earth! I thank you, O God, You are not in the world, but you live. I pray to you because you perhaps hear me, and because, when the ocean separates a mother from her child, he can still think of her with love and gratitude and mentally confide to her his joy and griefs[1]."

The pantheistic illumination that restored Mrs Pa. to hope and happiness after the loss of her husband, offers some instructive points of similarity to the theological illumination of Mme D. Their problems, seen at the root, are the same even though they assume different forms. Both seek the removal of inhibitions and contradictions and thus, a release of pent-up energies. Mme D. is enmeshed in a dilemma involving her peace of mind and her moral welfare. Mrs. Pa's tragedy is the too common one of the loss of a loved husband about whom the whole life of the wife is centred. There was in both a long period of misery and a threat of moral shipwreck. To both salvation came suddenly. Mme D. was saved as she became convinced that the living God in whom she believed is absent from the world; Mrs Pa, as she realized God's presence everywhere and in everything. Carlyle, whose case follows in small print, found salvation in a still different idea. It is evident that one must look elsewhere than in these conceptions themselves for an explanation of what is effected in these persons.

The adolescent crisis of CARLYLE, related in sledge-hammer words in *Sartor Resartus*, bears some resemblance to the preceding instances :—" Full of such humour, and perhaps the miserablest man in the whole French Capital or Suburbs, was I, one sultry Dog-day, after much perambulation, toiling among the dirty little Rue Saint-Thomas de l'Enfer, among civic rubbish enough, in a close atmosphere, and over pavements hot as Nebuchadnezzar's furnace; when, all at once, there rose a Thought in me, and I asked myself : ' What art thou afraid of ? Wherefore, like a coward, dost thou forever pip and whimper, and go cowering and trembling ? Despicable biped! What is the sum-total of the worst that lies before thee ? Death ? Well, Death; and say the pangs of Tophet too, and all that the Devil and Man may, will, and can do against thee ? Hast thou not a heart; canst thou not suffer whatsoever it be; and, as a Child of Freedom, though outcast, trample Tophet itself under thy feet, while it consumes thee ? Let it come, then ; I will meet and defy it ! ' And as I thought, there rushed like a stream of fire over my whole soul ; and I shook

[1] Théodore Flournoy, *Observations de Psychologie Religieuse, Archiv. de Psychol. de la Suisse Romande*, vol. II (1903), pp. 342-7, abbreviated.

base Fear away from me forever. I was strong, of unknown strength; a spirit, almost a god. Ever from that time the temper of my misery was changed: not Fear or whining Sorrow was it, but Indignation and grim fire-eyed Defiance.

"Thus has the Everlasting No pealed authoritatively through all the recesses of my Being, of my Me; and then was it that my whole Me stood up, in native God-created majesty, and with emphasis recorded its Protest. Such a Protest, the most important transaction in Life, may that same Indignation and Defiance, in a psychological point of view, be fittedly called. The Everlasting No had said: ' Behold, thou art fatherless, outcast, and the Universe is mine (The Devil's); to which my whole Me now made answer: ' I am not thine, but free, and for ever hate thee!'

"It is from this hour that I incline to date my Spiritual New-birth, or Baphometic Fire-baptism; perhaps I directly thereupon began to be a Man."
—*Sartor Resartus*, Book II, Chapter VII.

We add two interesting instances. The first, drawn from a novel, may represent faithfully an actual experience of the author. As to Rousseau's ecstasy, it is said that he has greatly exaggerated its remarkable features.

GEORGE MOORE.—During the Boer War George Moore was conversing with friends about the chances the Boers had of winning the war. The discussion ended with the statement that even if they should win now, it would be the same in the end; the war would merely be prolonged. This idea shocked George Moore, a pro-Boer. At night his thoughts returned to the same topic. I quote: " I was lifted suddenly out of my ordinary senses. The walls about me seemed to recede, and myself to be transported ineffably above a dim plain rolling on and on till it mingled with the sky. An encampment was there in an hallowed light, and one face, stern and strong, yet gentle, was taken by me for the face of the Eternal God upreared after combat with the Eternal Evil. What I saw was a symbol of a guiding Providence in the World. ' There is one, there is one!' I exclaimed, ' It is about me and in me.' And all night long I heard as the deaf hear, and answered as the dumb answer. A night of fierce exultations and prolonged joys murmuring through the darkness like a river. ' For how can it be otherwise?' I cried, starting up in bed. ' Yet I believed this many a year that all was blind chance!' And I fell back and lay like one consumed by a secret fire. Life seemed to have no more for giving and I cried out: ' It is terrible to feel things so violently,' and on these words, or soon after, I must have dropped away into sleep."—*Hail and Farewell*—Salve, New York, 1912, p. 169.

We note in this instance that, after a profoundly moving discussion, George Moore, while in bed, conscious neither of the outer world nor of his own body, found himself occupied with the recent discussion. There seems to be sufficient evidence to class this experience with hypnagogic dreams. There came to the dreamer the sense of a great Presence who typified for him the Eternal Good and the triumph of the just cause. This presence was felt with absolute certitude and stirred in him indescribable emotions, just as in Miss X, Mlle Vé, and a host of other mystics. His anxious doubt dissolved; the solution of the Boer problem came to him: the cause of the oppressed race would ultimately triumph, for a just Providence rules over the world.

ROUSSEAU rose to fame as the author of a prize-essay upon a question proposed by the Academy of Dijon. An interesting rapture is connected with that question. It happened as he was going to see Diderot, then a prisoner at Vincennes. " I had in my pocket," writes Rousseau, " a copy of the *Mercure de France* which I was looking over as I was walking. I noticed the question of the Academy of Dijon which was the occasion of my first writing. If ever a thing resembled sudden inspiration, it was what happened in me at the reading of that notice: suddenly my mind was dazzled by a. thousand lights; a crowd of ideas presented themselves at once, with a power and in a disorder which plunged me in an inexpressible confusion; I felt a dizziness similar to intoxication. Violent palpitations shook my breast . . . . I let myself drop under a tree and spent there a half hour in such a frenzy of emotion that only on rising did I notice that my coat was wet with the tears I had shed."—From a letter of J. J. Rousseau, written January 12th, 1762, to M. de Malesherbes. *Oeuvres Complètes de J. J. Rousseau*, Paris, 1886, vol. 10, p. 301. The incident itself took place in 1749.

Extraordinary as was the event, Rousseau did not regard it as due to a superhuman cause. He was not in the habit of seeing God's action in human affairs, and probably assumed his own competency in the sphere to which these ideas belonged.

There is considerable analogy between the situation of Rousseau as he foresees himself winning the Dijon prize, and that of poor Jean imagining himself pronouncing a magnificent speech in the Chamber of Deputies. Rousseau, however, unlike Jean, had pondered long over social problems, and had discussed them ardently with his friends. We may suppose that, as the question awakened a swarm of ideas and fired his ambition, he saw himself acclaimed throughout Europe as the winner of the competition. In both cases ecstasy was conditioned, on the one hand, by the presence of physiological factors favourable to the production of a violent nervous discharge ; and, on the other, by ideas calculated to arouse powerful emotional tendencies centering about the idea of the self. The store of nervous energy was drained into the channels indicated by the rational mental activity.

In *First and Last Things*, London, Constable, 1908, p. 60, H. G. Wells speaks of moments of communion with himself and with something greater than himself as " the supreme fact " of his religious life.—Quoted by Pratt, *loc. cit.*, p. 343.

The instances of Mrs Pa. and of Mme D. recall such famous records as that of the Great Enlightenment of the Buddha Gautama under the Bow tree. Is that experience—supposing it to have taken place—susceptible of the same explanation as the preceding ? And what shall that explanation be ? We cannot agree with Mrs Pa. and Mme D. in regarding their saving illuminations as the logical, rational consequence of the ideas which unexpectedly appeared to them. That is not a sufficient explanation. We are rather inclined to see in these cases something similar to that which happened to M.E. and to the person viewing Paris from the Trocadero, namely, the action of non-rational factors interpreted in a specific way.

The present instances are complicated by the realization on the part of the subjects of a problem to be solved and by their general effort to find a solution. We may perhaps suppose that dissatisfaction and vague strivings result in, or contribute to, an accumulation of energy which at the proper moment is set off by a minimal stimulus (the ideas mentioned) which produces a condition better adapted to the situation of the individual. The quality of the changes which take place on the occasion of the saving ideas would thus be in a degree dependent upon the strivings—vague as they are—that have preceded the change.

The cases of Miss X. and of Mlle Vé will provide further opportunities for considering the rôle of desire in the production of moral transformations.

We might, of course, in order to cover our ignorance, juggle with words brought into vogue by the Freudian psychology. Those imbued with the theories of the Austrian physician will hold that in these and in similar cases a mental activity had taken place of which the subject was not aware and that the crises we have related represent the irruption into consciousness of that subconscious mentation. It may be so. But, for our part, if we do not doubt the possible continuation of *nervous* activity when consciousness ceases, we have not been able to convince ourselves of the existence of a consciousness of which the subject was not at the time aware.

In any case we are limited to the existing documents. These persons are available neither for psychoanalysis nor for the application of the methods of research used by Morton Prince in his attempt to prove the reality of coconsciousness[1]. Under these circumstances, we have deliberately resisted the recent fashion to scatter profusely through the discussion of mystical phenomena terms referring to the mysterious activity of a coconsciousness or sub-consciousness. An appeal to a subconsciousness, the detailed operations of which cannot be ascertained, would be as futile and unscientific as an explanation of any phenomenon by reference to " God." The foregoing remarks apply, of course, not merely to the immediately preceding instances of illumination, but to almost all the facts considered in this book.

* * *

Among the more striking raptures coming together with, or following upon, the solution of practical moral problems, are those connected with Christian conversion. These sudden alterations of belief and behaviour are so fascinating to the psychologist that, if space permitted, we would introduce here several instances. The following one cannot be regarded as entirely typical of Christian conversion, but it is well adapted to our purpose.

Miss X., professor of a branch of natural science at an American College :—This is a pathetic chapter in the life of a lone woman. Her experience reaches far beyond our present topic, and we shall, therefore, have to pass over without comment several features of deep interest, in particular the devastating workings of primary, instinctive forces of which social life, as it existed for her, did not permit the natural expression, and also the demonstration which her case provides of the possibility for some people—one must insist upon the " some "—of using effectively the conception of a loving God in the absence of a rational conviction of his existence, yes, *in spite* of the recognition that all our knowledge opposes that belief.

[1] *Coconscious Images, Jr. of Abnormal Psychol.* 1917.
    An Experimental Study of the Mechanism of Hallucinations, British Jr. of Psychol., Medical Section, vol. II, 1922, pp. 165-208.

Miss X. soon lost her early faith in God. I quote[1]: "I came to believe that what men call God is the impersonal first cause of the universe. This state of mind lasted for about fifteen years, during which I went through various experiences of sickness and loss of friends without feeling in the least the need of belief in a personal God. It culminated in a physical breakdown and a moral crisis in which I first lived a life of deception, and then by reason of some tendency still utterly inexplicable to me, found myself obliged to fight and conquer the temptation. It is impossible to state too strongly my feeling of being the creature of an outside force both in the yielding and the conquering. It seems as if my own consciousness were literally only a spectator, while some deeper race or instinctive self held the stage.

"Then one day I found myself holding as the very centre of my life an ideal which suddenly appeared to be monstrous, to be filled with tendencies to wrong action. I realized that I was in truth little better than when I had yielded, since I lived in thought the same life of deception and continued to set before myself an ideal unattainable by any honourable means. I saw clearly enough that I should have to give up that ideal or become openly bad, and while I shrank with horror from the sin that lay open to me on one side, I shrank almost equally from the nothingness awaiting me if I uprooted the ideal. What a shrivelled, repressed nonentity my personality would become!

"Two factors especially contributed to my despair. The first was the feeling of my own insignificance or uselessness in the world of people, and the second was the paralysis of much of my emotional and intellectual self which followed upon the removal of my old ideal. My thoughts and feelings were constantly turning towards and groping for this loved and customary object. When they did close upon it, shame and remorse followed; but when they found only nothingness, the sense of being baffled, of stepping off into the darkness, was indescribably painful.

"During this time, my attention was called to the possibility of a new sort of belief in God. I felt that if I had belief in a personal God, it would serve as the focus for my thoughts, and would also remove the feeling of my worthlessness; but it seemed to me utterly futile to attempt to demonstrate the objective existence of such a God. No philosophy had ever proved more than the existence of a first cause, and science was emphasizing at every point that this cause was impersonal."

[1] Amy E. Tanner, *An Illustration of the Psychology of Belief*, Psychol. Bull., vol. IV, 1907, pp. 33-6, abbreviated.

She reflects, however, that, " if living demands the assumption of a personal God, then it is reasonable to make that assumption; but does it demand it ? Here I remained for some time, I questioned whether I could not in time conquer this desire as I had others, but I found myself standing on the brink of the abyss again and again, and I became so harrassed and at last so afraid that I was forced to admit that I could see no way of relief unless there were a Something to help me.

" But then came the question of whether I could use the concept of a personal God without belief in its objective existence. Could I try it as a mere working hypothesis and expect to get any valuable results ? If one can get strength and comfort from talking to God as if He exists, it makes no practical difference even if the sense of His love and help is an illusion created by one's own mind. It seems almost ludicrously self-evident that in either case one will not lose practically though one may be wrong theoretically.

" Therefore I deliberately set to work to reacquire the sense of God's presence which I had not had for nearly twenty years. I reinforced my reason by reiterating my reasons for assuming such a personality, and I prayed constantly after the fashion of the old sceptic : ' O God, if there is a God, save my soul, if I have a soul.'

" Then one night, after a week of this sort of thing, the old sense of God's presence came upon me with overpowering fullness. I cannot express the sense of personal intimacy, understanding, and sympathy that it gave to me. I felt the thing—whatever it was— so close to me, so a part of me, that words and even thoughts were unnecessary, that my part was only to sink back into His personality —if such it were—and drop all worries and temptations, all the straining and striving that had been so prominent in my life for years and years. Then, as I felt consolation and strength pouring in upon me, there came a great upwelling of love and gratitude towards their source, even though I was all the time conscious that that source might not be either personal or objective. It felt personal, I said to myself, and no harm would be done by acting as if it were so.

" This experience lasted for two days in nearly its original strength. Every time that attention relaxed from my tasks, the presence was there, and it was the last at night and the first in the morning in my consciousness. Gradually it became less vivid, but at times it still recurs with its original force.

" On the practical side its value up to now—after a period of three months—has been permanent. I find my thoughts falling back upon the idea of this presence as soon as I get into any sort of trouble or perplexity, and the invariable effect is to calm me and to enable me

15

to take a wider outlook. I am so curiously conscious of it as a person that I find myself checking certain thoughts and acts, just as I would check words if some one else were here, and I break out into conversation with it in the same incidental fashion as I do with a friend who happens to sit in the room where I am working.

" So far as the theoretical question is concerned, I cannot say that I am any nearer a solution than before, nor do I see any possibility of a solution. But I care less and less whether He exists outside of my own consciousness or not."

We have happened here upon a question that lies outside our immediate concern. We will, nevertheless, permit ourselves the remarks that it looms up omniously to-day in the Christian Church and that no religion asking of its votaries a *tour de force* such as is performed by Miss X., can possibly endure.

In this instance, as in ordinary Christian mystical experiences, the revelation took the form of an impression of God's presence—a presence as definite and convincing as sight or touch could make it. By that presence, the problem of Miss X. was solved: she had acquired the loving, guiding, all-sufficient friend she needed.

Let us observe, before passing on to what is probably the most remarkable of our cases, that Miss X. felt the impression of passivity, of being " the creature of an outside force," not only in connexion with the conquering forces but also with the others, the " yielding to temptation." This important observation, verifiable by everyone in his own life, should be remembered in the discussion of the psychology of passivity.

Mlle Vé, a Modern Mystic.—There exists probably no single account of mystical experience equal in scientific value to the diary published by Professor Flournoy of Geneva, under the title *Une Mystique Moderne*[1]. It owes its distinction to a rare introspective gift, a scientific curiosity, and a relative independence of traditional interpretation quite unusual among mystics. If it be added that Professor Flournoy has supplied explanatory notes and a penetrating critical discussion of many of the important questions raised by the document, the importance of this contribution to the literature of mysticism will be manifest.

[1] Th. Flournoy, *Une Mystique Moderne, Archives de Psychol. de la Suisse Romande*, Tome XV, 1915, pp. 1-224. In the quotations the italics are Mlle Vé's. See also H. Delacroix's comments, *loc. cit.*, pp. 338, ff.

In the section on the Sex-impulse we have already made use of certain aspects of Mlle Vé's diary. They will be merely referred to in the present connexion. The following pages dealing with Mlle Vé have already been published, almost as they stand here, in the *Jr. of Abnormal Psychology*, vol. XV, 1920, pp. 209-23.

We do not hesitate to set forth at some length information contained in this diary, for it is upon a full knowledge of the facts that a scientific understanding of mysticism, as of any other topic, depends. It is placed here, last in order, mainly for the reason that it brings up again, and in a particularly illuminating way, the central problems of mysticism that are to be discussed in subsequent chapters: the conviction of divine Presence and of illumination, and the nature of the mystical trance itself.

Mlle Vé is an unmarried woman of good education. In spite of a strong tendency to mental dissociation, her health is robust. She was brought up in a somewhat severe Protestant atmosphere. For a few years French governess in foreign countries, she became later head of a religious educational institution in her native land.

The salient facts of Mlle Vé's life, in so far as they bear upon our investigation, are the following:

1. A tenacious clinging to a high moral ideal and a persistent effort to realize it.

2. A dastardly assault of which she was the victim at the age of seventeen and a half, when yet ignorant of the sex-relation.

3. A conviction of unspeakable guilt, which for long years she thought attached to herself because of her misfortune.

4. The appearance, soon after her forcible initiation to sex-knowledge, of periods during which she was the shamed puppet of sex-desires. These periods, more and more sharply separated from the rest of her life, approached the appearance of a secondary personality. During these attacks, lasting several days and at times over a week, she retained sufficient control of herself to involve in them no one but herself, and to conceal them from everyone, even though alterations of her physiognomy and of the tone of her voice attracted the attention of her friends.

5. An intense need, always seeking and never obtaining satisfaction, for an intimate companionship of soul and body.

In 1910, at the age of forty-seven, she appealed to Professor Flournoy in the hope that hypnotic suggestion might become the means of her deliverance from sex-attacks that had recently become surpassingly distressing, and might also help her to break a morally dangerous friendship with a married man—a relation honourably begun, but in which her heart and her senses had become so far engaged that she felt herself powerless to resist longer. The writing-up of a detailed account of her experiences was suggested to her by Flournoy, in part as a means of exorcism.

In the Fall of 1912, as she was carrying out with success but not without struggle and a sense of desolation her resolve not to see M.Y.

any more, there came to her at night, before she fell asleep, a friendly presence. She calls it the Friend[1]. His approach was not made known to her through the senses. She felt him somewhere in space and yet within herself. She talked to him more than he to her. The Presence was soothing, purifying, and made no appeal whatsoever to sex; for the Friend, though "virile," was neither male nor female. Mlle Vé knows too much and is too keen an observer to mistake this creation of her heart's desire for an objective reality. She says, " I wish I was not so sure that he is merely a split in my personality, so that I might take it more seriously; but I see the ropes too clearly."

In March, 1913, something new and of much greater importance takes place for the first time. We shall call it the great Experience, or simply, the Experience with a capital " E." During the visits of the Friend she had remained self-conscious, but on this occasion her body became partly anæsthetic, and, later, all consciousness disappeared. On returning to herself, she was conscious of having been visited by a Presence other than the Friend. This trance, identical in essential particulars with that of the Christian mystics, was reproduced thirty-one times at irregular intervals between March 1st, 1913, and July 30th, 1914.

The Experience was for a while placed beyond possibility of critical examination by its amazing strangeness and overpowering violence. But soon Mlle Vé realized that the power was impersonal, whereas what she needed was the Christian God of Love. Later, a connexion between the Experience and sex was forced upon her unwilling attention. From that moment the charm was broken and a resistance, almost entirely involuntary, assisted very probably by certain external events, brought the Experience to an end.

Whoever considers carefully Mlle Vé's introspective account may convince himself that the Friend is a creation of auto-suggestion. She herself is aware of this. She saw the " ropes," to repeat her expression. We are all familiar with phenomena of the same type. Is it not something similar that happens to children when they play with imaginary persons; to the adult when he lives over again in imagination happy moments spent with a loved friend; to the bereaved mother who, in the obsession of sorrow, feels and hears the departed child? Mlle Vé was struggling against a passion that had marred a beautiful friendship. The dear friend had to be given up. But she continued to yearn with the energy of a famished soul for

[1] In the elaboration of the Friend the thought of her father, for whom she had a profound admiration and affection, played an interesting part. The Friend appeared usually in the early stage of sleep, as she hovered between self-consciousness and sleep.

the companionship of a worthy and tender friend. If dreams may be regarded as creations of desire, the apparition to Mlle Vé, between sleep and waking, of an ideal friend is sufficiently accounted for.

Her great Experience is, in some of its aspects, the product of desires ; and, in others, of organic factors operating independently of consciousness. The probable causes that brought the Experience to an end (the discovery of the impersonal nature of the Power and of its connexion with her sexual life had greatly disappointed her) indicate clearly enough the presence of conscious factors. These observations coincided with a decrease in the frequency of the Experience. When the Great War broke out, it stopped altogether. The war began early in August, and her last Experience took place on the 30th of the preceding July. Taking all the circumstances into consideration, there seems to be here more than a coincidence. Shall we not say that the tragic events that were riveting the anxious attention of the whole world liberated her from constant thought of her little, suffering self and canalized her energies into new paths ? Moralists and physicians tell of profound transformations due to the pressure of dramatic events far inferior to the Great War in their power to arrest the attention.

*   *   *

The three interrelated problems to which the diary of Mlle Vé calls our attention are these :—

Why does she regard her Experience as a manifestation of an impersonal, superhuman power ? Why does she insist upon the divineness of that power ? Why does she claim absolute certitude regarding her " revelation " ?

The mystics have always claimed a noetic value for their experiences. " It is," they have said, " a revelation " ; and, they have added, " its certainty is unassailable because it is not a deduction nor a generalization from facts ; it is itself a datum, an immediate experience." In this they have had at all times the support of a number of philosophers. Their case has recently been stated by William James in words that have gained popular success: " Mystical states usually are, and have a right to be, absolutely authoritative over the individuals to whom they come. . . . They break down the authority of the non-mystical or rationalistic consciousness, based upon the understanding and the senses alone. They open out the possibility of other orders of truth[1]."

In order to ascertain how far the experiences of Mlle Vé countenances this widespread opinion, we must transcribe with some

[1] *The Varieties of Religious Experience*, pp. 422-3, abbreviated.

fulness her account of the first one. It began with the sense of the presence of the Friend, a presence of which she had been deprived for some time. On the 1st of March, 1913, she had just gone to bed when, not feeling inclined to sleep, she wished the Friendly Presence would manifest itself. " I concentrated my thoughts and my will upon that object, remaining motionless, the eyes closed, and trying with all my might to avoid distraction. A fairly long time passed. I was beginning to find the effort very exhausting and I was on the point of giving up, when I felt a shiver and languor. I could no longer move, nor could I will with any definiteness and energy. (She compares this paralysis and sense of well-being to what she once experienced after taking morphine.) But my thoughts remained active and even very lively in the circle in which I was interested— I felt the Friend coming from the door to my bed. When I felt him there, and could commune with him, it seemed to me that I was but a soul without body—I had the impression that my spiritual being was free from the bonds that connected it with matter and that it had entered another world. I did not hear a dialogue nor a mono- logue, but I had the feeling of a kind of *liberation* because *he* had come, and I was no longer aware of my limited self, circumscribed by matter. I was passively conscious of *another essential and immutable reality*. The words of St Paul came to my mind, ' I was caught up to the third heaven, whether in the body or out of it, I cannot tell. God knows.' I saw nothing, heard nothing ; I was neither asleep nor in a swoon, and yet I was *elsewhere*, I was *changed*. [According to her own account she lost, at this point, entirely consciousness.] When I regained possession of my ordinary self, I felt very weak, as when upset by a very strong emotion, and found it very difficult to realize and to formulate what had happened. I got hold of it only by the impression that remained, a sort of *absolute assurance of the reality of the Divine*.

" It seems to me that to-day [the day after the experience] it is easy to endure life with fortitude because I have realized as never before that this life is not all, that it is but a part of the final reality."

Three days later (March 5th), she added the following informa- tion. " How long did that experience last ? Perhaps one minute, an hour, or longer. I came back to the world as one comes back from a swoon, but without any unpleasant feelings, except a cold sensation which came later on. As soon as my moral self began to reflect upon what had happened, I had the conviction that there had been an irruption in me *of the divine*. But, almost at the same time, I felt the *impossibility of formulating* that which had been

communicated to me.   An influx of spiritual life has certainly
taken place, but not in the form of a new dogma or an intellectual
conviction.   It was a living contact, producing life.

" I need hardly say that, now, biblical expressions crowd upon
my mind in order to express or explain that which I have experienced,
because throughout my life every religious experience has taken a
biblical form ; but at the time—apart from the fact that I have
very soon given the name *God* to what had surrounded me—I did
not have the impression that it was one of the regular religious experiences.   It was in any case much deeper, greater, more overpowering,
and less precise than anything I have so far considered in my life
as a religious experience.   Especially, I played a much less definite
rôle, or rather I did not play any rôle at all, since I had the feeling
of having completely disappeared, of *not existing*."

The Friend never reappeared, but in the course of the following
seventeen months the great Experience reproduced itself thirty-one
times and Mlle Vé had an opportunity of verifying her initial
description and of indicating alterations or new features.   This she
did with a power of introspection equal to that of St Theresa and a
critical ability far beyond hers.

With every ecstasy she struggled anew for a definition of the
" Divine."   The most significant of her utterances on this point
follow in chronological order :—

April 2nd.   " It is not easy to come closer to that Divine
Experience which I have had the privilege of undergoing four or
five times.   In several respects it upsets my best established notions
of the meaning of the Divine.   It is more vague and especially less
personal than that which I have so far regarded as the Divine.   As I
wrote yesterday, it really soars *beyond good and evil*."

April 16th.   " It is now only that I realize how narrow, dogmatic,
anthropomorphized my conception of the Divine was.   I had
elaborated a God residing altogether in the moral sanction, and
revealed altogether in the Father set forth for us by the Christ of
the Gospels.   I have at times felt all conception of God not modelled
upon Christ or leading back to Him as blasphemous."

" The Divine of which this Experience gives me glimpses, surpasses in grandeur and in directness everything I have been able to
imagine so far.   It is a God who surrounds and envelops me, lifts me
up, illuminates and purifies me.   But it is also a God that destroys
me ; to enter into contact with me He requires the complete sacrifice
of my self-consciousness.   This, the impossibility of the Divine and
of the human self to exist simultaneously, is something new to me.
But, then, what is this Divine that I do not apprehend as a person,

which engulfs my personality and afterwards communicates to it a living force ? "

Whatever perplexing queries may arise, Mlle Vé continues to feel for a while after each Experience " the absolute conviction " of a Divine intervention. On the occasion of the Ninth Ecstasy, she remarks, " I felt most of all my weakness, my powerlessness, and the uselessness of any attempt at resistance ; and also that curious impression of being surrounded by something at once violent and tender. I understood now that the mystics of the middle ages could compare their ecstasies, altogether spiritual, to the enjoyment and embraces of human love. Those are certainly the symbols (could I bring myself to use them) which best fit, not the Experience at the moment of contact, but the sensations that follow or precede it and that ultimate impression of the aim reached, of utter fulfilment."

On May 9th, on the occasion of the Tenth Ecstasy, she asks : " What is it that makes connexion with me in those instants ' in my body or out of my body, I do not know. God knows.' I have never had the impression that it was a manifestation of Christ; it is too impersonal, too elemental. And yet, afterwards, it has for my soul the value of a meeting with God and I feel vivified."

Visitation by an impersonal, elemental power, however entrancing and beneficial it may be, is not enough for her. On the 12th of May, after the Eleventh Ecstasy, she writes : " And, nevertheless, I need something else. I must find again the personal God ; the God-Power-and-Light does not suffice me. I hardly dare write this—there is something almost sacrilegious in asking for more than I have received, but I cannot do otherwise. Not even this contact can satisfy my soul, thirsting as it does after the living and loving God."

Certain important aspects of this trance must be emphasized. On the night of the first great Experience she had to make an especially vigorous and protracted effort of mental concentration before the Friend appeared. The account transcribed above indicates that she fell into a trance in which she was unable to move, although at first she remained conscious. The sensations of touch and pressure ordinarily present disappeared. This anæsthesia was in itself sufficient to induce the impression of being altered and of being " elsewhere," liberated from the weight of the body[1]. The Friend came, but there was no conversation with him. Mental inertia was apparently already too deep. Suddenly, consciousness disappeared totally. When she returned to herself, she realized

[1] See the following chapter for a discussion of this illusion.

the total eclipse; she felt weak, confused, not knowing at first what had happened to her.

It seems that no particular meaning attached to the Experience while it lasted. A person not imbued with ideas about mysticism present in Mlle Vé's mind and not in dire need of divine assistance, would probably have let the adventure pass as a surprising fit, an unusual swoon, or night-mare. Not so Mlle Vé; she could not afford to entertain angels unawares. There were, as she saw it, reasons for believing that she had been the subject of a divine visitation. In retrospect—on this fact of retrospection she insists—she becomes conscious of " a sort of absolute assurance of the reality of the Divine." On the following days, as her " moral self " began to reflect, she endeavoured to formulate her Experience. But, look back as hard and as often as she might, all she could say was, " An influx of spiritual life has certainly taken place "—something " producing life."

That she had been the object of the manifestation of a great superhuman power was for her, in her situation and limited as she was in knowledge of physiology and psychology, a natural, probably an unavoidable conclusion. When, independently of your will, you find yourself unexpectedly and in rapid succession the seat of unusual sensations, deprived of the use of your limbs, stripped as it were of your body, and finally deprived of the sense of existence itself, yet restored to normal consciousness a moment later, what explanation seems more natural than that some Great Power, external to yourself, has acted upon you ? That Mlle Vé could not regard it as personal, is the very logical result of the absence in this seizure of the kind of response on her part that is ordinarily elicited by the presence of a person. This explanation is confirmed by her Twelfth Ecstasy. It had seemed to her on that occasion that she had felt a Power "more personal, less elemental." Why that impression ? She provides the answer when she adds, " I had an impression of divine *sympathy*." " Nevertheless, there persisted that sense of the infinite which surpasses our limits and our measures." But this impression was an exception, and her final conclusion is that a Force which manifests itself in overpowering personality, instead of eliciting a personal, emotional response, is not a personal Power, still less the God of Love.

We now understand why she interprets her Experience as the manifestation of an impersonal, superhuman power. But why does she insist upon the divineness of that power ? Had she been more familiar with certain diseases, epilepsy for instance, with its aura of strange feeling and of disordered external perceptions, followed by a momentary loss of consciousness, she might have found it very difficult to speak of a divine power. But since, when reflecting upon her Experience, no comparable phenomenon such as would offer itself to the mind of a psychiatrist occurs to her; and since, instead, " biblical expressions crowd " upon her mind " in order to express or explain " that which she had experienced, she has but one alternative: the Power was either divine or satanic. Why did she choose the former ? There was no reason for regarding herself as the object of the action of satanic powers, unless it were the connexion of her trances with the forbidden sex-passion. This connexion, however, was not immediately realized by her. When it was realized, it suggested " the most radical doubt as to the nature of the Experience." On the other hand, the peculiarly strong need of help that she felt on that day, her habit of seeking assistance in prayer and divine communion, and her belief that divine powers might, and, in certain cases, do, manifest themselves in strange phenomena (she was familiar with the ecstasies of the Christian mystics), inclined her to regard her Experience as the expression of a good, a divine, power.

How strongly she was incited to make the best possible use of whatever happened to her, appears in the determination with which, even before she had become quite clear as to the nature of the Experience, she resolved that it " should have moral results." This compulsion to turn to moral account the puzzling doings of the Power was felt anew with each returning manifestation of it. This resolve was greatly strengthened by the conviction of the divineness of the Experience. Expectation, in things of the mind, creates the expected; she is strengthened, comforted; an " infusion of life " takes place just as if a divine power had interfered. And this consequence of belief in divine action reacts on the belief itself to confirm it; thus, a circular action is established.

Mlle Vé did not accept willingly the impersonal character of the Force which, she thought, acted upon her. She wanted communion with a loving personal God. Now, if, on the one hand, the Experience lacked traits which would have characterized the manifestation of a personal being; on the other, the practical effects of the ecstasy were not those to be expected of a brutal, unconscious power. This train of conflicting thoughts came to a head in reflections following the Fourteenth Ecstasy. I quote :

" In this divine contact I gather strength, light, a sort of vivification of my moral being, all things which, it seems to me, can only come from a personal Being. I do not see how these forces could come from a blind energy. Am I not justified in ascending from the work to the Workman ? " She concludes that an " act of faith " is legitimately required of her. " I believe, then, that I have the right not to stop at mere observation, but for the sake of my moral life, to add the conclusions of my unshakeable faith in a personal God."

We may observe in passing that this bit of reasoning is common to-day to all those—among them are found distinguished theologians—who base their religious faith upon "inner experience." They, as well as Mlle Vé, pass, as I have shown elsewhere[1], from an influx of energy, directed toward the realization of their ideal, to a personal God as its cause.

Fortunately or unfortunately for Mlle Vé, she is too keen-witted to rest satisfied with this argument. A little later, two months before the last Experience, she writes :

" I am disturbed by that which takes place in me at the time of the Experience. I think of it almost constantly and I see less and less clearly into it. This Experience, so frequently repeated, has remained for me inexplicable. Each time it possesses a living value for me. It is as real as any other inner experience, and each time it gives me the same impression of contact with a something outside of myself, yet within me, that reaches beyond me and envelopes me. And now, when I think of it, I no longer find God, or at least not the God able to satisfy me, the God of Jesus Christ, and I almost come to the conclusion that I have allowed myself to be deceived by my imagination, that there is nothing in it outside of my own self." " I am compelled to observe," she wrote a little earlier, " that alone the meaning I give to it, instinctively and retrospectively, is religious and divine."

When these thoughts had once found lodgment in her mind, the great Experience was doomed. As a matter of fact, however, additional reasons already mentioned contributed to its cessation. From now on, communion with Christ, in a state resembling the stage named " contemplation " in the classical Ascent of the Soul to God, replaced the Experience as source of affective comfort and moral energy.

*   *   *

One of the curious points insisted upon by all mystics is the invulnerability of their experience, and therefore the right to absolute assurance in the truth of their revelation. What light does the account of Mlle Vé throw upon this problem ? After the first Experience she affirmed an absolute certainty of the action within her of a divine and impersonal power. No one need deny that at the time she felt absolutely certain. But that is a fact of very little

[1] *A Psychological Study of Religion*, chapter XI, pp. 207-77.

significance. More important are the serious doubts concerning the divinity and even the objective existence of the Power that arose in her after full acquaintance with the Experience. Must not these doubts be accepted as proof that her assurance referred not to a fact of immediate experience, but to an interpretation by her own mind —and, apparently, a wrong interpretation ?

In the present instance, the only unassailable " revelations " appear to have consisted in the following classes of phenomena :

1. Various feelings of cold, of quivering, etc. ; i.e., disturbances of sensory and motor innervation, coming and going with considerable swiftness and violence.

2. Various ideas awakened by these sensations, and their accompanying emotions.

3. A total and usually startlingly sudden loss of consciousness.

4. On recovering of consciousness, various feelings similar to those characterizing the first phase, and a sense of fatigue or exhaustion.

5. Various emotions and ideas connected with her present and past experiences ; in particular, the idea of a divine power as the cause of the present experience.

6. A change in her mood and moral attitude. This change seems to consist essentially in a disappearance of irritating tensions and of worrying impulses and cravings. Thus a greater degree of unification of the self is attained ; and, correlated with it, a mood of greater optimism and energy.

That all these things happened to Mlle Vé is, of course, incontrovertible. But her claim of absolute certainty refers not to mental contents, but to the *objective reality* of an external power that is thought of as their cause or object : she claims absolute assurance of the existence of a transcendent, divine Power.

The derived, interpretative nature of that conviction is established by the appearance in her mind of doubt as to its truth. She could not have doubted her feeling of cold, or of fatigue, or her greater hopefulness ; but she could and did doubt the validity of her causal interpretation of these facts. We shall have to consider more fully elsewhere the ground for the widespread belief that a revelation of God or of the Absolute is given in mystical ecstasy.

*　　　　　*　　　　　*

III. Mystical Ecstasy in English Poetry.

Among the propagandists of the belief in the transcendental and revelatory nature of mystical ecstasy, great poets hold a dominant position. Their faith in an Invisible World is anchored on ecstatic trance-experiences, and it is under the indelible impression of these mysterious adventures that they bear testimony to the age-old claims of man that he is immortal and that he need not wait for death in order to be initiated into celestial existence.

The clearest description of ecstatic trance with which I am acquainted in English poetry is found in " Tintern Abbey," where Wordsworth in unforgettable words speaks of

> " That serene and blessed mood
> In which the breath of this corporeal frame,
> And even the motion of our human blood,
> Almost suspended, we are laid asleep
> In body, and become a living soul :
> While, with an eye made quiet by the power,
> We see into the life of things."

Similar words in the *Prelude* describe apparently a similar experience :

> " Gently did my soul
> Put off her veil, and, self-transmuted, stood
> Naked, as in the presence of her God."

Tennyson was familiar with trance-ecstasies and was influenced by them perhaps even more deeply than Wordsworth. In the conclusion to the Holy Grail the following words are placed in the mouth of King Arthur :

> " Let visions of the night or of the day
> Come as they will ; and many a time they come.
> Until this earth he walks on seems not earth,
> This light that strikes his eyeball is not light,
> This air that smites his forehead is not air
> But vision—yea, his very hand and foot—
> In moments when he feels he cannot die,
> And knows himself no vision to himself,
> Nor the high God a vision, nor that One
> Who rose again : Ye have seen what ye have seen[1]."

Every one of the features which we have learned to regard as characteristic of ecstasy is mentioned or implied in these passages— the disappearance of the external world ; the loss of bodily control and of the consciousness of the existence of the body ; an impression of limitless extension of the self, growing, it seems, in proportion to the removal of the limitations imposed upon the self by the

[1] See also *The Mystic*, in *Suppressed Poems of Alfred, Lord Tennyson*, London, 1910.
The hero in " The Princess " is afflicted by
> " Weird seizures, Heaven knows what.
> On a sudden in the midst of men and day,
> And while I walked and talked as heretofore,
> I seemed to move among a world of ghosts,
> And feel myself the shadow of a dream."

Sir Crichton-Browne, who quotes these lines, is of the opinion that they describe in outline an attack of *petit mal*—such " dreamy mental states " being often the prelude or accompaniment of Epilepsy.—*Cavendish Lecture, Lancet,* June 6th and 13th, 1895.

realization of the presence of the external world and the body; a sense of lofty and clear illumination which, however, refuses to let itself be put into words; and, finally, an incomparable delight.

Wordsworth claimed—I quote Miss Caroline Spurgeon—that " he had discovered a way to effect the necessary alteration in ourselves which will enable us to catch glimpses of the truths expressing themselves all round us[1]." I do not know what his method was. Tennyson was more communicative; in a letter to a friend, he wrote:

" A kind of waking trance I have frequently had, quite up from boyhood, when I have been alone. This has generally come upon me through repeating my own name two or three times to myself silently, till all at once, as it were out of the intensity of the consciousness of individuality, the individuality itself seemed to dissolve and fade away into boundless being, and this not a confused state, but the clearest of the clearest, the surest of the surest, the weirdest of the weirdest, utterly beyond words, where death was an almost laughable impossibility, the loss of personality (if it were so) seeming no extinction but the only true life. . . . This might be the state which St Paul describes ' Whether in the body I cannot tell, or whether out of the body I cannot tell.' " And he adds: " I am ashamed of my feeble description. Have I not said the state is utterly beyond words[2]? "

The poet seems not to have known that he was using a time-honoured method. Hindoo mystics have long ago taught us that in order to escape the delusion of the senses, to see into the real life of things, and to become one with the All, one needs only to repeat a mysterious syllable. Long search and practice have made the Hindoos proficient far beyond our great poets in the production of mystical trances. They are acquainted with several successful methods, some of which, I imagine, would have appeared unseemly to the Poet Laureate of the British Empire—this one, for instance: " While holding the body, head and neck motionless, look at the tip of your nose, with a tranquil self, devoid of anxiety or fear, and, adhering to the rules of Brahma Karnis, concentrate the mind on Brahma[3]."

The trances of Tennyson do not seem to have reached complete unconsciousness, but in other respects they are quite similar to those of Symonds and of the Yogin. They bear, moreover, essential

---

[1] *Mysticism in English Literature*, Cambridge, 1913. p. 63.

[2] Alfred, Lord Tennyson, *A Memoir by his Son*, New York, 1897, vol. I, p. 320.

[3] On Yoga practices, see chapter II of this book.

similarity to the drug-intoxication regarded by non-civilized peoples as divine possession. Let it be added that they may be reproduced at will and without the assistance of drugs by most or all of those who may care to do so, provided they be possessed of some patience.

James Russell Lowell passed through at least one ecstatic experience. It came upon him in the course of a discussion of spiritism. There are few topics better able to raise spinal shivers and to prepare the mind for hallucinations. Under date of September 20th, 1842 (he was then twenty-three years old) he wrote to a friend :—

" I had a revelation last Friday evening. I was at Mary's, and happening to say something of the presence of spirits (of whom, I said, I was often dimly aware), Mr. Putnam entered into an argument with me on spiritual matters. As I was speaking the whole system rose up before me like a vague Destiny looming from the abyss. I never before so clearly felt the spirit of God in me and around me. The whole room seemed to me full of God. The air seemed to waver to and fro with the presence of something. I knew not what. I spoke with the calmness and clearness of a prophet.

" I cannot tell you what this revelation was. I have not yet studied it enough. But I shall perfect it one day, and then you shall hear it and acknowledge its grandeur. It embraces all other systems[1]."

With his mind full of invisible presences, Lowell felt the proximity of " something." " The air," says he, " seemed to waver to and fro with the presence of Something. I knew not what." Why, then does he permit himself, in the sentence immediately preceding, to say that he felt clearly " the spirit of God " and that the whole room seemed to be full of God ? It cannot, however, be said that there is anything unusual in this. Lowell is merely thinking and writing in the amazingly loose way that is tolerated in things mystical and religious. May we not liken the poet's " feeling of a presence " to the well-known feeling which, in the dark, makes us aware of the proximity of a " ghost " ?

---

[1] *Letters of James Russell Lowell*, ed. by Charles Eliot Norton, 1894, vol. I, p. 69.

Compare this instance, chosen from many in the religious life : " I also in my youth ardently pursued these subjects of knowledge and I even prayed God to help me to attain them in order that I might be more useful to my Congregation. After this prayer I once found myself inundated with a vivid light ; it seemed to me that a veil was lifted up from before the eyes of the spirit, and all the truths of human sciences, even those that I had not studied, became manifest to me by an infused knowledge, as was once the case with Solomon. This state of intuition lasted about twenty-four hours, and then, as if the veil had fallen again, I found myself as ignorant as before."—St. Francis Xavier, as quoted by Poulain, in *Graces of Interior Prayer*, p. 279.

As to the stupendous revelation, the poet never consigned it to paper. It was unutterable at the time, and we may assume that if ever he caught intelligible glimpses of it, they possessed no particular significance.

We may well pause a moment to comment upon the practical, significance of this fact : great poets, gifted with means of literary fascination, and thus insidious teachers of multitudes, find an assurance of the truth of ancient beliefs dear to them in trances which come spontaneously to many and which can be induced artificially in most persons. And thousands of our contemporaries, not lacking in distinction and knowledge but ignorant of psychology, fall under the spell of these dazzling teachers and say with Miss Spurgeon : " Wordsworth's claim is a great claim, but he would seem to have justified it[1]." Thus is raised and solved in a naïve way the profound question that continues to divide philosophers : Is there in mysticism an intuition, a direct knowledge of Reality, to which reason cannot attain, and, if there is, what is the value to man of that revelation ?

*   .   *   *

IV. Scientific Inspiration or Revelation.

There are few beliefs more widely entertained than that of the passivity[2] of the artist at the supreme creative moment. It is a common dictum that he must wait upon "inspiration." That word, so ready upon the tongue in connexion with artistic creation, points to the spontaneity, the unexpectedness, of this kind of mental production. A well-known saying of Goethe may be appropriately quoted here as it expresses very well the current opinion :—

" All productivity of the highest kind, every important conception, every discovery, every great thought which bears fruit, is in no one's control, and is beyond every earthly power. Such things are to be regarded as unexpected gifts from above, as pure divine products[3]."

Psychology would seek to penetrate deeper than Goethe into this great problem of apparent spontaneous creation. It would learn something of the relation of "inspiration" to purpose, effort, and knowledge—something that would give us a degree of control over the so-called "gifts from above."

[1] Loc. cit., p. 65. Other ecstatic "revelations" are reported in the following chapter.

[2] It need hardly be said that the sense of passivity of the artist and of the scientist is independent of the ethico-religious conceptions in which is involved the passivity of the Christian mystic. There is no question of a surrender of the egoistic will to the divine Will.

[3] Eckermann's Gespräche mit Goethe, vol. III, pp. 166-7, ed. Moldenhauer, Leipzig, Reclame.

There is in Longfellow's *Diary* the following entry :
" I wrote last evening a notice of Allston's poems. After which
I sat till twelve o'clock by my fire, smoking, when suddenly it came
into my mind to write the ' Ballad of the Schooner Hesperus,' which
I accordingly did. Then I went to bed, but could not sleep. New
thoughts were running in my mind, and I got up to add them to the
ballad. I feel pleased with the ballad. It hardly cost me any effort.
It did not come into my mind by lines, but by stanzas[1]."

George Eliot, positivist as she was in philosophy, declared that,
in all the writings which she considered her best, there was a " not
herself " which took possession of her and made her feel " her own
personality to be merely the instrument through which the spirit
acted[2]."

A similar affirmation is made by the *Goncourts :* " It is fate,"
they say, " that brings to you the initial idea. Then, an unknown
force, a superior will, a sort of compulsion to write commands you
and leads your pen ; so much so that at times the book you have
written does not seem to be your own[3]."

In not limiting revelation to artistic creation, but in extending
it to " every important " and " great " thought, Goethe was true
to the facts : science, as well as art, may be a beneficiary of
revelation.

We begin with an instance which shows essential features of a
revelation, and yet not far removed from the commonplace. Prince
Kropotkin, before becoming an anarchist, had for several years been
intensely interested in the physical conformation of Asia. In the
course of his labours—I quote from his *Memoirs*—he had " marked
on a large-scale map all geological and physical observations that had
been made by different travellers, and tried to find out what
structural lines would answer best to the observed realities." This
preparatory work took him over two years. " Then followed months
of intense thought in order to find out what the bewildering chaos of
scattered observations meant, until one day, all of a sudden, the
whole became clear and comprehensible, as if it were illuminated
with a flash of light. The main structural lines of Asia are *not* north
and south, or west and east ; they are from the south-west to the

---

[1] Longfellow's *Diary*, under date of December 30th, 1839, as quoted by
Samuel Longfellow in *Life of H. W. Longfellow*, vol. I, p. 339, Boston, 1886.

[2] John W. Cross, *Life of George Eliot.*

[3] *Journal des Goncourt*, Paris, 1888, as quoted by Lombroso, in *L'Homme
de Génie*, Paris, 1889, p. 468.
F. C. Prescott's *The Poetic Mind*, New York, Macmillan, 1922, contains
much of interest on the unconscious in poetry. See, in particular, chapter VI.

north-east. . . . There are not many joys in human life equal to the joy of the sudden birth of a generalization, illuminating the mind after a long period of patient research[1]."

Here the great joy, rising almost to ecstasy, *follows* the illumination as a rational consequence of its perceived significance. It is the ecstasy of Archimedes, running naked through the streets of Syracuse after having discovered the principle of specific gravity, shouting " eureka, eureka ! "

The great French mathematician, Henri Poincaré, provides us with far more unusual instances of scientific revelation. In an article on invention in mathematics, he made the surprising remark that the most striking feature of mathematical invention is " apparent sudden illumination." Of one of the greatest of his discoveries, the *fonctions Fuchsiennes* he wrote :—

" I had been endeavouring for two weeks to demonstrate that there could exist no function analogous to those I have since called *fonctions Fuchsiennes*. Each day I spent an hour or two at my working table . . . but I came to no solution. One evening, against my habit, I drank some black coffee. I could not sleep ; ideas crowded in my mind ; I felt them knocking against each other, until two of them hung together, as it were, and formed a stable combination. In the morning, I had established the existence of a class of *fonctions Fuchsiennes*. There remained merely to set down the results, and that was done in a few hours[2]."

This accomplished, he set about exploring systematically the new domain brought to view by the discovery. In the course of that exploration a problem arose which again stubbornly resisted solution : " My efforts served only to give me a fuller knowledge of the difficulty —that was already something gained. So far, my work was entirely conscious. Thereupon, I left for Mont Valérien, where I was to be during my military service ; my preoccupations became therefore very different. One day, as I was crossing the Boulevard, the solution of the difficulty appeared suddenly." He found himself in possession of all the elements for the solution. Nothing remained

---

[1] *Memoirs of a Revolutionist*, P. Kropotkin, 1908, p. 211.

[2] Henri Poincaré, *Science et Méthode*, Paris, 1920, pp. 50-1. The distinguished chemist, A. Kekulé, reported two important discoveries made by him under similar conditions. He concluded his account with these words " Let us learn to dream, gentlemen. Then, perhaps, we shall find the truth . . . but let us beware of publishing our dreams before they have been put to the proof by the waking understanding." *Berichte der Deutschen chemischen Gesellschaft*, 1890, vol. 23, p. 1306. I quote from the " Kekulé Memorial Lecture " in the *Journal of the Chemical Soc.*, London, 1898, vol. LXXIII, p. 100.

for him to do but to bring them together and to organize them. This he did, as he says, "at one sitting and without any trouble whatsoever[1]."

Of another mathematical discovery, made while out walking, he wrote that it came to him " with the accustomed traits : brevity, suddenness, and immediate certitude[2]."

An equally remarkable instance is that of the greatest discovery made by Sir Wm. Rowan Hamilton[3]. In a letter to Professor P. G. Tait, dated October 15th, 1858, he wrote :—

" P.S.—To-morrow will be the fifteenth birthday of the Quaternions. They started into life, or light, full grown, on the 16th of October, 1843, as I was walking with Lady Hamilton to Dublin, and came up to Brougham Bridge, which my boys have since called the Quaternion Bridge, that is to say, I then and there felt the galvanic circuit of thought close ; and the sparks which fell from it were the fundamental equations between i, j, k ; exactly such as I have used them ever since. I pulled out on the spot a pocket-book, which still exists, and made an entry, on which *at the very moment* I felt that it might be worth my while to expend the labour of at least ten (or perhaps fifteen) years to come. But then it is fair to say that this was because I felt a *problem* to have been at that moment solved —an intellectual want relieved—which had haunted me for at least fifteen years before[3]."

*   *   *

Whatever its explanation, the fact itself has to be accepted : in artistic as in scientific discovery ; i.e., both in the field of imagination and of rational construction, there come, after periods of mental striving or vague brooding, fructifying moments, effortless and unexpected, which give the impression of inspiration.

But if Goethe was right in including among the " gifts from above " not only poetical thoughts but also great thoughts of any

---

[1] Poincaré, *loc. cit.*, p. 53.

[2] *Ibid.*, p. 52.

[3] *Life of Sir Wm. Rowan Hamilton*, by R. P. Graves, 3 vols., Dublin, 1882, vol. II, pp. 434-6.
In a letter to his son, August 5th, 1865, the Rev. Archibald H. Hamilton, adds some interesting particulars showing how close to his attention was the problem when it was finally solved. Shortly before the discovery, " the desire to discover the laws of the multiplication referred to [this was the especial difficulty to be overcome] regained with me a certain strength and earnestness, which had for years been dormant." And, about the walk with Lady Hamilton when the discovery was made, he says, in the same letter : " Although she talked with me now and then, yet an undercurrent of thought was going on in my mind which gave at last a result, whereof it is not too much to say that I felt *at once* the importance." He then repeats the image of the closing of an electric circuit.

sort, he was wrong in limiting these gifts to great and important thoughts. *All* kinds of ideas, and ideas of all degrees of puerility and importance, appear in our minds under the conditions which we have found to be those of revelation. "The Ballad of the Schooner Hesperus," which flowed from Longfellow's pen by stanzas, without effort, does not embody any great thought. Mozart seems to have claimed that all, and not only his remarkable, musical compositions came to him unexpectedly.

But why look so far for illustrations? Almost every moment of conscious life provides everyone of us with similar facts. The common instances of "bright" ideas, of happy thoughts, which offer themselves when we have ceased to seek them, are disconnected from the train of thought of the moment and seem not the reward of effort but gifts from unknown sources.

Action also—not only processes of intellectual discovery—may be characterized by the inspiration-features. When in bed in the morning, we have probably all of us reasoned with ourselves about the desirability or even the necessity of getting up, without getting up for all that. And then, when the mind had returned to somnolent blessedness or had passed to another train of thought, suddenly we found ourselves on our feet. Nothing could be falser than to say that our actions are always the immediate and direct consequences of relevant trains of thought. There are persons who believe in the existence of evil spirits because, like Miss X., they have observed that they do not deliberately do the evil deeds of which they are occasionally guilty. They find themselves doing evil as we have, on occasion, found ourselves on our feet in the morning, and as we find ideas popping up into our heads when least expected. We are essentially creatures of impulse, of instinct, and of habit.

*   *   *

The facts of inspiration and revelation are explained to-day in three ways. They are referred to "God" as their cause; that, however, is not really an explanation but merely a displacement of the problem. Or they are referred to a mental (not merely a nervous) activity of which the person is not aware, *i.e.*, to so-called sub-conscious processes. Or, again, both these conceptions are combined : God is supposed to make use of the subconscious in order to produce revelations in the human mind. This synthetic explanation pleases those who like to keep the old and at the same time enjoy seeming abreast of the times. Unfortunately, this last hypothesis suffers from the disadvantages attaching to each of the conceptions which it combines. From the point of view of science, the second explanation offers no advantage over the first ; it also is an appeal to the unknown.

If we are not able to say how the creation or invention is formed, we can at least reduce the mysterious to the commonplace by showing that even in the most striking of the well-authenticated instances there is nothing more to explain than in ordinary thinking.

*   *   *

An examination of striking scientific revelations yields the following results. They take place only after a period of conscious work and they complete or continue something already begun. When the solution is complex, it does not come to the mind with all the details fully worked out. The key is at hand, but it has still to be used. Or, as Poincaré says of the principle that has been given, " *il faut déduire les conséquences.*" These revelations are rare, and, what is more important, discoveries just as remarkable are made in the more ordinary way, *i.e.*, in answer, as it seems, to continuous effort. Finally, if it is true that the solution of a problem may come unexpectedly and, at times, long after we have ceased to be actively engaged in its consideration, nevertheless there is no satisfactory evidence in support of the assumption commonly made that it ever appears after the person has ceased to be interested in it.

On the contrary, the solutions that come in the form of inspiration refer to problems which have not been finally dismissed, which have remained in the " back of the mind," ready to force themselves upon the attention. A problem in a quiescent stage may flash unexpectedly into the fringe of consciousness and be immediately and almost unconsciously repressed and dismissed, unless it should happen—as it occasionally does—that it present itself in a new light. Then interest and attention are aroused, and the problem is again taken up. In the new light, the way to the solution may be discerned.

Similar remarks apply also to mystical inspirations. The monitions and other revelations that come to the Christian mystics are about topics that have much engaged their thoughts. As to the quality of these revelations, it rarely surpasses the entirely commonplace, and, as far as our information extends, it never goes beyond what may be expected from the unaided effort of the person himself. The reader may be reminded here of the series of revelations vouchsafed to St Marguerite Marie and used with conspicuous success by Roman Catholic priests in the establishment of the devotion to the Sacred Heart of Jesus. Neither do the instances of scientific revelation with which we are acquainted transcend the apparent capacity of men who possess the knowledge and ability of the individuals who experienced them[1].

The preceding observations cast a grey tint upon the lurid colours in which the phenomenon we are studying appears at the first glance. The mental processes of inspirational invention and of ordinary thinking are essentially similar. It is a complete misrepresentation of thought to picture it as gaining its ends by a straightforward, uninterrupted flowing movement. Conscious processes are, on the contrary, full of stops, of breaks, and of sudden forward leaps. They are like a fire which seems to go out when blown upon, and which spasmodically flares up again when left to itself. It is often when the unproductivity of effort has compelled us to give up, that an illumination surprises us. The revivalist admonishes the repentant soul to let go, to surrender into the arms of Jesus ; then salvation may come. The mystic, likewise, seeks the Divine in passivity. Old Egyptian wisdom had already reduced the truth involved in these practices to an aphorism : " The archer hitteth the target partly by pulling, partly by letting go ; the boatman reacheth the landing partly by pulling, partly by letting go[2]."

Thought proceeds very much like the formation of the chain we have all seen coming into existence on the screen of a moving-picture theatre. Each link appears separately and jumps into place suddenly. There is no more continuity in thinking than in the formation of that continuous chain. For a time the strain of purpose seems to act as a centre which attracts to itself, as it were, the various elements of the problem. These elements appear most irregularly. There are moments when no progress is made; attention relaxes and turns in desultory fashion to other things. Suddenly a new link pops into consciousness and adds itself to the chain. Then the directing purpose may again be felt and the double process of effort and relaxation repeats itself. The interruptions may be so brief as to be unnoticed, and then, remaining under the impression of the effort, we assume that the idea has appeared during the attentive phase[3].

---

[1] For many years past the *Society for Psychical Research* has attempted to prove the appearance in the human mind of specific items of knowledge under conditions which would make their acquisition impossible by natural means. It does not seem to us that they have been successful in removing from their observations and experiments all the possibilities of error.

[2] From the instructions of Ptah Hotep to his son. Quoted by Hocking in *The Meaning of God in Human Experience*, p. 419.

[3] The reader acquainted with the chapter of Wm. James on the *Stream of Consciousness* should not think that, differing with him as we do in describing thought as a discontinuous process and not a continuous stream, we lapse into the psychical " atomism " against which he was setting himself.

The moments of interrupted attention are filled with nothing at all, or with thoughts and feelings belonging to another topic: we may simply look up, finger our eyeglasses, consult the clock, light a cigarette, and presto, the idea we had ceased to seek is present. Again, the arrested voluntary activity—the passive phase of the process—may be protracted, and the task given up for the present. A week or a month later, a constructive thought may suddenly and unexpectedly appear and may lead to a speedy solution of the problem.

How prone we are to overlook the return, in the penumbra of consciousness, of problems held in suspended animation, is an interesting fact classed by the psychologists together with the disregard of habitual and meaningless stimuli that fall upon our sense organs. Careful and timely introspection alone reveals their presence. When Poincaré remarks that during his military service he was occupied with matters other than mathematical problems, we are not to understand him as affirming that the problem of the *fonctions Fuchsiennes*, with which he had been long and profoundly engaged, never crossed his mind. Sir William Rowan Hamilton states that during the weeks preceding the revelation active interest in the problem of Quaternions had revived, and that as he was approaching the bridge, although he was talking " now and then " with Lady Hamilton, yet in his mind " an undercurrent of thought was going on " which suddenly flared up into the memorable equations. When these frequent undercurrents of thought—brief and weak as they often are—have no particular importance, nothing is easier than to disregard and forget them altogether.

The problem of inspiration, illumination, revelation—call it what you will—does not, then, refer only to very remarkable and rare occurrences. The traits by which revelation is commonly separated from ordinary, natural, human products are in various degrees characteristic of all thought and action. Unexpectedness, absence of effort, passivity (and also, as we shall see subsequently, clearness and certainty) may belong alike to the great and the small, the true and the false, the religious and the secular. The day is past when these traits may be regarded as pointing to a dualism in the origin and in the nature of men's thoughts and actions, stamping some as altogether human and others as gifts from above. Amazing experiences, in which, following upon unavailing mental effort, the solution of a difficult problem appears suddenly and unexpectedly, are merely extreme instances of the ordinary processes of purposive, rational thinking. In the startling instances, the problems are sufficiently momentous and the phase of passivity is long enough to arrest attention and to cause wonder.

*   *   *

We have so far merely described and classified the facts; we may now explain why a long break in the attention-effort is at times the precursor of a surprising forward movement. Certain well-understood facts will lead us to an hypothesis of some probability. Suppose that you have learned to sort, according to colour, a pack of cards into boxes placed before you. You have repeated the operation a sufficient number of times to establish the proper movement-habits, so that they have become more or less automatic. Now, you are asked to sort the same pack of cards into the same boxes, this time not according to colour, but according to figure, *i.e.*, you are to place all the aces in one box, all the kings in another box, etc. The habits previously established of sorting according to colour will conflict with those you would now like to form, and your progress will be impeded; it will be slower than if you had not previously formed the colour-habits.

Something similar happens when learning any art that involves movements—learning to typewrite, for instance. Here one makes at first many wrong movements and each wrong movement establishes a tendency to repeat that wrong movement. If one continues practising too long, without rest, the moment comes when no further gain is made. That point is reached when as many wrong movements as right ones are made.

Now it is occasionally observed that after a sufficiently long rest—several weeks or months—on resuming the practice, it seems that an improvement has taken place. As a matter of fact, improvement after a long rest has been observed under experimental conditions. W. F. Book reports the following observations:—

A subject practised typewriting until he made, during the last ten ten-minute practices, the average score of 1,508 words per period of ten minutes. After an interval of six months, he was tested ten times, ten minutes each time, under exactly the same conditions as those prevailing during the practice. The average score was 1,433 and the number of errors was greater than during the last practice series. He refrained again from using the typewriter, this time, for a whole year. Thus one year and a half elapsed between the cessation of the practice and a second memory test. During this second test, the average score for ten ten-minute periods was 1,611 words, and the percentage of errors was less than during the first memory test. "There seems," says Book, "to have been an actual increase in skill during the rest interval of one year and a half. How is this to be explained ? The increase in score shown by our second series was due, so far as we could make out, rather to the disappearance, with the lapse of time, of numerous interfering associations, bad habits of attention incidentally acquired in the course of learning, interfering habits and tendencies, which, as they faded, left the more firmly established typewriting associations free to act. Such hindering associations were developed in all stages of practice and at the ' critical stages ' in great masses, forming a serious impediment to progress. After the rest of a year and a half these conflicting associations and hindering tendencies had noticeably disappeared." The six months which elapsed between the last practice and the first memory test were not sufficient, in the opinion of Book, to permit the disappearance of the hindering associations, hence the lowered score. " A year later, during the second memory test, the absence of difficulties and the greater ease had become so prominent as to attract the attention of the learner. The errors have slightly decreased and the score is better than ever before. We, therefore, conclude that it was the disappearance of the interfering associations and tendencies naturally developed in the course of the learning which caused the increase in the score[1]."

This explanation may be presented in a simplified way. Suppose that during a practice period you have made the right movement ten times and another movement five times. The right movement is more firmly established than the wrong one ; nevertheless, there is a tendency to make the wrong movement, and that tendency interferes with the tendency to produce the right movement. Now, let a sufficiently long interruption in the practice take place. The moment will come when, as it is less deeply established, the tendency to the wrong movement will have died out, while that to the right movement will still be present. It is true that it will be diminished in intensity, but the more important fact is that tendencies to the wrong movement will no longer interfere with it. (Obviously, if the interval is long enough, both the right and the wrong tendencies acquired during the practice will have disappeared.) Hence, when you return to your practice, the chances are that it will be more perfect than at any

---

[1] W.F. Book, *The Psychology of Skill* : *with Special Reference to its Acquisition in Typewriting, University of Montana Publications in Psychology,* Bulletin No. 53, *Psychological Series* No. 1. This experiment is summarized in Thorndyke's *Educational Psychology*, vol. II, pp. 311-17.

Thorndike sees in this instance the possibility of another interpretation than that offered by Book, namely, that the learner had not yet reached his limit when the practice ceased, and that, as chance would have it, during the second test a spurt of progress took place. Nevertheless, the same author, in discussing the permanence of improvement (p. 301), admits that an interruption of practice may result in an improvement by the " weakening " of interfering habits.

previous time. You have improved without practising. That improvement is not the effect of effort; it does not necessitate any selective activity of consciousness at all. The prevalent tendency to ascribe gains such as this to the activity of a subconsciousness, justifies whatever emphasis may be placed upon the preceding remark.

How one may pass from the above instance of improvement in typewriting to the explanation of scientific inspiration, it is easy to see. Thinking, as well as typewriting, involves a neuro-muscular mechanism. Our thoughts assume a verbal form, even when they are not expressed in audible speech or in writing. The merely " mental " formulation of thought does not take place without incipient innervation of the speech and of other mechanisms.

We may therefore say that thinking, like typewriting, involves false moves. As we repeat the unprofitable thinking, while exploring blind alleys, the production of the right thought becomes increasingly difficult. We all know that under certain circumstances is seems as if the mind had become limited to wrong directions; it goes round and round in the same vicious circles. If at such times we let go, thus producing a condition that will make possible a weakening or a disappearance of the unprofitable thought-movements, and subsequently return to the problem, we stand a better chance of striking a new path—and the new path may be the right path.

Thus, we may understand why the scientist, the philosopher and other persons are at times surprised by the appearance of fruitful ideas which strenuous efforts had failed to produce. Has the effort been useless ? Certainly not. Or, let us rather answer, *some* of the effort, and perhaps all of it, was necessary. Had not the problem been examined in every possible way, the solution would not, so far as the facts can be read, have been secured after relaxation.

Possibly it is not useless to repeat that remarkable inspirations of this sort are very rare, and that usually a return of the problem does not lead to a solution : wrong movements may again be made.

It might be remarked that, strictly speaking, it is not the thinker who returns to the problem ; it is rather the problem that suddenly and unexpectedly returns to the thinker. And it is usually impossible to say why a problem reappears at any particular moment. But it is quite sufficient for our purpose to point out that there is nothing unusual in that aspect of scientific revelation. We have frequently not the slightest indication of the reason why we find ourselves suddenly thinking of a particular thing—that is the way of the mind.

* * *

The description of scientific revelation has disclosed to us its fundamental identity with the mental processes of ordinary productive thinking. Whatever differences exist are differences of degree, and, on the whole, unimportant. We have also obtained what seems to us a satisfactory explanation of the way—or at least one of the ways—in which relaxation, passivity, and rest favour the appearance of new thoughts.

There remain the more difficult and fundamental problems of the origin and of the formation of new thoughts. Whence do they come, how are they created, and why do they appear when they do ? These are essential problems of mental production which we shall make no attempt to solve. In conclusion we may repeat that, with regard to specific problems, a necessary condition of their solution by "inspiration" is an antecedent, general preparation sufficient for their solution and, moreover, a direct consideration of them. The revelation of the *fonctions Fuchsiennes* and of the Quaternions came to great mathematicians who had worked long at the problems[1].

Poetical inspiration follows the same fundamental law : Poems do not flow out from the pen and eloquent speeches from the tongue, of persons who are not in the habit of thinking poetically or eloquently ; and the substance of extemporized poems and speeches is dependent upon previously acquired knowledge.

[1] The interesting post-hypnotic experiments of Morton Prince, in which an arithmetical operation apparently requiring attention (consciousness) is performed without the subject's awareness, disclose phenomena similar but not identical to those which we have called scientific revelation. Morton Prince's explanation is that the arithmetical operations are carried out by a sub-consciousness or a coconsciousness. Obviously, the principle of explanation set forth above does not fit this class of phenomena.—See Morton Prince, *The Unconscious*, pp. 167, ff.

CHAPTER X

THE MAIN CHARACTERISTICS OF TRANCE-CONSCIOUSNESS AND CERTAIN ATTENDANT PHENOMENA, IN PARTICULAR THOSE PRODUCING THE IMPRESSION OF ILLUMINATION

THE dictionaries correctly single out the main peculiarity of trance when they define it as a "state in which the soul seems passive, or to have passed out of the body; a state of insensibility to mundane things." But there are degrees in the depth of trances, *i.e.*, in the loss of mental activity and in the concomitant sundering of the soul from the outside world and the body. It is only when all consciousness has disappeared that the trance is complete.

Entire agreement reigns among the mystics regarding this, the basal characteristic of their mode of worship. The description (Chapter VI) of the Ascent of the Soul makes a long argument in support of that affirmation superfluous. It will be sufficient to remind the reader of Santa Theresa's descriptive classification. In the Second Degree (Orison of Quiet), the understanding and memory act only at intervals. When the will is active it "works in a marvellous way without the least effort." In the Third Degree, the mental quiescence has become deeper : "The powers of the soul are incapable of occupying themselves with any other object than God . . .; the soul feels herself dying to the world." If, in these two stages, the soul "is able to indicate, at least by signs, what she experiences, in the Fourth Degree (Ecstasy or Rapture) the soul is absorbed in enjoyment[1] without understanding that which she enjoys." "The soul seems to leave the organs which she animates" (levitation). Finally, all consciousness may disappear and, on waking, the soul may say in the words of Francis of Sales, "I slept with my God and in the arms of the divine Presence and I knew it not."

Most mystics believe, moreover, that the "suspended" intelligence is replaced in the trance-state by a supernatural understanding ; thus they would account for the conviction of revelation.

[1] We have accounted for the ordinary enjoyment characteristic of most Christian mystical trances as being mainly the natural consequence of the focussing of the mind upon a God of love.

What justification there may be for that belief, we shall see presently.

The partial or total suspension of the sensory and intellectual functions or, more generally, of mental activity, is the fundamental trait of all trances, whether religious or not, and whether produced naturally or artificially. It is accompanied by a great variety of phenomena, the more important of which we must now describe.

Disturbances of time and space perception, etc.—The comparative study of trance-states has shown that they may include as primary facts, or as products of expectation or suggestion, almost every possible modification of sensation and motility: hyperæsthesia, anæsthesia, analgesia, contracture, paralysis, hallucination, etc. The visions, auditions, and other similar phenomena of the drug-addict, as of the religious mystic, may be due directly to physiological factors (the coloured arabesques of mescal, the sensory disturbances in certain epileptic auræ, in mystical trances, etc.) ; or, they may take shape under the influence of desire or aversion (a desire to see Christ as he appeared after the Resurrection, a fear of the devil, a wish for guidance in a particular situation, etc.[1]).

The perception of time may be greatly modified. Events may pass amazingly quickly or be incredibly drawn out. The world of space also may be altered ; distances and sizes are changed, the body seems to expand enormously or to contract to nothing ; it loses weight and becomes like air, it floats through space, etc.

Certain observations upon the effects of ether and nitrous oxide made under experimental conditions by four persons, including the writer, may be introduced here. One of the subjects who became quickly unconscious, and on that account found introspection difficult, remarked, however, that it was very much like going to sleep. Disturbances of sensation were observed by all ; prominent among these were, at various stages of the intoxication, an unusual, pervasive warmth, a numbness of the skin, a feeling of bodily enlargement or extension (by three of the subjects), accompanied in two cases at least, (one under nitrous oxide, the other under ether), with distension and, in one of these (ether), by what seemed increased pressure of the body upon the couch. In all four cases sensations seemed to come from an abnormal distance ; the voices of the attendants became faint and receded. One of the subjects observed

---

[1] Madeleine entered into her ecstasies thinking of Christ crucified, and her feet assumed auto-suggestively, as far as the circumstances permitted, the position of those of Christ on the Cross : she stood on tip-toe ; contractures of the leg muscles were induced.

the reverse phenomenon on recovering consciousness: " The first words heard appeared to come from a great distance and with each succeeding word his voice became nearer and louder, ending in what seemed to be a shout." In one case there was a well marked impression of greater distance of the bodily extremities. This illusion of distance is probably the consequence of the decrease in the intensity of the sensations—a decrease which leads to their total disappearance. An impression of levitation was clearly realized by two of the subjects and another described something similar as a " floating " which followed upon the impression of being " blown up " and " becoming very light."

The subjects had been requested to indicate by lifting a finger that they heard and understood certain signals. This response became gradually slower and feebler and finally failed altogether. One of the subjects was aware of the request when she was no longer able to move her finger. Another was much surprised to hear on awakening that his last finger-movement had been long-delayed and feeble, for he had thought to himself at the time that he would astonish the attendants by the promptness and energy of his response. This last fact is interesting as a minor illustration of the consequence of the lessened vigour and accuracy with which the mind performs its functions. One of the subjects to whom a problem had been given endeavoured in vain to solve it ; she could not grasp the whole of it ; when she thought of the first part, the second vanished, and *vice versa*. This person had, nevertheless, the impression that " ideas were there in profusion."

Confirmation of most of these observations may be found in the experiments of Elmer Jones[1], and Jacobson[2], and of others quoted or mentioned in the preceding chapter.

[1] In a description of the effect of chloroform upon himself, Elmer E. Jones mentions slight hyperæsthesias during the earlier stage : " The colours in the spectrum appear a little brighter, letters and figures somewhat clearer." Hearing was disturbed by roaring sounds. " All movements made appeared to be much longer . . . . and much slower than they actually were." With increased anæsthesia the strangeness of the modifications of consciousness increased also. Sounds appeared to come from nowhere and the intonations of well-known voices became unfamiliar. " At one stage of the experiment, when the foot was touched with the point of an instrument, it seemed so far away that the subject wondered if it were possible that his whole body was in a single room." The body seemed to be nowhere, " simply floating in space." It is a most ecstatic feeling."—*The Waning of Consciousness Under Chloroform*, *Psychol. Rev.*, vol. XVI, 1909, pp. 50-2.

[2] Edmund Jacobson, in his *Consciousness under Anæsthetics*, observed that, before sight was entirely eliminated, perspective disappeared ; his field of view became entirely flat. This might be expected to follow upon the impairment of the visual functions of accommodation and of convergence.—*Amer. Jr. of Psychol.*, vol. XXII, 1911, p. 334.

Similar disturbances have been observed in spontaneous trances. Unfortunately for us, the religious mystics were too little interested in exact descriptions, and too utterly fascinated by the unearthliness, the wonder, and the incomparable delights of their experiences, to provide satisfactory accounts of sensory perturbations. Here and there, however, we glean some information. Mlle Vé, for instance, observed that "the impression of the sequence of things, of time, disappeared[1]," and she mentions a number of unusual sensations and feelings. Suzo speaks of a "heavenly taste." Tennyson remarked that, in his artificially induced trances, time seemed no longer to exist, and several classical mystics mention levitation.

*   *   *

Photism.—Few of the lesser trance-phenomena are more striking and incontestably wholly physiological in origin than a peculiar appearance of light or brilliance which may be called *photism.* The word " light " is frequently used by the mystics, but it is not always possible to know whether they use it in a symbolical or in a realistic sense. In a great number of instances, however, the perceptual quality of the experience cannot be doubted.

Jonathan Edwards, the great New England metaphysician and third President of Princetown University, relates how, after his conversion crisis, " the appearance of all things was altered ; there seemed to be, as it were, a calm beautiful appearance of divine glory in almost everything : God's excellency, His wisdom, His purity and love seemed to appear in everything : in the sun, moon and stars ; in the water, in all nature, which used greatly to fix my mind[2]." Similarly, the Rev. J. O. Peck writes, also after a conversion crisis, " I have a fresh recollection that when I went in the morning . . . into the field to work, the glory of God appeared in all His visible creation. I well remember, we reaped oats, and every straw and head of the oats seemed, as it were, arrayed in a rainbow glory, if I may so express it, in the glory of God[3]."

When describing visions during ecstasy, St Theresa makes frequent use of similar brightness-terms. Of a vision of Christ she says : " The beauty of the whiteness of His hands surpasses entirely everything one could imagine " ; and, concerning a dove, " its wings seemed formed of scales of mother-of-pearl which threw off a vivid

[1] First Ecstasy.

[2] *The Conversion of President Jonathan Edwards*, published by the American Tract Society.

[3] From a sermon by the Rev. J. O. Peck, delivered in Brooklyn, October 21st, 1883.

splendour." At times she sees " flames." Suzo and several other mystics speak of perceiving brilliant lights.

There has come into my hands a particularly valuable instance of photism, that of a University teacher, a doctor in philosophy, free from the traditional religious preconceptions and in the habit of assuming a critical attitude in the presence of ecstatic phenomena. When about twenty-four years old he fell in love (at the time of the writing quoted below he was about thirty). It was not his first love affair, but never before had he been so deeply in love. He proposed marriage to the lady. Here we may quote from his letter :

" She said she liked me and permitted me to try and win her love. I spent most of the day in her company, but had to leave early in the evening as I had some fifteen miles to walk to catch a steamer that was to leave at five in the morning. The weather was fine and still, the moon was full or almost so, and my way lay through a most magnificent landscape. I had just had a fortnight of rest and was in perfect health and good training and enjoyed the walk as much as I had ever enjoyed one. I came very late to the little village, and went to bed at once. I slept very well for three or four hours till I was called at four o'clock in the morning. I got up at once, feeling fully reposed, and looked out of my window to see where the steamer was lying. Then it was as if the world had changed during the night : everything had become new and fresh, and I specially remember the garden of my hotel, the road under the mountain-side, the lake and the mountains, and above all the sun. It was as if it were the first time I saw real sunshine, everything I had seen before being pale and lifeless as compared to that sunshine. I thought I discovered the real life and beauty of the varied colours of the fields and meadows and mountain-slopes as they had never been discovered before. It seems to me now that I never doubted a moment that my new world was the real one, the old one being somehow defective though I remember asking myself on my way to the steamer whether the feeling of newness would last or not. It did last, not only that day, but the following days and weeks as well. For days and weeks I lived as in a dream, though I think I did my daily work rather better than worse than habitually. I slept only four or five hours every night for a long time, but never felt tired or sleepy—only my eyes ached a little just as they do when I have had too little sleep.

" I do not think I ever for a moment interpreted the change in the appearance of things as an objective change, though everything did look quite new. Neither did I interpret it in a religious way— I was and remained an atheist or agnostic."

This is doubtless the very phenomenon described by Jonathan Edwards, the Rev. J. O. Peck, and a host of others, who regarded it as a divine intervention : objects, apparently *all* visible objects, gain added brilliance and are perceived with peculiar delight.

Without venturing upon any suggestion regarding the physiological explanation of this phenomenon, we shall merely note that it appears as a sequel to profound dynamic disturbances affecting the very springs of life. The person last quoted remarks upon his " intense joy in life " and notes that for a long time after the birth of love he got along well with only four or five hours of sleep a day[1].

Increased delight, if not the hyperæsthesia, may appear in other fields than that of vision. After ecstasy Madeleine found that bread and water had a new, delicious flavour ; the very odours of the hospital were delightful[2]. Victor Robinson, in *An Essay on Hasheesh*, made similar observations : " In the morning [after taking twenty minims of cannabis indica] my capacity for happiness is considerably increased. I have an excellent appetite, the coffee I sip is nectar, and the white bread ambrosia. I take my camera and walk to Central Park. It is a glorious day. Everyone I meet is idealized. The lake never looked so placid before. I enter the hot-houses, and a gaudy-coloured insect buzzing among the lovely flowers fills me with joy[3]." The enthusiastic expressions of Weir Mitchell, when he

[1] There is literally no end to the number of instances of photism under great excitement, in ecstatic trances, and in certain specific disorders, such as epilepsy. The following references may interest the reader.
Myers, Gurney, and Podmore, *Phantasms of the Living*, vol. I, pp. 550-1.
The Welsh Revival, *Proc. Soc. for Psyc. Research*, vol. XIX, 1905, pp. 128, 139, 145-61.
P. Janet, *Névroses et Idées Fixes*, case of V. K., p. 98.
Interesting information may be found under "Glory" in Hasting's *Dictionary of the Bible*.
The burning bush of Moses, the Tongues of Flame at Pentecost, may have had their origin in photisms.

[2] Pierre Janet, *Une Extatique*, p. 230.
We have been told that at the beginning of recovery, in diseases characterized by a sudden turning point, an appearance of newness and an unusual delightful brightness of the visual field are sometimes observed.

[3] *Medical Review of Reviews*, New York, 1912, p. 73.
We do not intend to convey the impression that wonderful feelings may arise only in trance, *i.e.*, under obvious limitation and degradation of consciousness. Perhaps any unusually rapid metabolic change produces them. We recall the miracle worked in Tennyson by a mutton-chop eaten after a long meat-fast. Feelings of sexual origin contribute to the wonderfulness and ineffability of the experiences of many of the great Christian mystics. The feelings of unfathomable mystery with which the growing adolescent gazes upon himself and the world partakes of that double origin.
Sir Crichton-Browne observed that in many instances certain disturbances of consciousness, similar to those that have occupied us, " persisted only while cerebral and mental development was going on actively (during early adolescence) and vanished when maturity was attained."—*Cavendish Lecture, Lancet*, June 6th and 13th, 1895.

attempted to describe the pleasure given him by the mescal-visions, have already been quoted.

This phenomenon interests us here mainly as a sign of a more or less widespread modification of the nervous dynamism, a modification which may have important practical consequences. In some religious conversions, these alterations are durable enough to permit the establishment of new habits.

*   *   *

The impression of levitation.—We shall now see how, in three different circumstances (the impressions of levitation, of increased moral energy, and of illumination), the disappearance of ordinary feelings or the production of unusual feelings may become the starting point for convictions which may or may not correspond to reality.

We have seen that the entranced (whether under the effect of a drug or not) is at times under the impression that his body has lost weight and is being lifted above the earth, or that his soul has been liberated from the body and that he has become a pure spirit. In her description of rapture Santa Theresa wrote, " Often my body would become so light that it lost all weight ; at times this went so far that I [no longer felt the floor under my feet[1]." She was aware of the presence of forces that " lifted her up[2]." Suzo mentions the impression of " floating."

This impression may arise independently of any religious preconception. In our own experiments with ether and nitrous oxide, two of the subjects had the impression of levitation. Elmer Jones reports that when under the influence of chloroform, " with the disappearance of the tactile sense and hearing, the body has completely lost its orientation. It appears to be nowhere, simply floating in space. It is a most ecstatic feeling[3]."

The trance need not be very deep in order to produce this impression. Pratt quotes one of his correspondents as follows : " It is a singular feeling or sensation which comes to me when I pray, that while I pray I feel my body is lifted up from the floor and I feel light and floating, so to speak, in the air. Though my eyes are shut, I see objects far below and yet I feel my arms on my bed (as I usually kneel down beside the bed). . . . I feel no weight of body and my body becomes as light as a feather[4]."

[1] *Life*, XX, p. 226.
[2] *Ibid.*, XX, p. 218.
[3] *The Waning of Consciousness under Chloroform, Psychol. Rev.*, XVI, 1909, p. 52.
[4] Pratt, *loc. cit.*, p. 421-2

Lydiard H. Horton, in his observations upon relaxation naturally produced, reports that " of twenty subjects who retained consciousness after they had completely relaxed, eight experienced the illusion of levitation[1]."

This illusion has been studied in connexion with certain forms of insanity, and of psycho-physiological alterations which precede death. Piéron has reported four instances of death-bed impressions of levitation. The illusion often takes an elaborate form : the dying person thinks that he is being carried to heaven by angels ; others, presumably burdened with an evil conscience, are being dragged out of their beds by demons and resist with all their remaining energy[2]. In all these cases a benumbing of tactile sensations, and a decrease of the intensity of the sensations dependent upon the tonus of the voluntary muscles and of the vaso-motor system, constitute, most probably, the basis of the illusion.

Perturbations of sensations in themselves are, however, not sufficient to produce this illusion ; a general lowering of the mental level is, in addition, required. As a matter of fact, the loss of sensibility before death is accompanied by the beginning of a general *mental* breakdown, and both the use of narcotic drugs and the religious method of producing trance reduce mental life to a condition resembling that of partial sleep. In dreams we suffer similar illusions, for instance, the illusion of flying, and for similar reasons. When we are awake, various ideas contradicting the dream come to our mind, and we say that it was impossible. We realize that the body is heavier than air, that its weight cannot be overcome without adequate means ; and we have, moreover, fairly definite ideas about what would constitute adequate means of flying. But in dreams, when these ideas do not present themselves, we have no reason for rejecting as false the belief that we are flying. A thing can seem absurd only to a mind that perceives contradictions. When contradicting ideas are absent, either because the mental activity is reduced or for other reasons, then the impossible thing is necessarily accepted.

* * *

The impression of increased moral energy.—If the phenomena so far discussed in this chapter, marvellous as some of them may seem, have on the whole ceased to be regarded by educated persons

---

[1] *The Illusion of Levitation, J. of Abn. Psychol.*, XIII, 1918-9, p. 50. His method was to seat his subjects in easy chairs and to ask them to relax completely, as if to go to sleep. He ascribes the illusion (without sufficient reason, it seems to us) mainly to vaso-motor dilatation.

[2] H. Piéron, *Contribution à la Psychologie des Mourants, Rev. Philos.*, 1902, vol. LIV, pp. 615-6.

as in any especial sense divine manifestations, the accession in Christian mystical worship of moral strength, of increased courage, hope, and altruism, continues to be looked upon as a token of direct divine action. To-day it is upon facts of that class that the belief in ·a God-Providence mainly rests[1]. In this respect Mlle Vé's argument is typical: "In this divine contact, I gather strength, life, a sort of vivification of my moral being, all things which it seems to me can come only from a personal Being. I do not see how these forces could come from a blind energy."

In an effort to draw a distinction between mystical experiences which are divine and those which are not, a leader of contemporary religious mysticism writes similarly: "To the mystic himself the experience is evidence enough. It lights his lamp and girds his loins for action; it floods him with new power; it banishes doubt and despair as sunrise banishes darkness. He no more wants arguments now to prove God's existence· than the artist wants arguments to prove the reality of beauty, or the lover does to prove the worth of love . . . such experiences minister to life, construct personality, and conduce to the increased power of the race—energy to live by actually does come to them from somewhere[2]." We shall see in a later chapter that no less a philosopher than William James offered this same argument in support of the hypothesis that super-human powers intervene in ecstatic trance.

Nevertheless, we will venture the affirmation that a line of demarcation between influxes of moral energy which are from God, and those which have an ordinary, natural origin, has never been satisfactorily drawn. It would be useless to seek such a separation on the ground of the quality or of the persistence of the accrued energy. Regarding persistence of energy, it is well known that the ordinary worshipper, as also the great mystics, must return to God periodically to replenish energies scattered under the assault of the evil tendencies that are within or without him. As to quality, that

---

[1] See the XIth Chapter of *A Psychological Study of Religion*.

[2] Rufus Jones, *Studies in Mystical Religion*, preface, pp. xxix-xxx.
One of Pratt's correspondents remarks in a similar manner: "Under great spiritual uplift I have stopped and asked, is it possible that this intense feeling, this spiritual joy, is subjective? But I could not believe it possible to exteriorize the peculiar experience without a divine presence."—James B. Pratt, *loc. cit.*, p. 348.
Numerous instances of this conviction, similarly produced, have been provided earlier in this book. In a thesis (Henri Suzo, *Essai de Psychologie Descriptive*, Genéve, 1908), which probably reflects the teaching of the theological seminary of Montauban, Georges Barlement exclaims: "We declare them to be divine (the mystical phenomena) when they impose themselves upon us with the kind of superior authority we are compelled to call divine, when they uphold the individual and increase the power of action.".

depends upon the purpose of the man himself. A glass of wine may exalt the exalted and debase the base. Accretion of strength from any source, be it a mutton-chop or the stimulation of the self-affirmation or of the sex-instincts, may, according to the dominant tendencies of the person, be directed to noble or ignoble ends.

The argument that would find, in sudden intellectual and moral exaltation, a proof of the action of a God-Providence should be considered in connexion with facts already sufficiently set forth in this book and with others that are or might be familiar to everyone. In the chapter on drug-mysticism we saw how, in the very infancy of the race, men learned by means of narcotics to secure a sudden increase of well-being, of hope, of happiness ; and how they returned thanks to the gods for those blessings. In subsequent chapters we learned how, finding it necessary to relinquish the drug-method, men discovered other means of procuring that which drugs had given them. With regard to narcotics, it will be sufficient here to repeat that if certain drugs are considered divine, it is largely because of the impression of liberation, of power, and of happiness which they bring. In *Braves Gens*, Richepin, that keen observer of human nature, speaks of occasional drunken bouts as " good baths of forgetfulness out of which one arises done up (*moulu*) and yet renewed (*retrempé*) ; a great purge of alcohol which scours, as with fire, body and soul[1]."

Neither drugs nor mystical experiences are necessary in order to purge the soul of at least a part of its burdens. A young man told us how on a certain occasion he had been obsessed and made miserable by sex-desires and how, much to his surprise, he found himself free from the temptation on leaving a theatre where he had been deeply moved. The setting-up of nervous activity in other channels had side-tracked or drained off the sex-impulse. In a comparable way, cupping relieves a congested region of the body by drawing the blood where it does no harm.

Fear of the trivial should not induce one to avoid, in this connexion, the mention of coffee, of tea, of a hot bath, and of other commonplace means of physical and moral refreshment. Nothing is trivial which alters so radically mood and outlook as a cup of tea sometimes does. There are neuropathic persons who describe their transformation after a cup of tea in terms which fall little short of those fittingly used to characterize the effects of a religious ecstasy. A hot bath improves not only the general well-being but also the moral

---

[1] Jean Richepin, *Braves Gens*, Select Collection, Flammarion, p. 24.

On the moral effects of alcohol, see G. E. Partridge, *Studies in the Psychology of Intemperance*, New York, 1912.

attitude : restlessness, mental dispersion, irritability, malevolence, pessimism, may vanish and be replaced by peace, mental unification, benevolence, optimism. These changes follow upon the removal of a mass of unpleasant sensations—some of them from the skin, others from contractions and tensions in the external muscles and in the viscera. There can be no peace, no contentment, no generosity, while one is submitted to a hundred and one pin-pricks.

Simple (non-mystical) trance or healthy sleep may work like an effective hot bath. The mystical trance itself often ends in a peaceful, sleep-like state from which the mystic awakens as he might from an ordinary sleep, physically and morally refreshed.

Persons subject to more or less periodic fits of anger feel, in the intervals, as if causes of anger were accumulating. They become increasingly restless, cantankerous, and generally intolerable, until the fit breaks out and they are relieved ; then, life is resumed in peace and hopefulness. It is customary in this last class of experience to ascribe the beneficial results to a belief that " justice has been done, judgment executed, the truth spoken, the basis for new and better understanding laid, etc.[1]" These and similar ideas doubtless exert a considerable influence, but they are not the primary cause of the happy mental change. In their absence the person would still enjoy some relief ; his feelings and his moral disposition would still be improved. We do not know what it is that accumulates in the interval between the fits, but here, just as in the case of the restless, discontented condition from which a person might be relieved by a hot bath, the fit of anger removes the primary cause of the abnormal condition.

A similar remark may be made in connexion with a class of facts illustrated by one of Morton Prince's patients, who, on coming out of the hypnotic sleep, exclaimed : " Something has happened to me. I have a new point of view. I don't know what has changed me all at once ; it is as if scales had fallen from my eyes ; I see things differently. . . . You have given me life and you have given me something to fill it with[2]." Credit for the changed outlook upon life and the return of happiness might be due to suggestions made by the hypnotizer. We must hold, however, that even in the absence of any suggestion a trance *may* work physiological changes which bring about the impression and the moral attitude described by Prince's

---

[1] G. S. Hall, *A Study of Anger, Amer. Jr. of Psychol.*, vol. X, 1899, p. 572.

[2] *The Unconscious, Jr. of Abnor. Psychol.*, 1909. For instances of increased, enlarged life, see also " The Dissociation of a Personality," chap. XXI, pp. 334, ff., and Appendix L and R.—especially the latter part of R. Also, Boris Sidis, *Studies in Psychopathology*, pp. 62-6.

patient. In support of this affirmation we refer to the instances already given where suggestion in any form is out of the question.

The rôle of love, in which organic and psychical factors combine to vivify and transform one's outlook upon life, should be recalled in this connexion. The reader will remember the instances of Nadia, of the University teacher, and in particular of Madame Guyon[1].

In the different classes of experience to which we have now referred, sources of energy are liberated, either by the removal of disturbing, inhibitory factors of trivial origin, or in connexion with the stimulation of the self-affirmation or of the sex-instincts, or yet otherwise. This energy, for a while at least, lifts man up above his usual level of courage, optimism, benevolence and happiness. In some of these experiences the vivification has no psychical cause. In others, mental causes are obviously present, but even then physiological forces,—those forces that achieve the purging in alcohol drunkenness, in irrational fits of anger, in a hot bath, etc.—frequently play a rôle whose magnitude is rarely suspected.

In the Christian mystical experiences the mental factors enhancing life are aroused mainly by the belief in the intervention of divine beings: God, Christ, the Holy Virgin, the Saints. We have endeavoured to show in another chapter how these experiences gain vastly in significance and in value through that belief, quite independently of its objective validity.

There remain to be considered certain phenomena particularly potent in the production of the impression of ineffable revelation.

*   *   *

Other roots of the conviction of ineffable revelation.—The real solution by so-called "inspiration" of definite problems has already engaged our attention. We are now concerned with a very different phenomenon, abundantly illustrated in the preceding pages and singularly interesting both to the psychologist and to the theologian, namely the assurance of *ineffable* revelation. Jonathan Edwards, whom we have already quoted in connexion with photism, provides a remarkable instance of an anguishing question which suddenly lost its power to disturb, as if by the discovery of a solution formulable in conceptual terms.

"From my childhood up," wrote Edwards, "my mind was full of objections against the doctrine of God's Sovereignty, in choosing whom He would to eternal life, and rejecting whom He pleased; leaving them eternally to perish and be everlastingly tormented in

---

[1] See in Janet's *Médications Psychologiques*, vol. III, p. 168, interesting information regarding the sthenic effect upon neurasthenic or psychasthenic persons of marriage engagement and of love.

hell. It used to appear like a horrible doctrine to me. But I remember the time very well when I seemed to be convinced and fully satisfied as to this Sovereignty of God, and His justice in thus eternally disposing of men, according to His Sovereign pleasure. But I never could give an account how, or by what means, I was thus convinced, not in the least imagining at the time, nor a long time after, that there was any extraordinary influence of God's Spirit in it[1]."

Here is a second illustration of the same phenomenon: A theological student had heard a paper on the authorship of the Gospel of John, in which the writer had come to the conclusion that St John was not the author of the Gospel bearing his name. This information set loose a storm in the student: " For three days the wild tide swept and surged past and around me. I felt I must give up the Gospel of John and, if so, my Christian faith also ; and with this the universe would go. . . . I yielded myself to what I conceived to be Higher Guidance. . . . At the close of the period I found myself at one with all things, Peace, that was all. . . . When I looked at myself, I found that I was standing on the old ground, but cherishing a toleration of doubt and a sincere sympathy with doubters such as I had never known before. I could take the logical standpoint, and could see that they (the arguments) were quite convincing, and yet my inward peace of belief was in no way disturbed[2]."

One could not be more categorical : the logical arguments that had prevented belief remain unweakened, and yet they now leave him indifferent. As for Edwards, although he knew of no logical reason for the change, he found himself accepting a doctrine which until then had seemed abhorrent. Later, he concluded that it was the effect of an extraordinary action of God's spirit[3].

[1] *The Conversion of President Jonathan Edwards.*

[2] Privately communicated.

[3] A similar experience happened to a prominent Ritschlian theologian : " I came into the presence of the traditions of the Church. These seemed strange. They belonged to a past age. I found a protest arising within myself at the very thought of believing the supernatural account of things. Then, something happened. The words which had been said to me were transformed into living power ; their complexity was changed to simplicity. I did not bring this about myself, and no man was the cause of it. The will of God in His omnipotence penetrated into my heart."—R. Seeberg, *Zur Systematischen Theologie*, as quoted by G. B. Smith, in *Amer. Jr. of Theology*, 1909, p. 96.

Cardinal Newman was familiar with and welcomed these irrational convictions : " I have never been able to see a connexion between apprehending those difficulties (of the Christian Doctrines), however keenly, and multiplying them to any extent, and on the other hand doubting the doctrines to which they are attached." *Apologia*, new ed., 1904, p. 148.

Amazing as these facts may seem, they are in their essence commonplace enough. Have we not all, at times, noticed in ourselves a difficulty or an inability to be rational? This disquieting phenomenon is particularly in evidence when desires are intense and emotions run high. It then becomes impossible to ascribe to arguments contrary to our desires the weight belonging to them; they may even be completely disregarded. Why should it be otherwise? The mere recognition of logical consistency has no efficacy; abstract truth has in itself no driving power. It derives whatever influence it exerts from its agreement with desires. Truth is powerful in the measure in which it agrees with things loved, or disagrees with things hated. It may possess the power of habit; but the habit of being swayed by truth has itself become established in society because of a more or less clear perception of the relation of truth to the ultimate realization of desire.

The experiences of Edwards and of the theological student are striking examples of the ordinary action of overpowering desires and attraction. Both these men had just passed through a conversion crisis. The photisms experienced by Edwards indicate how profound the physiological disturbance had been. Both ascribed the event to God and interpreted it as a loving manifestation of his Power. They felt themselves as clay in the hands of the Divine Potter, his to use as he pleased. Under these circumstances, it was not possible for arguments against the Almighty and his Revelation in the Bible to obtain a fair hearing. Love and criticism are in the main incompatible; and when the object of one's devotion is the Creator of heaven and earth, actually made present to one's heart and mind in a wonderful experience, what logic may urge against his existence or his Revelation ceases to matter. The logic of the argument against hell-torments or against the Johannine authorship of the fourth Gospel may still be recognized as good logic, but the tendencies or desires it would antagonize are now too strong: the truth can no longer arouse fear or apprehension. "The inward peace of belief is," as the student says, "in no way disturbed."

But disregard of logical truth and assurance in that which they wished to believe had, in these instances, still another origin. God had been made present to these persons in a wonderful way; they had "felt" him just as convincingly as if they had touched him. This particular "sense of presence" will form the subject of special consideration. At this point we shall simply remark that after an experience such as theirs, while one may continue to recognize the truth of an argument proving that God does not exist and while one may even wish that he should not exist, conviction of his existence cannot be shaken, for one is now in the presence not merely of an abstract argument but of what seems a concrete, perceived reality : God has been experienced. The only thing that could have destroyed the conviction of Edwards and of the student would have been an adequate appreciation of the existence of causes able to produce an illusory " sense of presence," and of the inhibiting influence of intense desire upon antagonistic logical arguments.

The term " revelation " is almost aptly used when applied to the experience we have described, for in it an intimacy, a sympathy, an *understanding*, are established between God and the worshipper. Now he sees his way, he knows what to do. When one sees or knows, without having gone through the cogitations that ordinarily precede knowledge, how is one to avoid believing in a superhuman illumination ? The alterations of conduct and the transformations of character which, at times, follow upon crises such as those just reported, may also be spoken of, without greater looseness in the use of words than is generally permitted, as the outcome of a revelation.

The case of Mrs. Pa., already reported, is similar to the preceding. On a beautiful spring morning, she awakened from a restful sleep and recalled Drummond's words about the presence of God in all things. That idea came to her with a new, marvellous meaning ; she saw or felt the divine Presence all about her. Her own self and the universe were transformed : faith and courage replaced, discouragement and pessimism. We have found reason to ascribe this illumination in large part to a non-rational process such as that which took place in Janet's patient when she saw everything transformed—a process not very different from love at first sight.

Photism particularly tempts one to the use of the term " illumination." Does not the world appear illumined ? Do not things stand, as it were, revealed in an unwonted light ? And yet, nothing is given in a conceptual form ; the revelation is ineffable.

*   *   *

There remains at least one other important root of the belief in unutterable divine revelation, quite different from those so far considered. It has already come to light in many of the descriptive passages of this book. Trance frequently generates feelings and emotions described as " exalted," " grand," " stupendous," and the like. We recall the " *sensations sublimes et solennelles* " of certain neurasthenics, as well as of normal persons, when in the presence of fairly commonplace scenery. Of his experience with nitrous oxide gas, Sir Humphrey Davy says : " My emotions were enthusiastic and sublime[1]." This effect has been observed by many not only with nitrous oxide, but with other narcotic drugs, notably with opium by de Quincey.

Similar feelings and emotions are not of very rare occurrence in the dreams of ordinary sleep. Masefield writes of a dream: " Words in it had seemed revelations, acts in it, adventures, romances; but judged by the waking mind, it was unintelligible, though holy like a mass in an unknown tongue[2]." Words to the same purport are used by scientific experimenters to describe their impressions during the drowsy state which precedes sleep.

Careful observations of the drowsiness preceding ordinary sleep have not been numerous or very thorough, but, such as they are, they indicate that the normal near-sleep condition involves the production of mental alterations similar to those characteristic of the early stage of abnormal and artificial trances. Imagination, relieved of the shackles imposed upon it by perception and by logical requirements, weaves, under the spur of external and internal impressions and of desire, fantastic pictures and non-logical trains of thought. The relative freedom of the mind from external direction and from rational guidance, favours the production of impressions of weird " otherness," and of " feelings of exuberance, buoyancy, confidence, and eager enthusiasm." In many instances " when a chain of reasoning is involved, all projects are [seem] fertile and all outcome expansive . . . The drowsiness experienced in the case of the present observers at least, resembles that following upon the inhalation of diluted nitrous oxide gas,' the mental symptoms consist in convictions of emancipation, relief, and happiness, in grand and sublime ideas which in their expansion seem to break down all barriers of doubt and difficulty[3] '."

Even a conviction of revelation may appear in ordinary drowsiness. In *Le Subconscient Normal*, Abramowski, speaking of his own observations before sleep, says : " In that state one gets at a certain juncture the impression that something important has happened ; one wakes up and feels very distinctly that a thought has taken place (*une pensée vient de s'accomplir*). That thought seems usually of great value and of a special interest : at times it seems almost a revelation. When I endeavour to get hold of that thought,

---

[1] *Lancet*, June 6th and 13th, 1895.

[2] John Masefield, *Multitude and Solitude*, London, 1909, p. 44. Compare this with the quotation from de Quincey, p. 20, of this book.

[3] H. L. Hollingworth, *The Psychology of Drowsiness : an Introspective and Analytical Study*, Amer. J. of Psychol., XXII, 1911, pp. 109, 111. The inner quotation is taken from the lecture of Crichton-Browne mentioned above.

I discover that I know nothing about it ; I find it impossible to put it down in words, even fragmentarily ; and, at the same time, I still feel an affective trace, very distinct, of its passage[1]."

If we seek to understand that which takes place in a simple partial trance produced by the repetition of a name, we find that the word soon ceases to bring up any of the ideas, images, or other references to which it owes its meaning. Dissociations have set in, and the mind remains on the sign, *i.e.*, on the visual appearance of the letters, instead of passing to the things signified. Consequently, the word appears as an unfamiliar thing ; it is no longer apprehended, it has become meaningless ; or rather, we should say that it has acquired a new, weird, puzzling, not-to-be-formulated feeling-significance[2].

But why should the feeling or emotion suggest in this case that something "important," "of great value," has taken place and, in other instances, that there has been a wonderful discovery, an "ineffable revelation"? Before proceeding further, we are to observe that a feeling or an emotion cannot in its own right be great, noble, or sublime. The emotions that come to be called "great" or "noble" are those arising normally in connexion with great or noble purposes or achievements.

The cause of noble or great emotion which first suggests itself, and the only one which may seem possible to the unsophisticated in matter psychological, is that, somehow or other, they are the accompaniment of great or noble achievements, thought of or actually realized, even though it should be impossible to tell what the achievements are. There are, however, other possibilities :

1. Feelings and emotions may take place without any mental cause, *i.e.*, may result from a purely physiological activity. We have already had occasion to record certain remarkable affective and emotional conseqences of brain-storms. There are prodromes of epilepsy which include "sublime" emotional states ; and there are other conditions, such as that of morbid anxiety, of pathological anger, etc., which are marked by emotions of a definite quality—this quite independently of any intellectual cause. There exists,

---

[1] Edouard Abramowski, *Le Subconscient Normal*, Paris, 1914, p. 201. Comp. Tennyson's trance induced by repeating his name.

[2] Comp. Abramowski, *Le Subconscient Normal*, p. 201, and the following from Wm Hocking : "' *Ineffableness* ' in mystical experience is largely if not completely due to the fact of disconnexion alone, not to any inherent mysteriousness or unnaturalness in the content of experience. Psychologically mystery is felt whenever there are two bodies of experience not in perfect communication, quite apart from the question whether the one or the other is inherently wonderful or weird."—*God in Human Experience*, p. 398.

however, much more commonplace illustrations of this phenomenon. A person who has dined well does not owe his good-nature and magnanimity, his increased self-confidence and optimism, to new knowledge or understanding. Alcohol and food produce these effects directly through their action upon the body. Music also may determine, directly, fairly well characterized emotional states.

2. Great or noble emotions may have as primary cause mere alterations of sensibility *which are interpreted* as signifying something great or noble. We have, for instance, been led to regard certain sensory perturbations as responsible for the impression of levitation. When that impression leads to the thought of the independence of the spirit from the body and to the various sacred beliefs commonly connected with that conception, noble and sublime emotions will be generated. Similarly, as in the instance of Jonathan Edwards, photisms suggest "God's excellency, His wisdom, His purity and love." The interpretation of any or of all the phenomena of ecstatic trance as divine manifestations, is obviously, among the religious mystics, the more general cause of the production of "exalted" emotions.

Emotions generated in this manner do not indicate the production during the trance of any remarkable understanding or revelatory conception, or any other stupendous achievement. They result from disordered sensibility interpreted in a naïve manner general among the non-civilized and civilized.

3. The primary cause of the kind of emotion with which we are concerned might actually be great or noble deeds, purposes, or thoughts ; for instance, the comprehension of mysteries beyond the grasp of the unaided human mind, or the disclosure of some divine purpose regarding the subject himself. The inability of the experiencer to clothe in conceptual form the achievement claimed by him would be no sufficient reason for disbelieving him. For it is well known that on awakening from ether-sleep or artificial trance nothing at all may remain in consciousness of a mental activity that has actually taken place. In other instances nothing persists after awakening except an emotional condition and dominant tendencies.

It happens, for instance, that we wake up from an ordinary sleep shaken by a more or less definite affective disturbance, the cause of which escapes us. Presently, however, we recall a dream which, because of its nature, we take as the undoubted cause of the lingering emotion. Proof of the dissociation of an emotion from its conceptual cause or object may be given experimentally. If a scene charged with emotional significance be described to a hypnotized person and the suggestion made that on awakening he will not remember the scene, the subject, on coming to himself, may feel the emotion although its cause cannot be recalled.

In his protracted study of Miss Beauchamp, Morton Prince has more than once had occasion to observe the survival of feelings and emotions when the ideas which had called them forth had disappeared. Once, on awakening from an ecstasy in a church, Miss Beauchamp found herself in the enjoyment of feelings of " lightness of body, of physical restfulness, and well-being, besides those of exaltation, joyousness and peace." Morton Prince was able to ascertain that these feelings and emotions were not due to any mysterious sub-conscious incubation and maturation of motives, " it was simply that the emotions of the trance-state persisted after waking as a state of exaltation[1]."

The persistence of feelings and emotions, after their causes have been partly or entirely forgotten, is a frequent phenomenon of everyday life. Tom, a talkative imbecile, will tell you with great enthusiasm that he has had a perfectly splendid dinner ; but if you ask him what he has eaten, he becomes speechless[2]. The pleasant feeling is still there or is reawakened by the mention of dinner, but he is unable to think of anything that was on the table. It is not necessary to be mentally deficient in order to find oneself in Tom's predicament. Psychology has set it down that emotions not only may continue but also probably may reappear in consciousness after an interruption, without being accompanied by the intellectual contents with which they originally came into consciousness. The Freudian and the medical literature dealing with war-neuroses contains numerous and striking illustrations of this fact.

* * *

We are now prepared to return to the problem as it appears to the religious mystics. They affirm that, even though they cannot formulate it adequately, divine knowledge comes to them during the ecstasies and determines the emotional and volitional changes of which they are aware on returning to their senses. That belief in an ineffable intellectual revelation cannot be accepted unless its truth be demonstrated by something more objective than the mystic's own conviction, for we have just found out that the trance-experience is rich in phenomena able to produce the illusion of transcendent revelation.

[1] Morton Prince, *The Dissociation of Personality*, Longmans, Green and Co., 1913, p. 352. For a full understanding of this illustration, see the whole chapter. It may be remarked that the feelings and emotions named above might have been produced easily enough, in a person of changeable moods, as the direct consequence of a restful trance.

[2] Henry Goddard, *Psychology of the Normal and Subnormal*, p. 162.

Since the alleged revelation cannot be adequately expressed verbally, and since mere assurance is no proof of truth, the one remaining basis of proof is the behaviour of the subject after the revelation. He might be so altered in character and temperament as to compel the admission of superhuman action. But nothing that has happened to the mystics with whom we are acquainted goes beyond alterations and transformations referable to known natural causes, physical and psychical. In this connexion, the influence of *belief* in divine intervention must not be overlooked. The scope of this factor has been sufficiently indicated in the preceding pages.

Scepticism as to revelation grows into complete disbelief when we learn that under conditions realized in the ecstatic trance (whether artificial or not) insignificant and even absurd ideas may take on the appearance of intellectual greatness. The setting forth of that fact will constitute the final part of our demonstration of the illusory nature of the impression of intellectual revelation in mystical trance.

Jacobson, who intended to make whatever observations he might while under nitrous oxide gas, exclaimed, according to the record made at the time : " I have made a discovery ; I have made a discovery ! The secondary consciousness . . ." Here is his own statement made after return to normal consciousness : " It seemed as if I had said, ' the secondary consciousness is the primary consciousness,' and I intended to go on and say that the same *I* was present in both, . . . but I ceased, owing to the difficulty of putting the matter into words and owing to the lack of strength." The persons present stated that he had stopped after saying " the secondary consciousness." He had apparently, at the time or subsequently, merely thought the rest. He was furthermore under the impression that, as he was observing the dwindling away of consciousness, this thought had been in his mind : " Your personality must be psychological at its core, if you think of such things at this moment[1]." Now the persistency of the idea of the self, when the external world and even the body have disappeared or are on the point of vanishing, has no transcendent significance ; and the thought that personality must be psychological at its core is, under the circumstances, commonplace enough not to deserve any attention. And yet, while under nitrous oxide, Jacobson thought that he had made a great discovery.

Sir Humphrey Davy, who reported his own emotions as " enthusiastic and sublime," was also under the impression that he had made remarkable discoveries : " I endeavoured," says he, " to communicate the discoveries made during the experiment, but my

[1] Edmund Jacobson, *Amer. Jr. of Psychol.*, XXII, 1911, 335-6.

ideas were feeble and indistinct; one collection of terms presented itself, and with the most intense belief and prophetic manner I exclaimed ' nothing exists but thought, the universe is composed of impressions, ideas, pleasures and pains[1] '." This is not very different from the " discovery " made by Jacobsen, by Dunbar[2], and by many another.

In our own experiments with ether and nitrous oxide three out of four subjects made similar observations. As the loss of bodily control and of sensations from the body proceeded, one of them had a " superior feeling " that it would astonish people when she should tell them, later, that " the will is after all a separate entity." Two of the subjects were impressed by the enduring reality of the self in the presence of the vanishing organism. The last or one of the last thoughts of one of them was that " the ego is a definite and indestructible unity." Professor Hill, experimenting with chloroform and ether, observed that he never was more curiously aware of " the one indubitable fact—the consciousness of self-hood[3]."

When one considers that there is probably no idea more central, more deeply implanted in us than that of the self, and that, in trance, the obfuscation or disappearance of the physical world and of the body makes the idea of the self stand out by isolating it, the persistence of the impressions just reported ceases to surprise.

The reader may recall how Symonds, a disbeliever in divine intervention, was also occupied, in his trances, by the idea of the self; but it was the wonderful alterations it suffered and the fear of its extinction which held his attention.

Sir Humphrey Davy makes the significant remark that, in respect to the persons with whom he experimented, persons of intellectual training and distinction, " the thoughts are in nine cases out of ten connected with some great discovery, some supposed

---

[1] As reported by Sir Crichton-Browne, *Lancet, loc. cit.*

[2] Dunbar, in *The Light thrown on Psychological Processes by the Action of Drugs*, writes: " My own experience under ether I shall never forget. . . . In my mind thought seemed to race like a mill-wheel. Nothing was lost— every trifling phenomenon seemed to fall into its place as a logical event in the Universe. As in Sir William Ramsey's experience, everything seemed so absolute. It was either yes or no. Either this was reality or it was not . . . If it was not, then it seemed to me in the nature of things that I could never know reality. Then it dawned upon me that the only logical position was subjective idealism, and, therefore, *my* experience must be reality. Then by degrees I began to realize that I was the One and the universe of which I was the principle was balancing itself into completeness. All thought seemed struggling to a logical conclusion; every trifling movement in the world outside my consciousness represented perfectly logical steps in the final readjustment."—*Proc. Soc. Psychol. Research*, 1905, XIX, pp. 73-4.

[3] *Of the Loss and Recovery of Consciousness under Anæsthesia, Psychol. Bull.*, VII, 1910, p. 79.

solution of a cosmic secret," while in humdrum people the feelings, though pleasant, are "in no way remarkable." He might have added that the alleged discovery relates usually to a problem with which the person has been concerned. An anæsthetized patient interpreted the "peculiar thoughts," which he endeavoured in vain to formulate, as containing the explanation of his puzzling malady[1]. Awake from the "meaningless" dream already mentioned, John Masefield, full of unsatisfied yearnings for the dead Ottalie, "feels that he had apprehended spiritually the mysterious life beyond ours, and had learned, finally, forever, that Ottalie's soul was linked to his soul by bonds forged by powers greater than his[2]."

It is at times possible to observe somewhat minutely the defective mental processes responsible in trance for false or inadequate solutions. Among the dreams observed before complete sleep, Hollingworth reports one of especial interest in this connexion. H., the observer, was in bed with "grippe," tossing from side to back, then to the other side. His report is as follows: "As I tossed, the numbers 50, 2, 36, kept running in my head, appearing clearly visually as 5236, and auditorially as 'fifty-two—thirty-six.' Now these (50, 2, 36), were the combination numbers of my gymnasium locker which I opened by turning the knob left-right-left-right, four turns, very much as I now tossed in bed. In my tossing the numbers rang and rang in my head, the left side seeming 52, the right side 36, the back 5236. It seemed that if I could juggle these numbers into the right combination I could find a comfortable position[3]."

In this dream, H. was vaguely aware that certain numbers and turning movements were involved in the solution of a problem. But neither the exact nature of the problem (opening a locker), nor the nature of the necessary turning movements (turning a key in a lock), was clearly present to his drowsy mind. In the absence of these correct ideas, the "felt" potency of the numbers became connected with the attempt to relieve a general discomfort by changing the position of the body. The numbers and the actual problem of finding bodily relief became connected not because of any logical relation. They were probably related by a common feeling: the unpleasantness of failing readily to open the box, and now the unpleasantness of failing to find ease of body. A fully awake mind would have rejected that thought as irrelevant.

If, in this instance, the conviction of a solution was not formed, it was probably because the discomfort continued until the dreamer woke up entirely or fell asleep completely. Had a solution come, it would probably not have been accompanied by a sense of sublimity, for there was nothing in the problem itself that could have suggested, even to an uncritical mind, a great achievement; the weird, mysterious feelings commonly present in trances produced by narcotics were apparently lacking.

*   *   *

The causes of the impression of mystical revelation may be partly summarized as follows: In the condition of diminished and degraded mental activity characteristic of trance, certain sensations, or the disappearance of certain sensations, certain feelings and certain emotions—which in certain instances have a purely physiological origin—may give rise to the thought of a great achievement.

[1] *Of the Loss and Recovery of Consciousness under Anæsthesia, Psychol. Bull.*, VII, 1910, p. 79.

[2] *Multitude and Solitude*, p. 51.

[3] *The Psychology of Drowsiness, Amer. Jr. of Psychol.*, XXII, 1911, p. 102.

We refer in particular to the feelings of " extension," of " inflation," and of " enlargement," mentioned by some observers, the hyper-æsthesias best illustrated by photism, the loss of skin and of other sensations resulting in the impression of levitation, and certain emotional experiences called "emotions of greatness," "of sublimity," and the like.

These sensations, feelings and emotions may, and at times do, suggest ideas of things exalted or marvellous, as in the case of the idea of levitation; or they may give rise to the idea that great problems have received a solution. Regarding this last occurrence two things may happen : (1) A great problem is present to the mind but is not solved. Nevertheless the feelings and emotions determined by the problem itself, or present independently of the problem, are taken by the disorganized mind as signifying the adequate solution of the problem. (2) A solution is actually found acceptable to the entranced, but it is discovered by the fully awake mind to be woefully inadequate. It proves to be a solution such as come to all in the dreams of sleep, or in any other trance-state.

Of an adequate solution of a great problem, forgotten on awakening, no satisfactory evidence has come to our knowledge.

The conviction is, therefore, forced upon us that we are here in the presence of one of the most widespread, tenacious, and potent of the many illusions to which man is subject.

*　　　*　　　*

The clearness and certainty of ineffable revelation.—The attention of the reader has probably been caught by the insistency with which the terms *clearness* and *certainty* recur in connexion with ineffable trance revelation. There is something puzzling in the connexion of unusual clearness with something baffling expression. It will be useful to preface the brief remarks we wish to make on this subject by bringing together a few of the illustrations scattered throughout this book.

During a nitrous oxide trance Sir Humphrey Davy attempted to communicate a discovery he thought he had made : " One collection of terms," he wrote, " presented itself, and with the *most intense belief* and prophetic manner, I explained that nothing exists but thought."

In our own experiments with ether, one of the subjects reported her discovery thus : " With *perfect lucidity* the thought came to me that the anti-introspectionists (the behaviourists) had never seen things as I was seeing them now. . . . It was so plain, I could examine minutely thoughts passing in review before me, etc."

Dr Weir Mitchell, after taking mescal, had " a certain sense " of the things about him as " *having a more positive existence than* *usual*[1] " ; and Hollingworth in his description of drowsiness states that " in the drowsy state, as in dream-life, images seem to *exceed by far in intensity the clearest images of the waking state.*" Tennyson, in trances induced by repeating his own name, felt that " the individuality itself seemed to dissolve and fade into boundless being, and this not a confused state, but the *clearest of the clearest, the surest of the surest* . . . utterly beyond words.*" Lowell " inspired," late one evening, " spoke with the calmness and *clearness of a prophet.*" Nevertheless, his philosophical constructions never saw the light of day. Madeleine understood with *absolute clearness and certainty* a variety of mysteries among them those of the Trinity and of the Immaculate Conception[2].

If in these descriptions the term " clearness " is used as involving exact, detailed, and complete perception or understanding, we would say that it is misused. In trance, the impression of exactness and fullness of perception or understanding is usually an illusion. The best observers among the Christian mystics have noticed this, even though they have not been able to understand its full significance. Santa Theresa discovered with surprise that she could not gratify the desire of her friends who wished to know the colour of the eyes of Christ. All her efforts to see served merely " to cause the vision to disappear." She made a similar observation on the occasion of a brilliant vision of the Virgin : " I was not able to note anything particular in the face of the Holy Virgin ; I saw merely in general that it was admirably beautiful[3]."

The same thing is true of the visions of the pre-sleep state. Bernard Leroy reports this interesting observation : " When I was studying anatomy, I was fairly frequently subject to an hypnagogic hallucination familiar, I believe, to medical students. While in my bed, the eyes closed, I would see, with great definiteness and a perfect sense of objectivity, the anatomical preparation with which I had been occupied during the day : the likeness was exact, the impression of reality and, if I may express myself thus, of intense life which emanated from it, was perhaps more intense than if I had been in the presence of a real object. It seemed to me also that all the details, each artery, vein, muscle insertion, all the various features which during waking life I had so much trouble to remember and to recall visually, were there before my eyes. . . . This hallucination

---

[1] Fernberger, in *Observations on Taking Peyote, Amer. Jr. of Psychol.*, XXXIV, 1923, pp. 269-70, was very much struck by the clearness—not the intensity—of the kinæsthetic and of other sensations.

[2] P. Janet, *Une Extatique*, p. 234.

[3] *Autobiography*, chap. XXXIII, p. 426.

having taken place many times, I was able to come to a definite opinion about it. Already at the second or third repetition, I gained the certainty that the abundance of details, the wealth of the vision, was merely an illusion. Despite the first impression, the hallucination included much less details than do the voluntary recalled images of the waking life[1]."

This illusion of completeness of detail—usually called clearness —takes place not only in the mental life of trance but also, in certain persons at least, in the ordinary waking life. There are persons who think that the recall of what they have seen is as clear as their actual perceptions. And yet, if such a person be requested, for instance, to describe in detail his mental picture of a building, or merely to count the windows in it, he will usually find the task impossible.

The peculiar clearness of the conceptions or perceptions in trance depends not upon fulness of detail but upon simplicity, isolation, and intensity. The simpler and the more isolated a thing is, the more clearly it is seen. Great intensity of stimulus is not necessary to clear perception ; yet, up to a maximal limit, increased intensity produces increased clearness.

The first two of these conditions of clearness, and often also the third, are in trance realized in an unusual measure. The reduction and degradation of the mental life simplifies and isolates the objects of thought ; and the benumbing of the higher (the " intellectual ") centres, tends probably, at a certain stage of the trance, to increase the intensity of the sensational and affective processes.

Regarding the dependence of certainty upon clearness, it is to be said that clearness is not the only condition of certainty : a proposition that is or seems perfectly clear may be or seem contradicted by another equally clear. Yet clearness makes for assurance, and it is no doubt because of this relation that these two terms are so frequently found together in the affirmations of the mystics.

---

[1] Bernard Leroy, *La Nature des Hallucinations, Rev. Philos.*, vol. LXIII, 1907, pp. 605-6.

In a remarkable article upon " *Visions Intellectuelles*," the same author treats briefly of the ineffable revelation which he includes as one of three classes of " intellectual visions." The illusion of understanding is produced, according to him, when certain " intellectual sentiments " which normally accompany every intellectual activity, are produced in the absence of that activity. The illusion depends upon a mechanism similar to the one by means of which he has accounted, in an earlier article, for the illusion of having-already-seen something which in reality has never been seen.

This suggestion, valuable though it is, cannot be regarded as exhausting the explanation of the phenomenon.—" Interprétation Psychologique des ' Visions Intellectuelles ' chez les Mystiques Chrétiens," *Rev. de l'Histoire des Religions*, vol. LV, 1907, pp. 1-50. See pp. 17-25.

The conditions of clearness set forth above are also conditions of assurance. Mental simplification, by eliminating contradictions or complexities that might be the occasion of doubt, tends to produce assurance as to what remains in consciousness. With only one simple idea in mind, uncertainty about it would betoken a pathological condition. But the downrightness, the cocksureness, of certain drug-intoxications, of alcohol[1] for instance, is not due to a mental simplification only ; it is in part the outcome of an increased intensity of the motor excitation : the " will " to act involves the " will " to believe.

The preceding considerations lead, it seems, to this proposition : the clearness and certainty of that which is experienced in trance-states bear no unequivocal relation to truth or objective reality. Mystical assurances of clearness and certainty need not weigh heavily upon us ; that to which these impressions are attached is to be regarded as true only in so far as experimentally verified or in so far as in agreement with established knowledge[2].

* * *

The Hypothesis of a higher intelligence in trance.—One of the important generalizations which forces itself upon us is that narcotic trance, suggestion trance and disease trance, and sleep are similar in that they involve a limitation and a degradation of the mental life.

The lower intellectual processes are affected first. When the perception both of the outer world and of the body has ceased, ideas may still be present and may even possess a striking clearness. They vary with the circumstances and reflect dominant preoccupations or concerns. They may be about lofty subjects, such as the soul, its independence from the body, its immortality, God, etc. But whenever the thinking itself can be observed, it proves to be of a simplified, rudimentary sort ; it proceeds in its inferences and

---

[1] There are narcotics which produce, apparently at every dose, diffidence and hesitation, but these do not induce an increased motor activity as does, for instance, alcohol.

[2] Regarding the weight which must be ascribed to the certainty felt by the mystic, we find ourselves in agreement with Delacroix (*Etudes d'Histoire et de Psychologie du Mysticisme*, pp. 380-1), and with George A. Coe (*The Sources of the Mystical Revelation*, Hibbert Jr., 1907, vol. VI, pp. 359-72) ; and also, if we understand him correctly, with Pratt. In the following passage, in which the latter is at pains to show how profoundly rooted is the belief in God, I take him to describe a subjective, psychological experience without affirming its validity : " This belief is not the result of an argument based on an emotional experience ; it is an immediate *experience of belief*. It is an organic, a biological matter, and hence has a strength and certainty that puts its possessor quite out of the region of doubt. This absolute certainty is characteristic of the Religion of Feeling in all times and in all creeds."—*The Psychology of Religious Belief*, p. 295.

conclusions upon data surprisingly incomplete and distorted. This impoverishment increases with increase in depth of the trance, and finally thinking and feeling may end in total unconsciousness.

In one of his sermons the mystic Tauler spoke thus : " Unto this house (his innermost soul) must man now go, and completely desist from and abandon his sensations and all sensible things, such as are brought into the soul and perceived by the senses and the imagination. And he must also put away all ideas and forms, even the conceptions of reason, and all activity of his own reason[1]." And Santa Theresa, the favourite guide of most Roman Catholic writers on mysticism, says : " If you ask me how it is possible that with all our powers and all our senses so much suspended that they are as dead, we nevertheless hear and understand something, I answer that that is a secret understood perhaps by no creature[2]." Further confirmation of this feature of trance has been provided in the biographies and in the chapter on Methods.

Nevertheless, the mystics hold that in the ecstatic trance the mind attains to a divine intellectual activity, and they speak of an " illumination of the understanding." They believe that an intelligence of a higher sort miraculously takes the place of the ordinary, or they say with Poulain that " full plenitude of the understanding is retained during rapture," or even that " during true ecstasy the intellectual faculty grows in a surprising way[3]." This

---

[1] Tauler, as quoted by Hocking in *The Meaning of God in Human Experience*, p. 373.

[2] *Inner Castle*, Sixth Dwelling IV, 431-2. Comp. this with the amusing passage quoted on p. 166 of this book. See also *Life*, XII, 135 ; XVIII, 199 ; etc.
  In a paper on Mescal which has just come to our notice, S. W. Fernberger reports that he attempted to test a " notable " impression of increased ability, only to become convinced of the reverse.—*Observations on Taking Peyote*, *Amer. Jr. of Psychol.*, XXXIV, 1923, p. 270.
  Elmer Jones states (*Psychol. Rev.*, XVI, p. 52) that, in the early stages of chloroform intoxication, " the deeper conscious states are perfectly normal . . . . memory is not impaired." If this is true at all, it holds only for the very lightest degrees of trance. Comp. the experiments with alcohol in Chapter VII of this book.

[3] Poulain, *loc. cit.*, p. 258. One section of his book is entitled " The Expansion of the Intelligence during Ecstasy " (277-281).
  The difficulties facing those who believe that in ecstatic trance God reveals himself and who, at the same time, know that in that condition the ordinary mental life comes to a stop, are illustrated in an interesting way in the following quotations from Sharpe :
  " ' Realisation [of God] in thought and feeling ' is not experimental [immediate] knowledge of God ; thought and feeling may perceive *quod est— that* He exists ; but they cannot see *quid est—what* He is in His own absolute being " (26). In the ordinary way of speaking there can be no idea or thought in mystical ecstasy ; " it has nothing before it but an absolute blank." " But the void is filled by the divine presence and by supernatural agency." " The mind does not extricate itself but is taken out of its normal relations with

is hardly surprising since the mystics assume that the impressions of loftiness, of sublimity, of revelation, recalled when they return to full consciousness, signify the presence during the trance of a revelatory intellectual content[1].

Recent psychological students of mysticism, much impressed by the conviction of enlightenment and unable to interpret it as an illusion, have called to their assistance the conception of a sub or co-consciousness. They have said : " But the higher mystical flights, with their positiveness and abruptness, are surely products of no such merely negative condition. It seems far more reasonable to ascribe them to inroads from the subconscious life, of the cerebral activity correlative to which we as yet know nothing[2]." This opinion expressed by William James is also the one preferred by Flournoy[3]. It is fair to add that the latter embraced it without much satisfaction as the more probable of the theories available to him.

The necessity for the supposition of an exalted intelligence replacing the vanishing natural intelligence, or of an influence from a sub-consciousness, vanishes as soon as the impression of revelation can be explained as an illusion.

---

the external world by that very presence and influence which supplies their place. The mystical knowledge of God is, in regard to all natural knowledge and light, merely ' Ignorance ' and ' Darkness.' " (23-4).

The mental and bodily reactions resulting from the action of God in the soul freed from ideas and thoughts " need not differ essentially in character from those ordinarily set up by sensation." "There appears to be nothing impossible, or even irregular, in the idea that consciousness and intelligence may follow their normal course on a basis of supersensible ideas, presented to them, not by means of sense, but by supernatural and divine interposition . . . . It is at least quite conceivable that God may cause Himself to be apprehended as immediately present merely by stimulating the consciousness in the same way in which it is ordinarily stimulated by the idea abstracted from sense-impressions, which in this case may be given ready-made instead of being constructed by the intellect " (31-2).—A. B. Sharpe, *Mysticism : Its true Nature and Value*, London, Sands and Co., 1910.

[1] The progressive limitation and degradation of the mental activity, characteristic of all types of trance, may be referred to a progressive dissociation of the nerve elements, i.e., to the undoing of that which takes place when knowledge is gained. This hypothesis perhaps finds confirmation in the observations of physiologists, that narcotics—such as laudanum, ether, etc.,—toxæmia, " shock " and sleep effect a similar limitation and degradation of the reflex movements. They all bring about a reduction of that which Head calls " vigilance."—Henry Head, " The Conception of Nervous and Mental Energy," Report of the Intern. Congress of Psychol., Oxford, 1923.

[2] Footnote to p. 427 of *The Varieties of Religious Experience*.

[3] *Une Mystique Moderne*, pp. 178-81.

CHAPTER XI

THE SENSE OF INVISIBLE PRESENCE AND DIVINE GUIDANCE

" It is curious to speculate on the feelings of a dog who will rest peacefully for hours in a room with his master or any of the family, without the least notice being taken of him ; but, if left for a short time by himself, barks or howls dismally."—Darwin, *Descent of Man*, 2nd ed., p. 153.

ECSTATIC trance, as realized in religion, attains the substantial ends of worship by what is, in theory at least, the most perfect of means, namely, the intimate companionship or union with an omnipotent, righteous and loving Being. We have already had the opportunity of remarking that to love, and to be loved by, a good and all-powerful Person is the most effective way to vivify the human heart and to fulfil its essential yearnings. In that relationship the motives of Christian mysticism—which are no other than those of human life in general—come to free expression. The tendencies to self-affirmation, the needs for self-esteem, for affection, for moral perfection, for peace, and even for sensuous enjoyment find in an intimate companionship with divine Beings—God, Christ, the Virgin Mary or other saints—a complete satisfaction.

It has, of course, not been left to the Christian mystics to discover the satisfyingness of companionship with gods. The beautiful Hebrew psalm, " The Lord is my Shepherd, I shall not want. He maketh me to lie down in green pastures," etc., is an earlier expression of that discovery.

When belief in personal divinities has disappeared, there remains the craving for belief in a community of nature between us and the Universe. Man cannot abide the thought of utter isolation ; he will not live in an altogether alien World ; there must be some sort of kinship between him and the forces of the Universe. One might speak of that affinity as a cosmic gregariousness.

The distinction of the mystics is to have found and practiced a way of realizing the divine Presence with as much, nay with more, intensity than if actually present to the external senses. The definition of mysticism as the direct, experiential realization of God is incomplete but not false. Quakerism, for instance, the more important of the modern mystical movements, is said to have been

" first of all the proclamation of an experience. The movement came to birth, and received its original power, through persons who were no less profoundly conscious of a *Divine Presence* than they were of a world in space[1]."

Of the different categories of alleged proofs of the existence of a God-Providence, this immediate experience of him is probably the one which has so far suffered least from the introduction of science into the sphere of religion. The many instances of divine Presence contained in Chapter IX have already shown that the experience means much more than the mere thought of the presence of God. At the moment of the sudden theophany, M.E. was so violently moved that he could no longer stand ; it was as if the goodness and power of God were penetrating him. The realization of God by Mrs Pa. was so " wonderful " that for days she went in awe of that experience. Miss X. relates that the sense of God's presence came to her with " overpowering fullness." She was at a loss to express " the sense of intimacy, understanding, and sympathy " which the Presence gave her. It was so much a part of her that communion went on without words or even thoughts. She felt " consolation and strength pouring in " upon her. Another scientist, a woman also, in a similar crisis describes the consciousness of the presence of the Father, of the touch of his Hand, as being as strong and real to her as that of any bodily presence[2]. The writings of the classical mystics contain numerous similar instances. One of the best observed of the many reported by Santa Theresa, is the following :

" On the day of St Peter, as I was in Orison, I saw near me, or rather I felt—for I did not perceive anything either with the eyes of the body or with the eyes of the soul—I felt Christ near me and I knew it was He Who was speaking to me. . . . It seemed to me that He kept walking at my side ; and, as it was not a vision of the imagination, I did not know under what form, . . . but He was always on my right side, I felt him very clearly[3]."

Illustrations of divine Presence[4] might be indefinitely multiplied. I shall add but one more. After a Sunday School class a young man was being prayed for by the Class Leader : " In the midst of it there came an overwhelming sense of a Presence infinitely pure and true and tender, a Presence that broke through all preconceived notions

---

[1] R. Jones, *Social Law in the Spiritual World*, p. 161.

[2] *A Scientist's Confession of Faith*, a pamphlet published by the *Amer. Baptist Publ. Soc.*, Philad., 1898.

[3] *Autobiography* of Santa Theresa, XXVIII, p. 84.

[4] Several will be found in the *Varieties of Religious Experience*, 3rd Lecture, in Pratt's chapters on mysticism and in an appendix to my *Study of Religious Conversion*.

and revealed itself to my consciousness in such beauty and power that after more than twenty-five years it seems to me the only real thing in my whole life. . . . It has been the strongest influence in my whole life[1]."

*   *   *

It would be an error to suppose that this conviction of an impressive Presence, more concretely real than what the eyes see and the hands touch, occurs only in the religious life. It is no more in itself a religious phenomenon than ecstatic trance. Many are the persons who have experienced it outside of all religious connexions. From the collection I have gathered from contemporaries, I shall transcribe two instances :

Miss L. " A young woman was sitting in the drawing-room of her parents at half after eleven at night, waiting for her father's return. Her mother lay on a couch near her, dozing. She herself was reading a book in which she was utterly absorbed. No one else in the house was awake. As she read, she was slightly disturbed by the feeling that someone was in the room in the corner opposite her mother's couch. She looked up, expecting to see her father, but saw no one and began reading again. The same sensation came over her three or four times ; but, since each time she looked up and saw no one, she continued to read, being very deeply absorbed in her book. But suddenly she felt someone come over from the corner and cross between herself and her mother. She felt it so vividly that she even thought she saw something, but could not say what the something looked like, or describe it in any way. She was perfectly certain, however, that someone had crossed the room. Startled, she cried to her mother, ' What was that ? ' Her mother had seen and felt nothing—but the girl insisted that someone had passed and persuaded her mother to search the house with her. They searched the house in vain."

Miss J. " We had an early dinner as we were all going to a wedding. I was dressing in my room on the third floor, and the rest of the family were on the second floor. I could hear them talking, and I sometimes joined in the conversation, calling down the stairs. Altogether we were having a most hilarious time. Suddenly, for no reason that I know of, a sort of terror came over me. The electric

<hr/>

[1] Pratt, *loc. cit.*, p. 358.
    It is something which happened to Goethe in his relation with Frau von Stein. He writes to her : " It is as if you were transubstantiated into every object. I am very clearly aware of the various objects and yet I see you in each one of them—my mind is on my work and yet I am always in your presence, always thinking of you." From a letter dated April 9, 1782.

lights had not yet been turned on, and my bedroom, although not dark, was lighted only by the gaslight from my study and from the hallway. I seemed to feel a ' presence ' and it was in the air, moving quite rapidly about six feet from the floor. I did not look in that direction, but tried to quiet myself by thinking that such a thing could not physically hurt me, and that, if it were anything spiritual, I should be glad to learn what it had to say, and then I turned—of course, to find nothing. I was still nervous, and went downstairs as soon as I was dressed." The writer of this letter adds that, under ordinary circumstances, she is never afraid in the house.

The realization of Presences such as these, not having the testimony of the external senses and yet possessing the certainty of perception, is of fairly frequent occurrence. It is, moreover, so far from beyond the reach of scientific investigation that it can easily be produced under experimental conditions. We have ourselves attempted it successfully. Each subject, or, as we may call him, each observer, in turn was seated in a dimly lighted room with his back to the assistants, who sat silent some twenty-five feet away. His eyes were carefully covered, so as to exclude all light. He was told that someone might come in and stand near him, back of the chair, and he was asked to indicate whenever he became aware of a Presence.

At irregular intervals, someone would approach silently, walking on thick rugs, and stand for a number of seconds back of the chair of the observer, and then withdraw silently again. In about half the cases, the subjects did not perceive the approach of the person. In the other instances, some noise or air movement would indicate to him the approach, and he would signal his awareness of a presence. This inference was, however, not confused by the subject with the Sense of Presence. The subjects were requested to make careful introspective observations of their experiences and reported them immediately afterwards.

Of the seven observers who took part in the experiments, all of them graduate students in psychology, at least half experienced the Sense of Presence. We speak somewhat indefinitely because in some instances it was not clear whether or not we had to do with the Sense of Presence.

The following notes are extracted from the observations of one of the two subjects who took part in a first series of experiments. They had been requested to assume an attitude of passive expectancy.

Subject A. Observation II.—" Very suddenly there was a feeling that some one was near me ; there was no visualization except to the point of knowing that the person was large. I was very sure it was a person, and that he or she was behind my chair, a little to the left, about one and a half metres away. [No one was in the room, nor had there been any one there for about three minutes.] I had a slightly uncanny feeling. Almost immediately there appeared an intense desire to stand up and turn around toward the person so as to be facing him during a conversation I felt sure would ensue. I had no idea what the topic of conversation would be, or why it would take place. But the idea of "carrying on a conversation" and the necessity of standing (more to have better control of my mental faculties than anything else—it was not out of respect to another person) were very clear and insistent."

Observation IV.—"About two minutes after starting the experiment I felt a jar like a foot-fall, but I heard no sound. A little later there came a feeling of a vapoury substance near the ceiling, spherical in shape and very definitely localized. Apparently there were no motor reactions here, and this lasted only about two seconds. About two seconds later I had a *very* strong impulse to run downstairs and out of the house. This was accompanied by an image of myself running downstairs. At this point there was a sort of terror, but *still no sense of presence.* The impulse was much like a panic that immediately subsided.

"After an interval of about ten seconds of passivity and relaxation, there came a sense of presence not very clear. [Here she raised her hand as a signal that the Presence had come.] Then *It* became very clearly present. 'Bearing down upon me,' was the phrase that flitted through my mind. There was a growing feeling of terror tinged with awe. By this time there was a noticeable muscular tension all over, accompanied by an increased rate of breathing. Shortly after this I began to shiver, and later I had a feeling of cold not connected with the temperature of the room. The shivering ended in jerking all over. When the shivering began, I had the feeling of cowering in my chair. After a short time I could stand it no longer and I impulsively removed the bandage from my eyes, though I knew we had agreed that the experiment should last ten minutes."

In another series of experiments with five different persons, the following instances of the Sense of Presence were produced in B. and C.:

Subject B. "I felt as if I were enveloped, as if I were the centre of concentric circles closing in upon me. The feeling would come after the person was here. [She means after one of the attendants had come in and stood behind her chair.] I don't think I should have felt it if I hadn't been convinced from the noises that someone was here, and I argued with myself on this point. I had the impression of a rhythmic motion. It was rather a restful feeling. There was no particular emotion."

During the experience just related, noises had been made in order to suggest the approach of a person, but no one had come near the chair of the subject. At this point of the experiment noises were again produced and the subject tapped loudly to indicate her awareness of a Presence. Subsequently she described her impressions thus : " When I tapped I was just beginning to have that same sensation. It increased after I tapped—the conviction of a Presence grew stronger. I had the sensation of something being rather close. I neither heard not saw, yet was aware of it. The more the feeling of enveloping, of drawing in, increased, the more I felt someone there."

. C. " The sounds made by people approaching and retreating, the tick of the clock, etc., had no effect upon me, for I was attending to my own psychic processes. The atmosphere seemed thicker than usual and felt charged with what might be called latent personality[1]. Out of this more or less vitalized atmosphere I tried to form definite presences, locating them with reference to my own position—left front, right front, etc. I succeeded to some extent ; but the fact that I was consciously imagining these figures detracted from their reality.

" Finally, without any effort or force, I felt a Presence standing at the table to my right and a little behind my chair. It existed only in reference to me—that is, I had no visual or auditory imagery of it, but felt it only in so far as it was aware of me. It did not look at me, but as it turned toward me and put out its arms as if it were about to touch me, I was so overcome with terror that I lost the sense of its nearness and became aware only of my own tendency to shrink away —almost run—and of my quickened pulse."

The attitude of these persons was similar to that frequently found in the mystics when they realize the Presence of God, of Christ, or of some Saint. Our subjects also desired and expected the Presence, but their efforts seemed no more successful than those of the mystics. If the Presence appeared at all, it came unexpectedly, after they had ceased to attempt to visualize or otherwise to realize it. We did not observe many instances of the gradual passage or, development, of a visualized presence into a Sense of Presence. On the contrary, although expectation contributes indirectly to the appearance of the Presence, images voluntarily brought up seemed to be an obstacle to success. And all the observers agreed that the Sense of Presence, intense and definite though it was, did not include any image

[1] It is interesting to recall in this connexion the experience of James Russell Lowell, related in chapter IX.

except with regard to the localization of the Presence somewhere behind the subject. There are however clear indications in the records that at times the Presence assumed, for a moment at least, something of a visual appearance. Localization is also a peculiarity of the sense of Presence in religion.

With very rare exceptions our subjects found no difficulty in separating the inference of a presence, made on the basis of perceived sounds, from what they called a Sense of Presence. An inferred presence left our subjects more or less indifferent, while the Sense of Presence involved emotions varied in character and usually intense, and it carried with it also an intensity of assurance lacking in the mere inference. It must be emphasized that, however convincing the experience, the nature of the Presence remained extremely vague[1].

*   *   *

What explanation can psychology offer of this curious phenomenon? Ordinarily, when we are aware of the presence of someone, the experience is far from being limited to the perceptions coming through the external senses. What else enters into the experience is readily discovered if we attempt to trace the formation, of the conviction of presence.

The impression made upon a new-born infant by the sight of a person is something very different from the corresponding experience a few years later. At first the visual impression is practically meaningless: it calls forth hardly any movements, and only the vaguest of feelings, emotions and expectations. But, in the course of growth, the vision of the person—of the mother, let us say—becomes almost endlessly enriched. The babe sees her in a thousand different attitudes, sees her walk, stand, sit, etc., etc. More than that, impressions from the external senses, other than the visual, are added in countless numbers : the mother touches, holds, and fondles the infant in an indescribable variety of ways. Sounds also crowd upon the consciousness of the child as he sees the mother. Her steps and other movements produce noises, and she speaks and makes pretty sounds to the child.

But all this, one might say, is merely the picture from the outside. The child *reacts* to all these external stimuli ; *responses are made* to the sight, the touch, the sound impressions. Different, discriminating responses come to be made to many of these different

---

[1] One might conjecture that the inciting cause of the experience is some stimulation of a sense organ which escapes the attention of the person. Of this we have no proof. Were it so, our general conclusions would not be altered.

stimuli. And these responses turn out to be far more important for the assurance of the presence of a person than are the sensory stimuli themselves.

These reactions involve the whole bodily mechanism ; first of all, the external voluntary muscles, *i.e.*, those under control and whose play is visible—for instance, the large muscles of the legs and arms and the smaller muscles upon which depends the facial expression. They involve also the less obvious, but not less important, muscles not under voluntary control and upon which depend the great vital functions of nutrition, circulation and reproduction. The repeated presence of a person gradually determines in the babe more and more definite and specific modifications of respiration (breathing is, for instance, retarded, or accelerated, or suspended for an instant), of the secretory organs, of the digestive system (they are activated or inhibited ; salivation, for instance, is in some way or other affected). Even the reproductive organs may come to be involved in the total effect.

When the infant has reached maturity, his reactions to persons he knows, and even to those he does not know, have attained a complexity which beggars description. We need not attempt to rival the novelist when he seeks to portray the endless *nuances* by which the accomplished society woman indicates to each different person his or her relative place. The almost infinite variety of impressions made upon her by each individual appears in her correspondingly varied forms of address, intonation, attitude, and gesture. And yet that which is perceived by an observer is only a fragment of that which takes place within her. The formation of infinitely varied reaction—patterns to the presence of different individuals is one of the main achievements of social education.

We are stating merely a well-known fact when we add that knowledge of a person does not imply only, or even mainly, familiarity with the sensations produced by his looks, the sound of his voice, the feel of his hand. These are for us *signs* of the nature of the personality before us. Real acquaintance with a person means knowledge of his character, his habits, his ways of thinking, feeling and doing ; this knowledge means that his presence produces in our bodily organism specific modifications of the kind described— modifications which constitute in part an actual *expression* of our ideas and feelings, and in part a preparation to meet, with the proper responses, his anticipated behaviour.

The reactions elicited by a person known to us include a stable kernel, corresponding to his established, recognized character, and, in addition, elements varying according to the circumstances : we see him with enjoyment when we are at leisure, and with annoyance when he interrupts important business.

It is evident that the more essential elements in the effects produced by the presence of a person are not the external perceptions considered in themselves (sight, sound, etc.), but those which we have called the " reactions," i.e., the activities in the whole organism determined by these perceptions—activities of which the subject is aware in feelings, emotions, impulses, desires, anticipations, intentions, volitions, etc. We may go a step further and say that the *only* essential part of the experience of realizing the presence of a person is constituted by these reactions. The insufficiency of the external sensations is strikingly demonstrated in abnormal cases, when the organism does not respond in its wonted ways. Then, the vivid, intimate sense of a personal presence is weakened ; or in extreme instances, when the organic irresponsiveness is sufficiently complete, the person is not even recognized in spite of the testimony given by the external senses. This is what happened to the unfortunate neurasthenic mentioned by Masselon. In the presence of his daughter, despite the likeness which he recognized, he would say, " It seems to me that she is not my daughter, for if she were my daughter I would experience a great joy[1]."

It follows from the above considerations that the absence of the ordinary visible, auditory and tactile tokens of a particular person does not preclude awareness and full realization of his presence. In a room with a screen, we may " feel " someone on the other side of it with all the intensity and definiteness which usually come with sight and with hearing—and yet no one may be there.

*　　　　　*　　　　　*

At this point the question of the possible incentives to a conviction of presence must be raised. We know that the original incentives are seeing, hearing and touching the person, himself. But these sensations soon cease to be necessary. They may be replaced by other sensations which have been associated with them. The creaking of the opening door may, for instance, determine in the infant the reactions which, previously, only the perception of the nurse could produce. Any sensation or perception which frequently accompanies the presence of the nurse may become a sign of her presence and replace it, so that the infant on receiving the vicarious impression begins to act as if she were present.

[1] Masselon, *Les Réactions Affectives et l'Origine de la Douleur Morale, Jr. de Psychol. Normale et Anormale*, vol. II, 1905, p. 496.
On the contrary, two persons different in their visual appearance and in their voices would, nevertheless, be " felt " to be practically identical persons, should it be possible for them to produce identical organic reactions.

At a later stage of development, the thought of these signs is enough to bring to the mind the idea of the person. Names soon assume a conspicuous place among the signs representing persons and things. But, of course, the thought or idea of a person and his presence are far from being identical experiences. The " thought " of the presence of a person is not the experience of the effects which that presence would produce ; it is merely a *representation* of part or all of these effects. There is here the same difference as between an actual visual sensation and the thought of that sensation.

It is important for us to observe, however, that the sign or the thought of a presence may set off some, or all, of the various reactions which the actual presence would call forth. When that happens, the experience becomes more or less exactly equivalent to an actual presence. We are told, for instance, that certain novelists (Balzac and Flaubert among them) would become so completely absorbed in their heroes that it was as if they were actually conversing with them, and at times as if they themselves were the heroes. For days Flaubert had on his tongue the taste of the poison with which Mme Bovary ended her life. In so far as, and while, the novelist experiences sufficiently completely the reactions which the actual presence of the person would determine, he may be said to believe in his presence. Theirs were, however, voluntary illusions. As soon as the purpose to realize the presence of the hero, in order more truly to picture his behaviour, gives way to another attitude, the illusion of reality disappears. So that if, at the moment of greatest absorption, you were to draw the novelist out of his imaginary world and ask him if he now believes that his personages have actually been present with him, he would answer : " No, I am not insane."

It is, however, not necessary to be insane in order, after the event, to remain persuaded of a visitation. It is merely necessary that the event should have taken place *not* as the result of the experiencer's own initiative and effort, that it should have seemed to be imposed from without[1]. In that case, unless he belong to the small class of the enlightened and critical, the experiencer will probably believe that somebody or something has been actually present with him. Believers in the traditional teaching of religious mysticism and, more generally, in alleged spiritistic phenomena, are

---

[1] In an article on *La Nature des Hallucinations, Rev. Philos.*, LXIII, 1907, pp. 593-618, Bernard Leroy rightly insists upon the absence of voluntary attention in the production of hallucination : " A particular mode of automatic attention is substituted to voluntary attention that has become impossible." P. 618. " A condition of passivity or of semi-passivity, clearly abnormal, are the most favorable conditions to the appearance of visions or voices." P. 610.

not in a position to be sceptical. In the instances of the Sense of Presence scattered throughout this book, we have observed that this condition of passivity was realized. Even though the subject desires the experience, when it comes he seems to have had no share in its production. Mlle Vé describes very well her impression of being acted upon by a power external to herself.

We have thus far expressed ourselves as if the starting-point of the illusion of Presence was either the perception of something which had become closely associated with the person (his name, an object belonging to him, etc.), or merely the thought of him. This is obviously the case in a number of instances. But there are numerous other instances where the Presence assails the subject without apparent causal antecedents. A careful examination of a number of these instances reveals, however, that even then some sensation or feeling, or emotion, or thought, suddenly and incongruously appears in the mind of the subject and suggests the thought of a personal, or of a less well-defined cause. The thought once present awakens instantaneously some or all of the reactions the actual presence would determine, and thus the illusory Sense of Presence is produced.

One cannot in every instance identify with assurance the starting-point of a Sense of Presence, but possibilities are never lacking. Mlle Vé was conscious before the realization of the divine Presence of unusual and more or less remarkable sensations and feelings. In the instances of Miss L. and of Miss J., and also in the reported experiments, the situations were such as to be productive of the kind of uneasiness or fear almost unavoidable when one is alone late at night in a silent house or anywhere in the dark. Any sense-impression for which one does not find immediately another satisfactory interpretation may occasion the thought of an external agent. In this connexion one must not neglect the possible intervention of peripheral visual impressions, and, in general, of subliminal sensory stimuli which, as the psychologist knows, although they may not be clearly conscious, may, nevertheless, be influential.

The unanimous observation of our subjects, that the perception of foot-steps behind them led to the belief that someone had come in, but not to the Sense of Presence, and that the effort to visualize a person did not seem to result in a Sense of Presence, are not to be regarded as antagonistic to the rôle we are ascribing to an initial sensory stimulation and to the thought of a causal agent. These observers knew that at any time one of the persons present might come in and stand behind them. When that happened, they were not to let themselves be disturbed, but were to continue to expect something else. Consequently when they became aware of noises which were for them clearly foot-steps, the idea of a person behind them arose in the mind, but only the idea; for, the person actually present was to remain as non-existent for them, they were to disregard him.

The Sense of Presence appeared, in these observations, on the basis of queer impressions which challenged the subject's power of explanation. For a while he may have maintained a detached attitude towards them, or assumed the rôle of a disinterested scientific observer. So long as this lasted there was no Sense of Presence. If, again, some unaccountable feeling took place, the strangeness of which roused astonishment, apprehension, anxiety, or even full-fledged fear, the thought of an agent, personal or not, might instantaneously be formed, for it is an ineradicable habit of the mind to ascribe causes, and usually personal causes, to phenomena. In the peculiar circumstances in which the subjects found themselves, the idea of an external agent was not inhibited; it set off various reactions, awareness of which constituted the Sense of Presence.

The production of queer, mysterious sensations and the readiness with which these experimenters yielded to the personifying, or at least to the objectifying habit, is to be accounted for on the ground of the state in which the conditions of the experience had placed them. One cannot remain for a considerable length of time motionless, with closed eyes, in a noiseless room, without approaching the sleep-state. The surprisingly defective observations of competent witnesses in attendance at mediumistic seances, we take to have the same cause : a certain degree of mental dissociation occurs[1]. Our experimenters were, in fact, in a light trance while awaiting a rather weird phenomenon—the Sense of Presence. They were in a condition similar to that of Tennyson repeating his name, of Abramowski experimenting on dissociation, of Mme Guyon hoping, while in Contemplation, for the appearance of the Bridegroom, and, generally, of the religious mystics in orison.

But the Sense of Presence appears also in other circumstances. M.E., for instance (Chapter IX), was walking with companions in the Alps, when suddenly God manifested himself to him with such power that he had to sit down and let his companions proceed without him[2]. Here a brain storm, which may have to be classed with psychic

[1] One of our subjects thought she had dozed.

[2] In the presence of grand, or particularly beautiful, natural scenery, many persons " feel " the presence of God. As McDougall remarks, this is no doubt, because the main emotions evoked are those of admiration and reverence—emotions that involve negative self-feeling. Now, negative self-feeling is an attitude referring to persons. Thus, one is led to the thought of a personal power as the cause of the impression.—*Introduction to Social Psychology*, p. 130.

epilepsies, caused overpowering disturbances. These were interpreted as a divine intervention, and this interpretation itself resulted in the production of attitudes, feelings, emotions, and thoughts such as might be experienced in the presence of the Christian God of Love. The violence, the strangeness, and probably also the peculiar quality of the sensory disturbances, were so marked in this instance that, without the assistance given by a trance-state, the subject reverted to the naïve habit of personification.

Miss J., while in partial darkness, and in an excited state, did something similar on the occasion of much less amazing impressions. But she did not altogether assent to an automatic personification : she remained sufficiently mistress of herself to assume a critical attitude. Had she been in a trance-condition, the conviction of Presence would probably have been complete.

The essential processes resulting in a Sense of Presence are the same, whether they be determined by a brain storm or prepared-for by the slow process of orison, or by its equivalent as in our experiments, or determined by any other means.

The Sense of Presence may refer to a particular person or to an undefined person whose sex even is not known : it may, indeed, refer to a physical agent. These different types of the Sense of Presence are illustrated in an enlightening manner in the trances of Mlle Vé (Chapter IX). The Friend was a person, but his sex was obscure. Later the Friend was replaced by a divine Power, at first personal and subsequently impersonal. In the instances given in the present chapter, these three possibilities are also realized.

The nature ascribed to the Presence depends, in the first instance, upon the nature of the data which initiate the phenomenon, upon the mental habits of the subject, and upon the content of his mind at the time. It depends, in the second instance, upon the reactions set off by the initial thought of the Agent. The importance of the rôle played by the several factors, in determining the nature ascribed to the Presence, varies in each case. When Mlle Vé was yearning for a friend, the Friend came. She conversed with him and enjoyed the sweetness and comfort provided by the company of an assured and wise friend. When, later, the character of her trances changed and the manifestations she experienced seemed to her clearly beyond the power of man to produce, she thought herself the object of divine visitations. If, still later, she passed to the conviction that the Power was impersonal, it was because she no longer received the comfort or felt the sympathy with which, she knew, the divine Father, would have filled her. The more sceptical she became as to the personal nature of the Power, the less she experienced the reactions which a personal God would be expected to produce, and the more did her scepticism grow.

Our theory of the Sense of Presence is then, in brief, that the cause of strange impressions (sensations, feelings, emotions) whose origin is not perceived, is, according to a deeply ingrained habit of the human mind, automatically personified, or at least externalized in an Agent, and that the idea of this Agent sets off in the subject reactions which themselves contribute to the formation of the idea of the nature of the Agent and to the certainty of his presence.   The production of the phenomenon is much facilitated by a state of trance such as is induced in mystical worship.

When the Presence takes the form of the Christian God, the experience may acquire the incomparable significance and the value which Christians ascribe to his approval and his love.

NOTE ON THE SENSE OF PRESENCE IN CONTEMPORARY PSYCHOLOGY.

The main interest of James, when he wrote the *Varieties of Religious Experience*, was to find in religion facts which could be used to support his over-belief in a superhuman consciousness.   Nowhere in that book is he more completely dominated by that wish than in Lecture III where, under the comprehensive title, " The Reality of the Unseen," he discusses the Sense of Presence.

In that lecture the phenomenon is abundantly illustrated, but no attempt is made to explain it.   His purpose is not to analyse and to understand, but to set forth the wonder, and to declare the inadequacy of reason to cope with it.   He turns away from the problem with these remarks :

" Such cases, taken along with others which would be too tedious for quotation, seem sufficiently to prove the existence in our mental machinery of a sense of present reality more diffused and general than that which our special senses yield.   For the psychologists the tracing of the organic seat of such a feeling would form a pretty problem—nothing would be more natural than to connect it with the muscular sense, with the feeling that our muscles were innervating themselves for action.   Whatsoever thus innervated our activity, or ' made our flesh creep,'—our senses are what do so oftenest—might then appear real and present, even though it were but an abstract idea. But with such vague conjectures we have no concern at present, for our interest lies with the faculty rather with its organic seat[1]."

Instead of attempting to do the work that might be expected of the psychologist, James launched into a tirade against rationalism : " We have to confess that the part of it of which rationalism can give an account is relatively superficial.   It is the part that has the *prestige* undoubtedly, for it has the loquacity, it can challenge you for proofs, and chop logic, and put you down with words.   But it will fail to convince or convert you all the same, if your dumb intuitions are opposed to its conclusions.   If you have intuitions at all, they come from a deeper level of your nature than the loquacious level which rationalism inhabits."   " Something in you absolutely *knows* that that result must be truer than any logic-chopping rationalistic talk, however clever, that may contradict it[2]."

It is fortunate for science and philosophy that this passage does not represent William James completely.   It expresses only one, or perhaps two, of the several moods or attitudes of this gifted writer : the mood of the scientist

---

[1] *Varieties of Religious Experience*, p. 63.

[2] *Ibid.*, p. 73.

acutely conscious of defeat and limitation, and partly discouraged; and the mood of the romantic soul, lover of adventure and mystery. The first is the mood that enslaves men to Authority, the second is the mood of Superstition. That there will always remain unplumbed depths, is as certain for us as for William James, but this admission should not dispose us to heed the admonition to hold back from an examination of alleged "intuitions." Psychological knowledge has already gone far enough to deliver man from the belief that all the so-called "intuitions" that come to him with an assurance of certainty are therefore true.

It is perhaps not superfluous to remark that our own conclusion (the Sense of the Presence of a personal God is adequately explicable as an illusion) is not equivalent to a denial of the reality of any and every kind of Unseen.

*   *   *

In the *Psychology of Religious Belief*, Professor Pratt had already approached this problem. In the *Religious Consciousness*, he returned to it with especial reference to Professor Coe's article in the *Hibbert Journal*, mentioned elsewhere in this book. Pratt affirms, in opposition to Coe, that the Sense of Presence and the strength which comes from it often appear when the trance conditions are absent, and he argues that the explanation of Professor Coe is inadequate : "Education and suggestion (the principles of explanation offered by Coe) then, constitute a partial, but only a partial, explanation of the mystic consciousness. For a full and complete explanation we must go deeper than this . . . . But if it is ever to be fully made out, it must be sought pretty far down in the less superficial parts of our psycho-physical being. . . . The full explanation of it, if it is ever found, will involve not merely the acceptance of suggested ideas, but much of our emotional and volitional nature, the fringe region of consciousness, and perhaps also the unconscious and instinctive regions of·our being. It is hardly to be expected that such a complete explanation will be made out for several generations at the earliest[1]." Whether Professor Pratt has not exaggerated the difficulties is a question which the reader will have to decide for himself.

*   *   *

In a paper already mentioned in this book[2], Bernard Leroy cites several instances of the Sense of Presence, extracts their characteristic features, and attempts an explanation. It was, in so far as our information goes, the first serious effort to find a scientific solution of that puzzling problem. The explanation is of the same type as that given, in the same article, to the illusion of illumination. It may be summarized in three propositions :—

1. A group of specific emotions normally accompany the presence near us of a particular person.
2. This group of emotions may appear in the absense of the person.
3. The character of the person, felt as present, will vary according to the composition of the emotional complex which appears.

He introduces also in his explanation a volitional element, but only in an effort to account for the localization of the Presence.

This theory constitutes an important step in the right direction. It is, however, too incomplete and too general to be acceptable as adequate. The psycho-physiological effects of the presence with us of a person is by no means limited to the production of a specific complex of emotions, and I know of no reason for limiting to the emotional life the processes to which the Sense of Presence is due.

It is also to be observed that Leroy brings no light to bear upon the origin or cause, of the "non-logical" processes which are responsible for the hallucination of Presence.

*   *   *

[1] *The Religious Consciousness*, New York, Macmillan, 1920, pp. 451-2, abbreviated.

[2] *Interprétation Psychologique des "Visions Intellectuelles" chez les Mystiques Chrétiens, Rev. de l'Histoire des Religions*, vol. LV, 1907, pp. 25-50.

We must draw attention also to an historical review and a critical discussion of this class of problems by Henri Delacroix, in a valuable appendix ("Hallucinations Psychiques—Sentiment de Présence ") to *Etudes d' Histoire et de Psychologie du Mysticisme.*

The Effects of the Impression of Divine Presence.—The Sense of the Presence of God greatly increases the far-reaching effects which the mere thought of him may have upon the worshipper; and when the divine Presence is felt during a state of increased suggestibility, such as trance, it becomes difficult to overestimate its possibilities. Our great mystics find in it the satisfaction of the needs and cravings for which they have entered upon the religious life Loved by the Christian God, their lives become unified and centred about him. Their energies are no longer dissipated in fruitless yearnings and conflicting tendencies; sources of energy until then dormant or inhibited are aroused to great activity. Thus their vital aspirations are fulfilled and their claims granted.

It is not necessary to insist upon the truth of these affirmations, for they are amply verified in the foregoing chapters, in particular in " Motivation of Christian Mysticism." It will be more instructive for us to turn to a comparison of the acknowledged effects of God's presence with the effects of man's presence when his ministrations are exercised under circumstances similar to those of the mystical trance.

In Chapter VI it was shown that, in its larger aspects, the hypnotic trance was similar to the religious trance of the mystics, the presence of the hypnotizer acting in the same way as the divine Presence. A particularly intimate relation of trust is usually established between hypnotizer and hypnotized. The hypnotizer is no ordinary man to his subjects; for him they would do almost anything. They express their feelings in various ways according to their age, situation, etc. A patient of Janet who was no longer young wanted to regard him as her son[1], and another one used to say that she had for him the same feelings as for the " *bon Dieu*[1]."

" The first obvious fact regarding many of these subjects is that during the period of influence, they think constantly of their hypnotizer." When they cannot see him daily, they fall into the habit of writing a diary for him, or of writing him interminable letters. " The idea of the hypnotizer manifests itself especially in connexion with the actions that have been forbidden during hypnosis. The subject no longer feels himself free, he thinks himself directed." One of them says, " I am a machine of which you are the spring "; another, " I am a jumping jack of which you hold the strings ";

[1] *Névroses et Idées Fixes*, vol. I, p. 447.

another, " It is your will that has taken the place of mine, it seems to me that I no longer belong to myself[1]."

" At times, the idea of the hypnotizer is conscious and obsesses the mind of the subject ; at times it is subconscious and manifests itself by automatic movements or hallucinations[2]."

It is only when there exists this intimate relationship with, and domination by the hypnotizer that the patients are profoundly transformed[3]. When, as invariably happens after a time, the thought of the hypnotizer has lost its power, the patient feels abandoned : *Vel.* says, " Oh, it is not nice of you to have abandoned me, to have left me alone. I am lost if you do not sustain me." And *Me.*, thus left alone and having no one to think of, falls again into despair and once more loses her head[4].

This description of the influence of the hypnotizer upon the hypnotized corresponds with striking exactness to that given by the mystics of their relation with God. It would be easy to draw from the biographical chapters, expressions parallel to those just quoted. They are God's favourite children, or they stand to him in a still closer relationship—that of the bride to the bridegroom ; it is no longer they who think and act, it is God in them. Their dependence upon him may become so complete that when he has not visited them for a space they complain of being abandoned, become restless, miserable, and fall into " dryness[5]." Automatic movements and hallucinations appear in the mystics also and are ascribed by them to the divine Presence.

But a person need be neither in a religious trance nor in hypnosis in order to undergo the unifying influence of a divine or human presence. According to the founder of psychoanalysis no cure is possible by that method—a method that does not include hypnotization—until emotional interest is transferred to the physician. By emotional interest he means the tender emotion, love. We need not attempt to say who or what was the original object of the emotional interest which is to be transferred. It is sufficient for our purpose to know that for Freud the condition of cure is such a transference to the person of the physician. The " transference may occur as a stormy demand for love or in a more moderate form ; in place of wishing to be his mistress, the young girl may be content to be adopted as the favoured daughter of the old physician ; or the

[1] *Névroses et Idées Fixes*, vol. I, pp. 447-8.
[2] *Ibid.*, pp. 451-2.
[3] *Ibid.*, p. 452.
[4] *Ibid.*, p. 454.
[5] The causal relationship may be the reverse.

libidinous desire may be toned down to a proposal of inseparable but ideal platonic friendship[1]." The male patients behave in a similar way; there is the same overestimation of the qualities of the physician, the same readiness to confide in him all their private affairs, the same jealousy, etc.[2]"

The facts observed should not be confused with the Freudian explanation of them. Practically all the physicians who treat neuropaths—whatever the school of therapeutics to which they belong—observe that an intimate relationship develops between the patient and themselves, and they agree in regarding that relationship as essential to success.

No one familiar with the disclosures of the great mystics will fail to notice that this relationship, as described by Janet or by Freud—whether the patient be hypnotized or not—is couched in terms similar to those of the mystics when they describe their relation with God. They also make upon God or the Virgin a " stormy " demand for love ; they also wish to be lovers or mistresses ; and, even though they have no thought other than that of an ideal, platonic love, nevertheless their sexual organism participates in the intercourse[3].

That human love, while it lasts, cures body and soul is perhaps nowhere demonstrated more convincingly than in the recent great work of P. Janet, *Médications Psychologiques*, to which we have already referred several times. The experience of Héloïse is not limited to psychopaths. She writes to her physician : " When an intelligent man chances to show me some interest, it sets my eyes so to sparkling that they dazzle the one who in kindness has paid me some attention. You won't believe it, but that is for me the best medicine[4]." " As long as I was in an atmosphere of tender and reciprocated affection, I was a ray of sunshine, a living and life-giving person. Now, I am a corpse who speaks and weeps. . . . As soon as I fall in love all my ailments are cured[5]."

Under the happy excitement of love, a man forty years of age recovered all the enthusiasm and all the facility of literary composition enjoyed during the war : " I was a marvel of love, of literary fertility and joy ; I felt as if I were a demi-god[6]." A woman

---

[1] *A General Introduction to Psychoanalysis*, Eng. trans., 1920, p. 382.

[2] *Ibid.*, p. 382.

[3] What is meant by this affirmation is indicated in the discussion of the sex motive.

[4] Vol. III, p. 206.

[5] *Ibid.*, p. 205.

[6] *Ibid.*, p. 168.

of the same age declares that the only thing which has always been successful with her are amorous adventures : " I have tried religion and philanthropy, but they are only makeshifts ; always I have to come back to the treatment that suits me best[1]." " Ec. (a woman forty-two years old) has gone through several great fits of depression ; for months she remained inert and groaning, complaining of digestive troubles, of insomnia, of anxiety, etc. ; then rapidly she appears to recover and her husband is delighted. These recoveries mark the beginning of a *liaison* with the husband of one of her friends : 'These secret assignations occupy and divert my mind, prevent me from thinking of my unfortunate marriage with a good fellow, but so prosaic. . . . When I had seen him (her lover) during the day, I digested very well and I slept all night.' This relation lasted three years, during which the patient had no relapse. Unfortunately her lover died and speedily the fits of depression returned. After many months of suffering, she thought of trying religion, went to a priest and formed the habit of seeing him every day. A new intrigue began, mysterious meetings followed, and the attack of melancholia came to an end. After one year of perfect health the patient is again miserable because the priest, fearful of being discovered, brought the relation to an end and left the country[2]." Love of God—platonic though not unsexual,—represented in succession by two priests, produced quite the same effect on Mme Guyon.

It might be objected that the remarkable instances of cure and vivification reported above refer to abnormal persons ; moreover, that they take place under the ministrations of professional medical men ; whereas, in religion, ordinary normal persons for whom baleful external circumstances have been too much, or whose only disorder is " spiritual," are healed not only physically, but also " spiritually " and without intervention of medical psychological science ; that, therefore, a power of another kind is manifested in religion.

But is it not a widely known fact that love, without the mediation of psychotherapy or of religion, performs spiritual miracles ? The great human loves are favourite topics of the poets. We shall content ourselves with the reproduction of a passage from J. S. Mill's autobiography, in which the loss suffered by the death of a beloved wife gives some idea of what she had been to the philosopher :

" Since then I have sought for such alleviation as my state admitted of, by the mode of life which most enabled me to feel her

[1] *Ibid.*, p. 169.
[2] *Ibid.*

still near me.   I bought a cottage as close as possible to the place where she is buried, and there her daughter (my fellow-sufferer and now my chief comfort) and I, live constantly during a great portion of the year.   My objects in life are solely those which were hers ; my pursuits and occupations those in which she shared, or sympathized, and which are indissolubly associated with her.   Her memory is to me a religion, and her approbation the standard by which, summing up as it does all worthiness, I endeavour to regulate my life."   " I endeavour to make the best of what life I have left, and to work on for her purposes with such diminished strength as can be derived from thoughts of her, and communion with her memory[1]."

In the class of cures illustrated above, just as much as in the instance of J. S. Mill, it is evident that the remedy reaches the very sources of life and for that reason heals body and soul together. The degree of perfection of the life which is generated by love depends upon the quality of that love and of its object.   It is obviously, in part, because of imperfections in the object of love, as well as in the ideal of the lover, that most of the transformations we have reported leave so much to be desired from the ethical point of view and that they are rarely permanent.

For persons suffering from the social mal-adjustments characteristic of the early life of our great mystics, sufficient as a remedy is any means which shall remove the inhibitions and repressions and shall tap the springs of life.   Whatever liberates the pent-up forces and provides normal outlets for self-expression will induce in the afflicted a transformation similar to that achieved by the love of God.   Of all the liberators, none equals love, whether of God or of man ; for the love-relation brings about the satisfaction of the most fundamental and irresistible of all physiological functions and innate cravings : the sex functions, the tendencies to self-affirmation and self-esteem, and the desire for the peace of inner unity and of affectionate trust.

*   *   *

The development of the mystical technique for the realization of a quasi-physical presence of the Perfect One constitutes the most remarkable achievement of religion in man's struggle to overcome adverse external circumstances, his own imperfections, and those of his fellowmen.   It is one of the outstanding expressions of the creative power working in humanity.   It is paralleled in the realm of reason by the development of science.   Both lead, if in different ways, to the physical and spiritual realization of man.

---

[1] J. S. Mill's *Autobiography*, New York, 1887, pp. 251 and 241.

CHAPTER XII

RELIGION, SCIENCE AND PHILOSOPHY

I. Science and the Belief in the Gods of the Religions.
It is a generally accepted proposition that science is not qualified to pass judgment on religion. It is said that science stands outside the lists in which the question of the existence and of the nature of God are to be decided, that these problems concern metaphysics. " Psychology neither rejects nor affirms the transcendental existence of the religious objects ; it simply ignores that problem as being outside of its field[1]."
This principle of the exclusion of the transcendent from the province of science, made repeatedly by authoritative philosophers and scientists, has been acclaimed with the keenest satisfaction by modern theologians as an impenetrable shield for their religions. They construed it as meaning that science, which has already shattered so many secondary religious beliefs, was impotent with regard to the central, the one necessary, belief of the organized religions, i.e., the belief in a God in direct communication with man, a God with whom the worshipper may commune and who under certain conditions will answer man's desires and supplications, either by suspending the natural laws or by altering them, or by inserting, as it were, his Will between the natural forces. They have rejoiced in this assurance and have found delight in directing their followers to utterances such as these : " Never be afraid of science. In particular do not fear its influence upon your faith, for science and faith are not of the same order. Science is neutral, silent, ' agnostic,' regarding the foundation of things and the final meaning of life. And so, never ask of it arguments favouring your convictions. But be equally certain that it does not speak in favour of antagonistic doctrines[2]."
But the principle of the irrelevance of science to the transcendent shields the cardinal belief of the established religions only if their gods are transcendental objects. In taking for granted that they are

---
[1] Flournoy, Th, *Les Principes de la Psychologie Religieuse, Archives de Psychologie*, vol. II, 1903, pp. 37-41.
[2] Flournoy, Th, *Le Génie Religieux*, a lecture to the Swiss Students' Christian Association, Sainte-Croix, 1904, p. 34. Abbreviated.

such objects, an error has been committed and grave confusion has been introduced in the discussion of the relation of science to religion.

If it should turn out that the beliefs in the gods which make possible the religions, as they have existed and as they exist to-day, come from the naïve interpretation of certain phenomena—whether physical or psychical—then *those beliefs* would disappear together with that interpretation. If, for instance, anyone should believe in the existence of a superhuman personal Power because of thunder and lightning, or because unaccountably to himself he has escaped a sudden danger, or because, after prayer, health has been restored and moral refreshment and strength have come to him—if that should be the ground of his belief in God, that belief would vanish should he become convinced that these facts are susceptible of an explanation in accordance with scientific principles.

Should the present belief in the gods of the religions have that source, the agreement of philosophers and of scientists regarding the limitation of science would in no way warrant the interpretation of the theologians, for the affirmation that science has nothing to say on the problem of God disregards the supposition we have just made.

The question raised by the affirmation we are discussing is that of the relation of science to the belief which makes the religions possible, i.e., the belief in a sympathetic God in direct communication with man. We affirm that a *belief* naïvely derived from the observation of phenomena would not be independent of science ; it would, on the contrary, be subject to its conclusions. Physical science declares that thunder and lightning are in themselves no proof of the existence of invisible superhuman beings in direct relation with man, and psychological science altogether discredits the attribution of healing and of the increased confidence and happiness following upon prayer to anything other than the operation of natural laws.

It is to be noted, however, that even if this conclusion be accepted, and the ground of belief of the average believer thus removed, it might still be possible to satisfy oneself as to the existence of some sort of God : the metaphysical method of proof would remain open.

Our argument leads to a question of fact : is the belief in God, or are the beliefs in gods which have made possible the historical religions[1] due entirely or essentially to an animistic interpretation of

[1] We are discussing the religions that are or have been, not those that might be ; for we should like to avoid the confusion arising from a favourite practice of liberal writers on religion. They are fond of speaking of religion in the abstract, of " Pure Religion." Of that non-existent, they find it easy to say the most admirable things ; and it usually happens, to the satisfaction

particular physical phenomena and of the phenomena of " inner " experience ?

It will be readily granted that neither the non-civilized nor the semi-civilized believe in gods because of metaphysical considerations, but because of a variety of specific experiences which, as it seems to them, point to the action in nature or in themselves of personal invisible superhuman Beings[1].

The present-day religions of civilized peoples are no more dependent upon metaphysical proofs of God for their existence than are those of the non-civilized. These proofs, as it is customary to call them, are known to only an infinitesimal number of the members of the Christian churches. Apart from the will to believe—and of this motive we are not now speaking—the really effective cause of whatever belief in God exists in our Christian churches is of the same kind as that of the belief in the divine Beings of the non-civilized.

If, among the educated, physical phenomena have almost ceased to be regarded as direct expressions of the will of God, the facts of " inner " experience, or at least the rarer and the more surprising of these facts, constitute the ground of the present-day vital belief, in the God-Providence. We refer to the " voice " of conscience, to sudden conversion, to the peace, the hope, and the courage produced by prayer, and to the various other striking phenomena of mystical ecstasy considered in preceding chapters. For additional evidences we refer the reader to an earlier book[2], from which we abstract the following passages :

Document 3.—A professor at the school of Protestant theology in Paris writes : " God is not a phenomenon that we may observe apart from ourselves, or a truth demonstrable by logical reasoning.

---

of almost everybody, that their readers understand them to refer to the particular religion of their adherence. I might quote distinguished names ; let me rather illustrate from a regular writer on religion for a great daily paper. He wishes to show that it is because of misunderstandings that science and religion seem opposed to each other. He affirms that " True Science and True Religion cannot be opposed."—Probably not, if we are concerned not with the religions as they exist, but with something else that does not exist ; and obviously not if " true religion " is sufficiently defined as he defines it : " The Art of living truthfully and well " !   But if we are concerned with reality, with the actual religion of the Roman Catholic Church, of the Protestant Episcopal Church, of the Methodist Church, etc., then it is foolish or worse to speak in that fashion. Of what relevance would it be to descant upon the high utility and necessity of business in the abstract ?   To speak usefully one should speak with reference to forms of business actually in existence or which might be established.

[1] As to the origin of the God-ideas, we have said what we could in *A Psychological Study of Religion*.

[2] *A Psychological Study of Religion*, New York, Macmillan, 1912, Chapter XI, pp. 205-77.

He who does not feel Him in his heart will never feel Him from without. The object of religious knowledge reveals itself only in the subject, by means of the religious phenomena themselves. . . . We never become conscious of our piety externally, we feel religiously moved, *perceiving, more or less obscurely, in that very emotion the object and the cause of religion,* i.e., *God.* Observe the natural and spontaneous movement of piety ; a soul feels an inner peace and light ; is it strong, humble, resigned, obedient ? It immediately attributes its strength, its faith, its humility, its obedience, to the action of the divine spirit within itself. Anne Doubourg, dying at the stake, prayed, ' Oh God, do not abandon me lest I should fall off from thee ' . . . *to feel thus in our personal and empirical activity the action and the presence of the spirit of God within our own spirit, is a mystery, as it is also the source of religion."*

" Truths of the religious and of the moral order are known by subjective action of what Pascal calls the heart. Science can know nothing about them, for they are not in its order[1]."

Document 4.—A leader of the liberal movement in the United States expresses similar views. " God is not an hypothesis which the minister has invented to account for the phenomena of creation. *He knows that there is a ' power not ourselves that makes for righteousness, because when he has been weak that power has strengthened him, when he has been a coward that power has made him strong, when he has been in sorrow that power* has comforted him, when he has been in perplexity that power has counselled him, and he has walked a different path and lived a different life and has been a different man because there is that power, impalpable, invisible, unknown, and yet best and most truly known[2]."

The entire self-sufficiency of the experiential basis of faith in God has nowhere been more boldly proclaimed than among the Society of Friends. " The fundamental significant thing which stands out in early Quakerism was the *conviction* which these founders of it felt, that they had actually discovered the living God and that He was in them. They all have one thing to say—' I have experienced God.' " " It (Quakerism) was first of all the proclamation of an experience. The movement came to birth, and received its original power, through persons who were no less profoundly conscious of a *divine presence* than they were of a world in space[3]."

[1] Sabatier, A., *Outlines of a Philosophy of Religion,* James Pott and Co., New York, 1902, pp. 308-9, 311.

[2] Abbott, Lyman, *Address before the Alumni of Bangor Theological Seminary, The Outlook,* June 25, 1898.

[3] Jones, Rufus, *Social Law in the Spiritual World,* p. 161.

From end to end of the Protestant world these "inner experiences" constitute the only argument actually relied upon for the belief in a God in affective and intellectual relation with man.

*   *   *

Should there be no ground of belief other than physical phenomena and inner experiences, then, for those who are acquainted with the modern scientific conceptions, there could be no belief in God. But philosophy knows, as we have already remarked, of another route to the belief in a God: the metaphysical route. As this is a scientific inquiry we can discuss neither the nature of the metaphysical arguments nor their degree of validity, but we may draw attention to two results of the metaphysical effort of the past centuries :

1. It seems that materialism, as a metaphysical doctrine[1], has few supporters to-day, while idealism and spiritualism in their various forms, are the dominant conceptions. These doctrines agree in affirming that the ultimate Reality, commonly spoken of as God, is of a mental, a spiritual nature.

2. The God to which this dominant trend of metaphysics points, is an impassible, infinite Being—a being therefore who does not bear to man the relation which every one of the historical religions assumes to exist and seeks to maintain by means of its system of creeds and worship. The direct address characteristic of the rituals of every existing religion would no longer be possible should the gods of metaphysics replace the gods of the religions.

A strenuous effort is made in liberal religious circles, supposedly in the interest of religion, to conceal the magnitude of the difference between the God of the Christian religion and the impassable, infinite Reality of metaphysics. It seems clear, however, that the passage from the former to the latter belief would mean nothing less than the disappearance of the religious worship of to-day. That another form of belief and practice, which might with some degree of propriety be called religion, would take the place of the actual religions, seems to us most probable, but that is not a question for discussion in this book.

It should not however be overlooked that even though metaphysics should establish the existence of the gods of the religions, the practical problem would not be solved, for the metaphysical proofs are accessible to but a few ; even for these, they do not provide a ground of belief comparable in power of conviction with the impression of a direct apprehension of God in " inner " experience.

---

[1] For a brief review of the metaphysical arguments adduced in support of personal immortality, see the author's *Belief in God and Immortality*, Chicago, Open Court Publ. Co. 1921, chap. V.

II. Mystical Trance and the Conception of God; the immediate Apprehension of God.

The influence of mystical trance upon philosophical systems would make one of the most curious chapters of the history of philosophy. Let us hope that some competent person will soon write that chapter. As for us, after brief remarks upon the Neo-Platonic philosopher, Plotinus, we shall do no more than examine with some care the teachings of two modern representatives of the mystical tradition, Wm. James and Wm. Hocking.

When one believes with the mystics that God, the Absolute, the Ultimate Reality—these terms and others are used interchangeably in this connexion—is directly experienced in ecstatic trance and nowhere else, it would seem to follow that knowledge of the trance-consciousness includes a knowledge of God.

The problem of the nature of the divine Power or Powers was hardly formulated in the mind of the uncivilized mystic. He was engrossed in enjoying and using his trances. He merely affirmed its transcendental significance, he did not speculate about it. But it was otherwise at the beginning of the Christian era among the possessors of Greek culture. There the problem of the nature of God had been definitely formulated and was eagerly discussed. The Neo-Platonists, Plotinus in particular, took up certain strands of Hellenic thought, woven, perhaps, partially and indirectly from Hindoo mystical metaphysics[1] (itself dependent upon the much older and cruder tradition of the uncivilized regarding ecstatic trance), and spun wonderful theories.

That the mystical theories of Plotinus (born 205 A.D.) had one of their roots in ecstasy, appears with satisfactory clearness in his writings, and nowhere better than in this passage from the Enneads :

"Now often I am roused from the body to my true self and behold a marvellous beauty, and am particularly persuaded at the time that I belong to a better sphere, and live a supremely good life, and become identical with the godhead, and fast fixed therein attain its divine activity, having reached a plane above the whole intelligible realm." "Now since in the vision they were not two, but the seer was made one with the seen, not as with something seen, but as with something made one with himself, he who has been united with it might, if he remember, have by him some faint image of the divine. He himself was one (in the vision), with no distinctions within himself

---

[1] An excellent brief exposition of the mystical metaphysics of the Upanishads may be found in Josiah Royce's *Gifford Lectures, The World and the Individual*, vol. I, Fourth Lecture, pp. 165-75.

either as regarded himself or outer things. There was no movement of any sort in him, nor was emotion or desire of any outer thing present in him after his ascent, no, not any reason or any thought, nor was he himself present to himself, if I may so express it[1]."

The theory that in ecstasy the self becomes "identical with the godhead and attains its divine activity" offers a special difficulty; for ecstatic trance is not a simple experience, uniform as long as it lasts. It consists, on the contrary, in a succession of mental states which grow more and more simple and end in total unconsciousness.

At which one of these stages is the deification complete? If at the final stage, the description of the Divine would be brief indeed, since that stage is characterized by complete unconsciousness. The practical Christian mystics, however, firmly anchored in the beliefs in Christ as Son of God, and in a personal and more or less anthropomorphic Father, can not possibly make God equal to unconsciousness. They select among the various and successive aspects of ecstasy those which are not too far removed from the traditional Christian conception. The phases of the trance in which ravishing love or peace and trust, in complete surrender to the Will of God, dominate are those which they regard as divine. We recall also that a condition of automatic activity, referred to Christ or God as the cause, is spoken of by some of the great Christian mystics as deification.

As to Plotinus, if he was not embarrassed by an anthropomorphic conception of God, he was influenced by other preconceptions, those familiar to the philosophers of his time. Hindoo as well as Greek philosophy regarded God as infinite, i.e., as in no way limited or conditioned. Therefore nothing could be predicated of him; for the possessing of specific qualities would be a limitation of his infinite nature.

Under the influence of considerations of that type, uncompromisingly logical minds might identify the Absolute with the final phase of ecstasy of which, as a matter of fact, only negations can be affirmed. That is what the philosophers of the Upanishads did. Certain German mystics, in particular Boehme and Eckhart, have yielded to the same temptation : " Alles Endliche ist ein Abfall vom Wesen. Im Wesen giebt es keinen Gegensatz, nicht Lieb, noch Leid, nicht Weiss noch Schwarz," said Eckhart. In this view, not even being or essence can be affirmed of the Absolute : "Nichts werden ist Gott werden[2]."

---

[1] Charles Bakewell, *Source Book in Ancient Philosophy*, New York, Scribner's Sons, 1907, pp. 386, 391-2.

[2] A. Lasson, *Meister Eckhart, der Mystiker*, Berlin, 1868.

If these Hindoo and German philosophers followed logic into a black hole, Plotinus was somewhat less radical. The delightful aspects of ecstasy, which are responsible for the warm, humane elements in the divine picture drawn by less intellectual mystics were not without influence upon him. He noted the marvellous beauty of his visions and believed that he was " living a supremely good life." He seemed to have identified God with a lingering consciousness of selfhood and with indescribable, yet desirable, feelings characteristic of an advanced stage of ecstatic trance.

However that may be, the non-civilized and the practical Christians under the influence of popular preconceptions identify God with a penultimate stage of ecstasy, while radical philosophers, slaves to logic, make him one with the ultimate phase, i.e., with complete unconsciousness. This means that for the former, not unity or simplicity, not the disappearance of individuality, of differences and divergences, but a plenitude of felt-life, a wonderful impression of free-power, realized in a variety of illusions and hallucinations, are the aspects of ecstasy which make it divine.

We wish to draw especial attention to the convergence upon the conception of the Divine of what is by many regarded as two co-ordinate sources of knowledge ; on the one hand, discursive think-ing ; on the other, the trance-experience, a source of " immediate knowledge,"—knowledge independent of fallible mental processes. Some speak as if reason *recognized* in a phase of ecstatic trance the Divine whose nature it had previously determined. Others speak as if the ecstatic experience *revealed* the nature of God, while the rôle of reason remained a subordinate one. What we are to think of this mystical " source of knowledge " will appear in the sequel.

*   *   *

Wm James and mystical ecstasy.—In a book in which religious life is searched for facts that would support his pluralistic philosophy and provide a basis for a religious belief, Wm James sets down these three propositions :

" Mystical states, when they are well developed, usually are, and have a right to be, absolutely authoritative over the individuals to whom they come.

" No authority emanates from them which should make it a duty for those who stand outside of them to accept their revelations uncritically.

" They break down the authority of the non-mystical or rationalistic consciousness, based upon the understanding and the senses alone. They show it to be only one kind of consciousness.

They open out the possibility of other orders of truth in which, so far as anything in us vitally responds to them, we may freely continue to have faith[1]."

The mystic's revelation is, we are told, invulnerable because, even though his senses are in abeyance, his experience is as truly a direct perception of fact as any sensation ever is[2]. He is in possession of " immediate " or " intuitive " knowledge, therefore of unassailable knowledge, since it is *given* and not secured by mental operations always open to error[3].

We agree with Wm James that whatever is " immediate," " pure experience," whatever has not been mentally elaborated, is invulnerable. There is here no room for difference of opinion. Disagreements may appear, however, over the problem of *what* is to be regarded in experience as " immediate."

In our opinion Wm James has erred, not in considering " pure " experience as unassailable, but in unwittingly regarding as such more than the " given." He has confused pure experience with elaborations of it. It is because of that error that he was a believer in mysticism ; or, one should perhaps say that he committed that error because he wished to believe in a mystical revelation.

But for what in mystical experience does James claim invulnerability ? The uncritical mystic believes that Christ, or the Virgin, or some saint, has manifested himself to him. Although these and similar experiences have at times, for the recipient, a " sensational " quality as compelling as that of true perception, James regards them as illusory because, when critically examined, when confronted with the rest of experience, they do not stand the test. They hold, however, he affirms, a kernel immediately given, intuitional, and, therefore, invulnerable. What is this kernel ? He answers that it consists in a feeling or conviction of vastness, of reconciliation, of repose, of safety, of union, of harmony[4]. In these terms, and in no others more explicit, does our distinguished philosopher define the kernel of unassailable truth revealed in mystical ecstasy. It is more than the Nothingness extolled by the

[1] *The Varieties of Religious Experience*, pp. 422-3.

[2] *Ibid.*, pp. 423-4.

[3] In a preceding section we have attempted to account for the impression of certainty which accompanies that " knowledge."

[4] " The key note of it is, invariably, a reconciliation." *Ibid.*, p. 388. The mystical states " tell of the supremacy of the ideal, of vastness, of union, of safety, and of rest." *Ibid.*, p. 428. Elsewhere he is much less definite, as when he writes that mystical ecstasy reveals " states of insight into depths of truth unplumbed by the discursive intellect. There are illuminations, revelations full of significance and importance, all inarticulate though they remain." *Ibid.*, p. 380.

Neo-Platonists. It bears closer affinity to positive happiness and intimates that there is ground for radical optimism.

It should not be forgotten that these alleged "truths" are revealed not only to a few lofty religious souls. Any and everybody may enjoy them. Nitrous oxide "stimulates the mystical consciousness in an extraordinary degree"; and alcohol "brings its votary from the chill periphery of things to the radiant core. It makes him for the moment one with truth[1]." Here James is certainly in accord with the facts as our investigation of drug-ecstasy has revealed them. However it may be produced, ecstasy is ecstasy, just as fever is fever whatever its cause. The truth-kernel of religious ecstasy is, as we have shown, no other than the truth-kernel of narcotic intoxication and of ecstatic trance in general.

There is no doubt whatsoever that the words quoted—reconciliation, repose, safety, union, harmony—describe the more general, fundamental impressions which come to most mystics. But it appears to us evident that everyone of these words implies an *interpretation* of "neutral stuff." Their meaning involves, as all meaning does, a relating of two terms. If, for instance, "reconciliation" and "union" have any meaning at all, it is that of the establishment or recognition of a specific relation between two or more terms. Now, unification may be attained in two ways: (1) An understanding of the two terms may be achieved which shows them to be subsumed under a general principle or included in a larger whole. That is the kind of harmony produced by the understanding. (2) The terms may lose their individual features and be degraded to a level of undifferentiated simplicity. That, as we have seen, is the mystical way of producing "harmony" or "unity." It is a way which does not secure any knowledge.

If by "union" James had merely meant to indicate that, as the trance progresses, the mystic notices the gradual disappearance of boundary lines between objects, the merging of ideas into one another, the fusion of feelings, and that he enjoys a delightful sense of peace, no objection could have been raised against the claim of unassailability. But it would have been an insignificant claim. What James means is that the mystical experience points to, or signifies, a union of the individual with Someone or Something else. Now, that is just as much an interpretation of immediate experience as the affirmation of the Salvation Army lassie that she has met Christ face to face. Before it can be accepted as true the alleged "immediate" experience in both instances must be tested according to the canons of scientific evidence, for the "perceptual" quality of

[1] *Loc cit.*, p. 387.

the experience no more justifies the mystic in placing credence in it than the absence of certain organic sensations authorizes the asylum patient to believe that the doctors have removed his viscera.

In a letter published in part in *Letters of Wm James*, one reads : " The intellect is interpretative and critical of its own interpretation, but there must have been a thesis to interpret, and that thesis seems to me to be the non-rational sense of a ' higher ' power." And, further on : " May not this mystical testimony that there is a God be true, even though the precise determinations, being so largely ' suggestive ' contributions of our rational factor, should widely differ[1] ? "

In this passage, the error which I have tried to lay bare is again clearly apparent. The thought of a " higher power " is not an " immediate " datum of consciousness. It is already a product of elaboration and interpretation ; it involves, in particular, judgments of relative " height " or value of powers. It is, therefore, no more entitled to claim invulnerability than any of the other, grosser and more obvious interpretations of the ordinary mystic.

The wide-awake, rational consciousness finds no difficulty in understanding why the " kernel " of the mystical experience is describable as reconciliation, union, peace, rest, and the like. Are these not the very terms which would come to the mind of a person who had undergone the mental simplification characteristic of ecstatic trance ? Would a person from whose consciousness the external world had disappeared, whose mental activity had been reduced to a vague general idea of the presence of a traditional God, whose affective life was on the point of peaceably dying out—would such a person describe his condition as one of internal *strife*, would he be impressed by the irreconcilable *multiplicity* of the elements of experience ? Of course not. He would be able to find no better terms than those actually used by the mystics, and, generally, by those familiar with certain aspects of trance-consciousness. Why, then, ascribe a metaphysical significance to that description ? Whatever contribution to knowledge may come from that aspect of trance-experience must proceed from the critical activity of the fully-awake mind working upon the whole range of human experience.

We are thus led to affirm that if James found it possible to say that " as a matter of fact and in point of logic " the claim of the mystic (reduced to the minimum we have been discussing) " escapes

---

[1] From a letter to the Author. I might take this opportunity of saying that when these *Letters* were published, none of my books had yet appeared.

our jurisdiction," it is, it seems, because he confused more or less automatic or habitual causal interpretations of sense-data with the sense-data themselves[1].

The " universality " of the mystical conviction is frequently offered in proof of its truth. But the truth of a belief is not proved by the fact that it is shared by all known men. Moreover, this conviction is, as a matter of fact, very far from common to all those who have experienced trances possessing the traits singled out by James as characteristic of mystical ecstasy (ineffability, noetic quality, transiency, and passivity). Most of the users of narcotics and many of the subjects of spontaneous trance regard its contents, just as they do their dreams, i.e., as having no other than a subjective validity.

The history of the philosophers' belief in mystical revelation seems to announce the disappearance of the belief.. At the beginning, ecstatic trance was held to reveal extensive " truths," concrete as well as abstract, for instance, the will of God at a particular juncture of events. With Wm James, the revelation has become limited to a sense of safety, of unity, and of harmony. With Wm Hocking it is attenuated still further and becomes a mere " That " of which nothing more can be said.

*   *   *

William E. Hocking and religious mysticism.—In the English language it is Wm Hocking who, since James, has most comprehensively and richly dealt with the philosophical problems of religious mysticism[2]. He is generally regarded as a champion of mysticism. Yet a careful examination of his latest utterances may leave one in doubt as to his present position. He complains that certain " immediate " qualities of the trance experience have unjustifiably been ascribed to God : " What I want to point out, is that these words, unitary, immediate, ineffable, which at all events apply to the mystic's *experience*, are precisely the words which the

---

[1] The argument against James' position contained in the preceding pages was urged in a criticism of the *Varieties of Religious Experience* in the *Intern. Jr. of Ethics*, vol. XIV, 1904, pp. 322-39.

Comp. George A. Coe's criticism of James and of others in an unusually substantial paper on the *Sources of the Mystical Revelation*, in the *Hibbert Jr.*, vol. VI, 1907-8, pp. 359-72.

[2] *The Meaning of God in Human Experience*, Yale University Press, 1912. *The Meaning of Mysticism as seen through its Psychology*, Mind, N.S., XXI, 1912, pp. 38-61. *Principles and Method in the Philosophy of Religion*, Rev. de Méta. et de Morale, XXIX, 1922, pp. 431-53.

As Professor Hocking's most recent utterances on this topic are contained in these last two papers, our exposition and criticism will be based mainly upon them.

metaphysician applies to the mystic's *doctrine*. And I suggest that the misinterpretation of mysticism here in question is due to the fact that *what is a psychological report* (and a true one) *is taken as a metaphysical statement* (and a false one). From the fact that one's experience of God has been ' one, immediate, and ineffable,' it does not follow that God Himself is merely ' one, immediate and ineffable '—and so a Being wholly removed from all concrete reality. It is true that this inference from the nature of the experience to the nature of its object is here of the closest order ; and it is also true that many a mystic has committed himself to that inference. But it is possible, and necessary, to reject it[1]." " An ' immediacy ' does not legislate about what is beyond itself either to deny it or to affirm it[2]." " I judge, then, . . . that the marks commonly attributed to the mystic absolute are in the first place so many contributions to mystic psychology[3]."

These passages mean that what is regarded by others (James among them) as an immediately given and invulnerable revelation of the nature of God, is really an inference and, therefore, authoritative only in so far as reason can make it so. For him the only *unquestionable* content of the trance is a " Something," a " That " about which nothing more can be said. Any knowledge whatsoever about it is the fruit of rational thought ; knowledge of God is not a revelation or an intuition, it is the product of intellectual activity. If the foregoing statements represent Hocking's position correctly, he repudiates mysticism and agrees with us. For we have held that, unwittingly, the savage infers identity of the Divine with the plenitude of delight, power and freedom that comes to him in the earlier phases of the drug ecstasy ; that, unwittingly, the Neo-Platonic philosopher *infers* identity of the Absolute with the ultimate period of the trance, and that James and others do likewise with certain feelings and attitudes prominent in a phase of that experience.

James and the mystics in general (including Bergson) have erred, according to Hocking, in placing mystical knowledge—intuition or the immediately given—in hostile opposition to conceptual knowledge. The relation is another one : " Intuition must be regarded not as a station, but as a *point through which* true knowledge must pass, . . . as a mode of cognition by which conceptual knowledge is not so much excluded as concentrated[4]." " Immediacy

---

[1] Mind, *loc. cit.*, p. 43.

[2] *Ibid.*

[3] *Ibid.*, p. 44.

[4] *Rev. de Méta. et de Morale, loc. cit.*, p. 447.

and idea are not disparate stuff ; they are different stages of the same stuff, the same meaning[1]." Both intuition and interpretation are necessary in order to attain truth. Intuition alone is empty. " With these two methods, the way is open for a hopeful resumption of metaphysical effort[2]."

When you have said, as Professor Hocking does, that the " That" of mystical ecstasy has no meaning until interpreted, that it is mind-stuff or " neutral-stuff," out of which in an active mind, knowledge issues, logic compels you, it seems to hold that the same is true of all the " thats " immediately given in any other experience. The immediately-given in ecstasy is no longer isolated as a unique phenomenon ; it is now properly classified together with the meaningless and yet potentially meaningful Something *which is at the root of every psychical experience whatsoever*. For, not only in mystical ecstasy but also in every perceptual or affective experience, something unassailable and ineffable is given. Thus, the metaphysical effort to find God is provided with a much broader intuitive basis than that of mystical ecstasy alone ; its basis includes the " given " in conscious experience generally. In the search for God no position of vantage may now be claimed *a priori* for the immediately given in trance experience.

To draw the above corollary of the propositions laid down by Professor Hocking regarding the mystical revelation is equivalent to a renunciation of the essential mystical position. But Professor Hocking does not draw that corollary, does not renounce mysticism ; for, notwithstanding the passages we have quoted, he holds that the mystical experience *reveals* God directly, authoritatively. Otherwise, what is the meaning of these utterances : " The mystic knows the Truth, so he assures us : but he seems to spin hopelessly about this point, and to come forward very slowly with any statement of its contents. May it be that the mystic is more sure *that* he is sure than of *what* he is sure—except that he is sure of God and of his own relation to God[3] ? " " Let the mystic, then, be certain of his ' the truth,' his ' God's truth,' and do not enviously require him at every turn to say what the truth contains[4]." " The mystic gives us the

---

[1] Mind, *loc. cit.*, p. 44.

[2] *Rev. de Méta. et de Morale, loc. cit.*, p. 451.
In his metaphysical search Professor Hocking is moved by a desire to establish the existence of a God conceived so as to fulfil human needs and aspirations, and he is of the opinion that metaphysics leads to such a God and not merely to the empty Absolute of Plotinus.

[3] *God in Human Experience*, p. 454.

[4] *Ibid.*, p. 455.

thing which is to be modified . . . But who else could have pulled down from heaven that substance[1]? "

It seems after all that Hocking holds, with James and the mystic philosophers in general, that the immediate in ecstasy does not remain meaningless until rationally interpreted; it is not on a level with the immediate in conscious experience in general, for it conveys a direct and truthful assurance of God and of the mystic's own relation to him; it is a divine substance known intuitively to come "from heaven." That first, immediate apprehension does not, it is true, lay hold on all the knowledge about God which we might like to have, but it suffices to lift man up above fatal doubt, and disbelief. Further knowledge must wait upon intellectual labour.

*   *   *

If we reject the mystical claim, even when it is limited as by Hocking, it is because the passage from sensations and feelings, whatever they may be, to the thought of "God," however understood, seems to us always an elaboration of the "given." To think

[1] *God in Human Experience*, p. 460.

In order to do full justice to Professor Hocking's argument for mysticism, it would be necessary to give an adequate abstract of several chapters of his book. The following quotations, although mere disjointed fragments, may stimulate the reader's curiosity.

"It may be that the more we press the conclusions of our position, the less we shall be able to recognise in any concrete characters of our own experience, the experience here described. We have made all social experience depend upon a conscious knowledge in experience of a being, who in scope and power might well be identified with God. We have been led by the successive requirements of logic to the position that our first and fundamental social experience is an experience of God " (295).

"God is known as that of which I am primarily certain; and being certain, am certain of self and of my world of men and men's objects. I shall always be more certain *that* God is, than *what* he is: it is the age-long problem of religion to bring to light the deeper characters of this fundamental experience. But the starting point of this development (which we shall have occasion to trace in some rough way) is no mere That Which, without predicates. Substance is known as Subject: reality from the beginning is known as God. The idea of God is not an attribute which in the course of experience I come to attach to my original whole idea: the unity of my world which makes it from the beginning a whole, knowable in simplicity, is the unity of other Self-hood.

"God then is immediately known, and permanently known, as the Other Mind which in creating Nature is also creating me. Of this knowledge nothing can despoil us; this knowledge has never been wanting to the self-knowing mind of man " (296-7).

"In applying the name of God to the Other Mind which in sustaining physical experience does continually create and communicate itself to us, we have gone indeed beyond our warrant. We have what must justify the animism of our ancestors—the inevitable animism of all mankind " (300).

"Man knows well that he is not alone; he does not so well know in what companionship he is. The knowledge of the presence of spirit beyond self is no conjecture; nor does this social experience ever *arise*. Man's world is from the first a living world, even a divine world; and primitive animism is in so far no mere theory, but a report of certain and intimate experience " (317).

See also the footnotes to pages 449-450.

of God—any kind of god—on the occasion of a sensory or affective experience, however unusual in intensity or quality, is to ascribe a cause to an intuitive, immediate experience. The confusion of this automatic assignment of a cause with immediate, intuitive, experience reveals how deeply ingrained is the habit of assigning causes. It begins to be formed at birth and soon becomes mechanical. When the uncivilized *hears* God in the thunder, he is subject to the same illusion of immediacy as is the Christian who *feels* God in an influx of moral energy when in ecstasy or ordinary prayer.

*   *   *

This book began with the examination of experiences regarded by uncivilized man as revelation of, or union with, the Divine. They were submitted to a critical analysis, and recently acquired scientific knowledge of the psycho-physiological effects of certain ecstasy-producing drugs was brought to bear upon them. It appeared that the early mystics owe their belief mainly to delightful impressions of limitless power and freedom, to altered self-feelings, to the impression that the soul is liberated from the body, to automatisms including wonderful sensory hallucinations. Now, every one of these impressions and beliefs can be satisfactorily explained as the result of psycho-physiological forces set in activity or inhibited by the drug. We then examined the mystical ecstasies of the Yogin and of a group of Christian mystics. Their own descriptions were compared with non-religious ecstasies—those of poets, of epileptics, of ordinary normal persons.

In all these ecstasies, the same fundmental characteristics were discovered, and we came to the conclusion that there need be no differences between religious and non-religious ecstasies other than those due to a different interpretation—the interpretation being itself the cause of important affective and volitional phenomena.

Particular attention was given to the impressions of ineffability and of illumination or revelation ; for they, perhaps more than any other feature, are responsible for the persistency of the belief in the divineness of ecstasy. Both these traits are frequent in trance— whether it be produced spontaneously or by drugs such as ether and nitrous oxide. They occur also in near-sleep conditions arising naturally. Any narrowing of consciousness or any dissociation of mental connexions, whatever the cause, may be accompanied by these strange impressions. We have offered a psychological explanation of the impression of illumination which to us appears sufficient.

Other features of the mystical trance to which philosophers have ascribed much evidential value (unity, harmony, and the sense of security which goes with them) have also received in the preceding pages an explanation which should relieve one of any inclination to appeal to a divine illumination ; they are unavoidable products of the psychological condition in which an entranced person finds himself.

Thus, our comparative investigation of trance-states with their impression of unlimited power and of passivity, their excitement and quietude, their hallucinations and exclusion of the world of sense, their absolute certitude and moments of doubt, their harmony and ineffability, led us to the conclusion that mystical trance contains nothing, no " sign " no " thesis," no " That," demanding, from the informed and reflective mind, belief in divine revelation—unless, however, one should take the term " divine " as designating merely the general ground of life ; or unless one should conceive of " God " as manifesting himself in those ways of physical and psychical nature of which the scientists find the laws. *Should one do so, then every part and aspect of conscious life would, as well as the mystical ecstatic-trance itself, be an expression of the Divine. But if the regular, law-bound nature known to science should be called the " Divine," then the essential claim of mysticism would be given up.*

In seeking intercourse with God in the disappearance of diversity, in the peace of utter surrender, in excruciating delights, in a sense of freedom and illumination, the mystics have followed a wrong way. These experiences reveal not the Christian God, but the lawful workings of our psycho-physiological organisms. In that respect the mystical experience is not of a nature other than that of the rest of conscious experience. It points to the same conclusions as conscious life in general.

One might speculate and suppose that when the higher mental life and the activity of the external senses have ceased, the primordial quality of organic sensations and feelings is revealed. On the brink of unconsciousness—whether it be the unconsciousness of sleep or of abnormal trance produced in any way whatsoever—consciousness is at its simplest ; it is continuity without parts, and, therefore, let us say, eternal and timeless. This might be spoken of as the *Urgrund*, to use a term of the German pantheistic mystics, and it might be surmised that it is in this form that consciousness began in the organic world. Thus far one might speculate. But what an incredible confusion it would be to regard the *Urgrund*, so disclosed at the vanishing point of consciousness, as a revelation of the nature of the Perfect God made flesh in Jesus Christ and worshipped in the churches !

*   *   *

Is it claimed that this investigation amounts to a proof of the non-existence of God ? It amounts in the author's opinion to no more than a demonstration of the total insufficiency of the ground on which rests, on the whole, the belief in the existence of the gods of the religions. Of other conceptions of God or gods this book speaks only incidentally, and without definitely offering any conclusion. We have not presumed to say how the *ultimate* source of the new energies by which the mystic is enriched is to be conceived. We have limited ourselves to the affirmation that there are in the human being innate sources of energy, customarily spoken of as innate tendencies or instinct and regarded as dependent upon or connected with the presence of physiological (neural) mechanisms. And we have added that physical and moral health, and with them happiness, depend upon an adequate stimulation and an harmonious manifestation of these sources of energy. We might have used the expression " subconscious sources of energy." But that would not have constituted an addition of real knowledge, nor would it have made anything clearer. When these and other things of the same purport have been said, the questions of the ultimate origin and of the nature of " God," as raised by the philosopher, remain unanswered.

*　　　*　　　*

It has seemed to us that, for the philosopher, the fact of greatest significance in religious mysticism is perhaps not the accession of energy but the direction it takes, i.e., the manifestation of a will to actualize an ideal, thought of as divine and involving the socialization of humanity. We have seen how great Christian mystics strove to establish the Kingdom of God on earth. Without regarding their social ideal as perfectly conceived, the Divine in them might be seen, if anywhere, in the unrelenting effort with which they endeavoured to realize in themselves and in others a lofty social ideal. In this effort they were not attempting to adapt themselves to the demands of actual society : they strove instead, with unconquerable tenacity, to create something to which the World opposes a stubborn and cruel resistance.

That direction of the mystical effort is perhaps the thing most worthy of notice. It might be spoken of as a manifestation of the Life-Energy, of the *Elan Vital*. But, then, let us not deceive ourselves. These words would be merely names for the designation of what has been observed. The important thing to do is to determine the conditions of the manifestation of the Life-Energy in order that we may control it more and more.

It is of course quite clear that, conceived in this way, the Divine does not manifest itself only, or even especially, in mystical ecstasies.

It is equally evident that this Life-Energy does not delight in praises and thanksgiving ; it is not the God worshipped in the Churches.

*   *   *

For the psychologist who remains within the province of science, religious mysticism is a revelation not of God but of man. Whoever wants to know the deepest that is in man, the hidden forces that drive him onward, should become a student of mysticism. And if knowing man is not knowing God, it is nevertheless only when in possession of an adequate knowledge of man that metaphysics may expect to fashion an acceptable conception of the Ultimate.

*   *   *

We find much satisfaction in being in agreement with Henri Delacroix and George A. Coe with regard to the illusory nature of the mystical claim. In the Hibbert paper already referred to, the latter writes : " The mystic acquires his religious convictions precisely as his non-mystical neighbour does, namely through tradition and instruction, auto-suggestion grown habitual, and reflective analysis. The mystic brings his theological beliefs to the mystical experience ; he does not derive them from it[1]." " We may even go so far as to say that all real religion consists ultimately in some mystical practice, namely, the making real to ourselves of that which we do not perceive. *Here is where the mystic's psychology falls short.* He will not admit that his certainty of spiritual things is self-produced ; he insists that it is infused[2]." " The tendency of this discussion is toward the view that the supposed mystical revelation is part and parcel of the general historical movement of religious life ; its sources are the same, and the *superior certainty and authority that it claims for itself are illusory*[3]."

The position of James B. Pratt is less sharply cut than our own or that of the two authors just named. The remarks added in fine print to the chapter on the *Sense of Presence* may interest the reader in this connexion.

[1] *The Sources of the Mystical Revelation, Hibbert Jr.*, vol. VI, 1907-8, p. 367. The italics are ours.

[2] *Loc. cit.*, p. 372.

[3] *Ibid.*

CHAPTER XIII

THE DISAPPEARANCE OF THE BELIEF IN A PERSONAL SUPERHUMAN CAUSE AND THE WELFARE OF HUMANITY

OUR purpose in this book has been to learn whatever we might about the mystical experience; our inquiry has, therefore, moved forward regardless of practical consequences. But we are loth to bring these pages to a close without some reference to a widespread opinion concerning the consequences of the loss of belief in a super-human personal Cause.

We shall not be primarily concerned with grand mysticism, not even with moderate mysticism, but with the traditional belief, wherever it may appear, in a personal, superhuman Will amenable to human intellectual and affective influences and regarded as a direct cause of " outer " or " inner " events.

As to grand mysticism itself, no one apt to read this book would be inclined to commend it to general emulation, either as seen in the Yogi who spend their lives in a state of *hébétude* entirely unfit for any human activity, or as seen in the Christian saint of the type of St Marguerite Marie, described by Mgr Bougaud, Bishop of Laval. She had been growing more and more incapable of performing the services expected of a nun : " They tried her in the infirmary, but without much success, although her kindness, zeal and devotion were without bounds, and her charity rose to acts of such a heroism that our readers would not bear the recital of them. They tried her in the kitchen, but were forced to give it up as hopeless—everything dropped out of her hands. The admirable humility with which she made amends for her clumsiness could not prevent this from being prejudicial to the order and regularity which must always reign in a community. They put her in the school, where the little girls cherished her, and cut pieces out of her clothes (for relics) as if she were already a saint, but where she was too absorbed inwardly to pay the necessary attention. Poor dear sister, she lived on earth in 1675 still less than in 1672, and they had to leave her in her heaven[1] " ! To love God in this way is to open the door to

[1] Mgr Bougaud. *Histoire de la Bienheureuse Marguerite Marie*, Paris, 1900, pp. 266-7.

some of the worst perversions and distortions possible to human nature.

* * *

The traditional opinion is that the loss of the belief in question would be calamitous. To this the answer may be made that if the scientific conception should be the true one, whatever dismay and discouragement it might produce at first in a limited number of persons, nevertheless, its acceptance would eventually be, on the whole, for the best. This general conviction in the superior value of knowledge may be supported in this instance by certain considerations and by specific information which we shall now set forth in part.

There was a time when it was wicked impiety to regard a storm as a phenomenon exclusively determined by physical forces. Among the educated that belief may be said to have almost entirely disappeared. Would anyone, for the good of humanity, return to the attitude of the heroes of the Iliad and of the Odyssey regarding the relation of the gods to nature, or, for that matter, to a genuine belief in the efficacy of prayer in the weather, as implied in our Prayer Books ? Was it a loss to replace the gods of the wind, of the storms, of the waves, etc., by orderly impersonal forces ? And is it impiety to refuse to see in these events the benevolent or wrathful hand of God stretched out to reward or punish ?

One of the gains—but not the only one—resulting from this changed understanding of nature is the recent strikingly rapid growth of the physical sciences. It is in part due to the unity of efforts made possible by the almost complete disappearance from the educated classes of a real belief in the divine personal causation of physical phenomena.

The same transformation is also almost completely achieved with regard to the causes of bodily diseases. Would any educated person say that, in matters of disease, the increased reliance on hygiene, on surgery, on serum treatment, and the corresponding decrease in genuine reliance upon God, betokens a loss to humanity ? Who, except the benighted, would to-day balance faith in God with vaccination for small-pox or typhoid ? What would the Chinese better give up—belief in superhuman personal causation of disease or the diffusion of medical knowledge now taking place in their country under the direction of the Rockefeller Institute ? There are those who would answer that they would better keep both. This solution will be considered presently.

With regard to divine personal causation in matters psychical, a corresponding change seems to be in progress. Here also, if much more slowly, the belief in the intervention of a personal God according to his good pleasure or in response to man's request, or desire, is giving way. The immaturity of psychological science accounts for the incompleteness of its present success in replacing in the mind of the educated the conception of personal causation by that of law. That accounts also for the keen apprehension still felt by many of these persons at the threat of the loss of the traditional belief.

One may, however, even now venture the statement that in the history of humanity the rise of that science during the second half of the last century will appear as a fact of greater practical importance than the far-reaching applications of the mechanical and of the biological sciences.

One of the first outcomes—not altogether desirable—of early scientific work in normal and abnormal psychology has been the production of mind-cure movements, monsters compounded of false religious beliefs and of scraps of ill-understood mental science[1]. In the wake of these hybrids have come other premature and often ill-considered systems of treatment by suggestion or auto-suggestion.

A more recent product of the same strands of psychology may be seen in the work of Freud, a Viennese psychiatrist of genius, but without any aptitude for exact science. His system of psychotherapy called "psychoanalysis," is so obviously lacking in accuracy and completeness that it may not long endure in the form given it by its author. Nevertheless, its success in forcing upon the physician and others a recognition of the effectiveness of psychical methods in the cure of a great variety of disorders of body and mind gives to the movement a real importance.

The most careful and comprehensive work in the field of psychotherapy has been done in France. To that country, mainly, belongs the honour of having initiated and developed the studies in abnormal psychology connected with the so-called " subconscious " and their practical applications to the restoration and increase of bodily and mental powers. William James' prophetic utterance that it was the most important movement of modern psychology may be said to have already been proved true. It is in Pierre Janet's work

---

[1] In certain of the established churches a better-informed effort has been made to utilize psychological knowledge together with religion. The false position in which these churches have been placed by having to recognize that the religious method has produced no cure " which cannot be paralleled by similar cures wrought by psychotherapy without religion " is most interestingly suggested in the recent report of the committee appointed by the Archbishop of Canterbury in accordance with Resolution 63 of the Lambeth Conference of 1920. This report on the *Ministry of Healing* has been published by the *Churchman* for February 16, 1924. The preceding quotation is taken from that report.

and especially in his monumental *Médications Psychologiques*[1] that one must look for the ripest knowledge and the finest art in this field.

The psychiatrist has come to regard his problem as being the finding of ways and means :

1. To save energy by simplifying life and by eliminating the waste due to inner antagonisms, contradictions, inhibitions, repressions—whether these be the result of intellectual insufficiency or of moral defects.

2. To stimulate sources of energy that have remained untapped and thus to lift life up to a higher psycho-physiological level.

3. To organize life on a basis of enduring interests and unifying conceptions and aims, and thus to complete the saving and stimulating of energy.

At the end of the chapter on the Sense of Presence, both the directing and the energizing influence of the physician have been illustrated. A psychiatrist in possession of the higher and finer psychological knowledge takes the place both of the physician and of the religious Director of the soul. He not only arrests waste and generates energy by physiological means but, as he is also a practical psychologist, he organizes and directs its manifestations by proposing goals and principles of conduct which it is quite proper to call " spiritual." Thus he may produce the happiness which comes with the peace of passivity and the peace of activity.

There is neither rashness nor impiety in affirming of mystics such as Suzo, St Theresa, St Catherine of Genoa, Mme Guyon and St Marguerite Marie, that the best psychotherapy of to-day would have saved them a great deal of physical and spiritual suffering, and that it would have led them along natural ways to an earlier self-fulfilment and to a degree of perfection in no way inferior, ethically or otherwise, to the one which they attained during the active phases of their lives.

The time is not far off when it will seem just as out of place to treat cases of social maladjustment by the mystical religious method, as it now would be to deliver for exorcism to the ministers of any religion certain unfortunate inmates of our insane asylums.

There are those who will exclaim in derision : " How could man ever take the place of God ? " It must be granted that man never could take the place of a god maintaining with man the relation assumed to exist by the religions. But if, as this book

---

[1] *Les Médications Psychologiques*, 3 vols, Paris, Felix Alcan, 1919.
It might be added that to France also psychology owes the first scale of mental measurements—the Binet-Simon scale.

seems to show, the Ultimate Power does not stand to man in that personal relation, the question is not one concerning the replacement of that God by man, but one concerning the replacement of an illusory belief in such a God by a more accurate understanding of the causes of whatever effectiveness is possessed by that belief.

*   *   *

It might be argued that even though there should be no satisfactory proof of the existence of the gods of the religions, a statesmanlike policy would continue to use both the scientific and the religious methods. For it will be truly said that, when God is conceived as a God of love and righteousness, there is assuredly in his worship an indirect, or, as some call it, a psychological source of intellectual steadiness, of character improvement, and of moral courage and happiness. No statesman worthy of the name would, however, formulate his policy in the matter without first seeking to ascertain whether the belief in a providential God entails also disadvantages, and whether the values it yields cannot be secured in totality or in part by other means.

John Keeble tells us that he wrote the *Christian Year* with the chief purpose of exhibiting the " soothing tendency " of the Prayer Book. He was apparently one of the tormented and wearied souls who above all yearn for peace. But the Prayer Book is, of course, not to be recommended because of its soothing effects without regard to what else it may do ; otherwise syrups for children and drugs for adults would advantageously replace that book. Before one may safely confirm mystical piety in the place of dignity which it has gained, *all* its consequences whether immediate or remote, direct or indirect—not only its desirable fruits—must be taken into account, and it must be clear that no other method can replace it advantageously.

The belief that the conception of God embodied in Christian worship corresponds perfectly to objective reality and that it " works " adequately is so profoundly rooted in the Christian worshippers that a mere hint of possible evil resulting from it will seem to them preposterous. Since the days of Pascal we have been told : " Better in any case behave as if God existed ; for if he should not exist you would lose nothing. Whereas, should you behave as if he did not exist, you would run the risk of losing eternal life." The modern World no longer sees the problem in this naïve way. It may be shown that the belief in a God who, according to the biblical saying, does not permit even a sparrow to fall to the ground without His Will, is open to serious objections

It is unfortunate that these objections are in the main beyond the unaided observation of the average man, and that the conception of impersonal cause, particularly with regard to certain " spiritual " experiences, does too much violence to habits of mind, older even than the race, to secure a ready hearing. For an instant the believer may grasp the truth, only to slip back the next moment to the habitual animistic interpretation. On the ground of that almost irresistible inclination, he justifies to himself his irrationality by repeating the comfortable saying that, in spiritual things, feeling is a safer guide than reason.

The harm done by false beliefs, such as the one under discussion, is not only that in various ways they impede and discourage the seeker after knowledge which would place in human hands a large measure of control of the psychical forces, but also that they obstruct the recruiting of scientific workers.

So long as the belief in superhuman personal causation was universal and supported by the irresistible prestige of the established religions it blocked any other conception, however fruitful it might have proved to be. And even when the conception of impersonal. regular, predictable, and controllable forces had become established in some minds, little progress could be made in the scientific understanding of human nature in the face of the opposition, active or passive, of a large and influential portion of society. The traditional belief in a God-Providence amenable to human influence, together with semi-magical beliefs and practices in physical and mental therapy, in social reform and in religion, continue to absorb, even in the most favoured nations, a large share of energy and wealth and to exert a paralyzing influence upon the progress of knowledge.

We are no longer in the dark concerning the prevalence of the two main traditional religious beliefs among the intellectual leaders. A careful statistical investigation carried out in the United States, according to accepted statistical methods, has yielded the following percentages of believers :

Believers in the God of the Christian Churches.	Physical Scientists.	Biologists.	Historians.	Sociologists.	Psychologists.
Lesser Men	49.7	39.1	63.0	29.2	32.1
Greater Men.. ..	34.8	16.9	32.9	19.4	13.2
Believers in Immortality.					
Lesser Men	57.1	45.1	67.7	52.2	26.9
Greater Men.. ..	40.0	25.4	35.3	27.1	8.8

These figures show that the belief in the God under discussion[1] is still widely prevalent among intellectual leaders in the United

[1] A God acting upon the physical world, or at least upon man, at man's request, desire, or desert, i.e., the God of the established Christian religion whatever form it may have taken.

States. Especially significant, however, is the discovery that unbelief is very much more frequent among the more than among the less distinguished, and that not only the degree of ability but also the kind of knowledge possessed is significantly related to the rejection of these beliefs.

" The correlation shown, without exception, in every one of our groups between eminence and disbelief appears to me of momentous significance. In three of these groups (biologists, historians, and psychologists)' the number of believers among the men of greater distinction is only half, or less than half, the number of believers among the less distinguished men. I do not see any way to avoid the conclusion that disbelief in a personal God and in personal immortality is directly proportional to abilities making for success in the sciences in question. What these abilities are, we shall see in the following chapter.

" A study of the charts, with regard to the kind of knowledge which favours disbelief, shows that the historians and the physical scientists provide the greater ; and the psychologists, the sociologists, and the biologists, the smaller number of believers. The explanation I have offered is that psychologists, sociologists, and biologists in very large numbers recognize fixed orderliness in organic and psychical life, and not merely in inorganic existence ; while frequently physical scientists recognize the presence of invariable law in the inorganic world only. The belief in a personal God as defined for the purpose of our investigation is, therefore, less often possible to students of psychical and of organic life than to physical scientists.

" The place occupied by the historians next to the physical scientists would indicate that, for the present, the reign of law is not so clearly revealed in the events with which history deals as in biology, economics, and psychology. A large number of historians continue to see the hand of God in human affairs. The influence, destructive of Christian beliefs, attributed in this interpretation to more intimate knowledge of organic and psychical life, appears incontrovertibly, as far as psychical life is concerned, in the remarkable fact that, whereas in every other group the number of believers in immortality is greater than that in God, among the psychologists the reverse is true ; the number of believers in immortality among the greater psychologists sinks to 8.8 per cent. One may affirm it seems that, in general, the greater the ability of the psychologist *as a psychologist*, the more difficult it becomes for him to believe in the continuation of individual life after bodily death[1]."

[1] *The Belief in God and Immortality*, 2nd Ed., Chicago, The Open Court Publishing Co., 1921. This book is made up of three parts, Part II (pp. 172-287)

But the pressure exerted by public opinion in favour of the traditional belief in God is vastly stronger in the United States than the prevalence of the belief among men of science would warrant. This appeared in several ways in the statistical investigation just referred to[1], and may be inferred from recent happenings in that country[2].

And yet the nation is assuredly not Christian in so far as a real belief in the government of men's affairs by a divine Person is a Christian belief. Statesmen trust in God no more than ward politicians. Their every step repudiates the idea that they regard God as in any degree a partner in the management of international relations or in municipal slate-making. In the conduct of petty business as in that of vast affairs of state there is nowhere any convincing hint of an effective belief in divine action. The meagre remnants of social tradition expressive of that belief seem now pitifully out of place. The prayers to the Almighty of the Chaplain of Congress, the Yearly Thanksgiving Proclamation, and the like, are now unbecoming formalism.

The maintenance of gestures and professions of belief, in the presence of persistent and detailed denial in action, works nowhere

---

is a statistical inquiry referring mainly to the persons listed in Cattell's *American Men of Science* and to college students. The classification according to distinction was made possible by the starring of the more distinguished names in that directory. How the selection was made under the direction of Cattell is stated in my book, foot-note, p. 248.

It is, of course, not to be supposed that disbelief in God, as defined, means a materialistic philosophy. The disbelievers in the God of the Christian Churches may, and it is known that many do, believe in a god otherwise conceived.

[1] See, for instance, the comparison of the signed with the unsigned answers, pp. 272-74. To admit disbelief in the God-Providence is, in the United States, to place oneself in a most unfavourable light in the eyes of most of those who control the finances of our colleges and universities, and, usually also, many of those who direct their educational policies.

[2] Scientific associations, in particular the *American Association for the Advancement of Science*, and the *American Association of University Professors*, have recently felt it necessary to protest against such actions as the following :
" In Kentucky a bill for suppressing all evolutionary teaching passed the House of Representatives, and was only rejected, I believe, by one vote, in the Senate of that State. In Arkansas the lower house passed a bill to the same effect almost without opposition, but the Senate threw it out. Oklahoma followed a similar course. In Florida, the House of Representatives has passed, by a two-thirds vote, a resolution forbidding any instructor ' to teach or permit to be taught atheism, agnosticism, Darwinism, or any other hypothesis that links man in blood relation to any form of life.' "—W. Bateson in *Nature*.
It is fair to observe that in the Southern states only has the agitation against the teaching of the animal descent of man been powerful enough to lead to official state-action. Nevertheless, the same influences in the Northern states are far from negligible.

more disastrously than in the churches. Unbelief in the God-Providence is, in churches and theological seminaries, fatal to intellectual honesty, and it is the main cause of their weakness. Their influence has waned because of the decline of faith in the fundamental Christian dogma[1]. As the rehabilitation of that belief seems to be made hopeless by every forward step of science, the recovery of the churches is to be sought in such a transformation of the conception of God as would make it generally acceptable to modern scientific scholarship. The beneficent forces to-day at cross purposes in humanity, and mutually destructive, would then find an harmonious expression. Religion and science would work hand in hand for the production of a better and a happier—a diviner—man[2].

*   *   *

The traditional belief in divine personal causation, strikingly embodied in religious mysticism, works perhaps nowhere so mischievously as in its implication that ethical knowledge and moral energy are in the custody of a personal Divinity and that this knowledge and energy are transmitted to man in consequence of a personal relationship with that God, in particular during mystical worship. The fear of losing that divine assistance accounts for much of the desperation with which the best among·Christians cling to the traditional belief. In Chapter XII of the *Belief in God and Immortality*, we have discussed the social origin of moral ideas and inspiration. The following extracts are taken from that chapter.

" Our alleged essential dependence upon transcendental beliefs is belied by the most common experiences of daily life. Who does not feel the absurdity of the opinion that the lavish care of a sick child by a mother is given because of a belief in God and immortality ? Are love of father and mother on the part of children, affection and

---

[1] Not the disbelief in the Virgin Birth, but unbelief in the kind of God-Providence implied in the worship of all the Christian churches, is the more profound cause of their palsy.

[2] It may be recalled in this connexion that the religions have never been protagonists of higher *scientific* knowledge. As soon as it became evident that science struck at the root of many of the dogmas officially regarded as essential to one or the other of the religions, most of their ministers and adherents became openly opposed to the development of higher scientific education, or at least regarded it with misgiving.

The past and present coldness, not to say active opposition, to higher scientific training among the sponsors of the organized Christian religion will of necessity continue so long as the conception of God set forth in creeds and books of common worship remains what it is. To-day, in the United States, the Fundamentalists are directly or indirectly, wittingly or unwittingly, hindering the development of the biological sciences, even though their great practical value has been convincingly demonstrated.

serviceableness between brothers and sisters, straightforwardness and truthfulness between business men essentially dependent upon these beliefs? What sort of person would be the father who would announce divine punishment or reward in order to obtain the love and respect of his children?

" The heroism of religious martyrs is often flaunted as a marvellous instance of the unique sustaining strength derived from the belief in a personal God and in heaven. And yet, for every martyr of this sort, there has been one or more heroes who has risked his life for a noble cause, without the comfort which these beliefs may bring. The very present offers almost countless instances of martyrs to the cause of humanity who were strangers to the belief in God and immortality. How many men and women have in the past decade gladly offered and not infrequently lost their lives in the cause of freedom, or justice, or science?

" Nothing could be more evident than that the approval of God and the assurance of eternal happiness are not original motives for the generosity with which man offers up his life. The fruitful deeds of heroism are at bottom inspired not by the thought of God and of a future life, but by innate tendencies or promptings that have reference to humanity. Self-sacrifice, generosity, is rooted in nothing less superficial and accidental than social instincts older than the human race, for they are already present in a rudimentary form in the higher animals.

" There is no simpler nor better statement of the origin of the love of God than the well-known Biblical passage : ' If a man say, I love God, and hateth his brother, he is a liar ; for he that loveth not his brother whom he hath seen, how can he love God whom he hath not seen.' In the education of the young, as well as in the reformation of the warped adult, the truth of this is ever seen anew. It is love of man that convinces child and hardened sinner alike of the love of God."

The evils bred by the traditional conception of God may be called by the general name of " other worldliness." It would be difficult to evaluate the harm done to humanity in the past by the conviction that the real destination of man is the World to Come, and equally difficult to estimate the harm done by the conviction that for its ethical improvement society is dependent upon a personal God. If these evils are of lesser magnitude now than in the past, it is because the traditional belief has lost some of its ancient potency, and because the sense of responsibility of the individual for the material and spiritual welfare of society has grown correspondingly greater. In order that he may come to a full realization that he and he alone is his brother's keeper, it is necessary that man should entirely give up the belief in personal, super-human causation. Divided responsibility works no better in religion than in business.

*   *   *

It will not be denied that by the acquisition of a wealth of physical and psychical knowledge, and by its applications to the satisfaction of physical and moral needs (both in the way of physical appliances and of social institutions), society has begun to fulfil the desires and aspirations insistently expressed to God in worship. Some degree of self-realization is now possible for all; and, as to the unfortunate, the sick, the aged, they may to-day, in the most civilized communities, place their trust in man with some measure of assurance.

It is customary in religious circles to limit to physical and intellectual things the improvement in the individual which may be expected as a consequence of the natural development of society. And yet, to raise man economically above the condition of a beast of burden, to free woman from servitude and to deliver both slave and master from the moral evil attached to that relation, to train and enlighten the mind, are certainly primary conditions for the spiritual flowering of human nature. The most serious of the indictments against the belief in a superhuman personal source of spiritual progress is that this belief stands in the way of making full use of the real source of spiritual discernment, i.e., the teachings and the training of social life.

The main problem raised by admirable characters refers to the sources of their excellences. The biological and the psychological sciences are now contributing to the solution of that great problem. And when it is considered that men in the ancient as well as in the modern world (a Buddha Gautama, a Socrates, a Marcus Aurelius), entertaining other conceptions of the Divine, have shone with a beauty similar to that of the great Christians, it becomes clear that belief in the particular conception of God with which we are concerned is an irrelevant circumstance. Innumerable believers in the traditional God grovel in spiritual darkness, while some who entertain a very different conception of divinity are among the beacons by which humanity has steered its upward course.

A blending of humility and self-confidence, sympathy with the weak and defective, abhorrence of weakness and vice, awe and reverence for the mysteries of life and death, the consciousness of being one with the Whole, the faith that the Universe is somehow rational, and the mental unity, strength, peace, and happiness which come to the possessor of these virtues and beliefs, are in no way exclusively bound to the conception of the personal God of the Christian books of worship.

*   *   *

It would be indeed surprising if in religious mysticism, a movement which began almost with the birth of man and has never ceased to engross the attention and to receive the unbounded admiration of many, there was nothing deserving a permanent place among the means of self-improvement. The traditional conception of the mystical Agent might be wrong, certain alleged boons of mystical ecstasy might be illusory or worse, and yet it might still be possible to vindicate it in some of its features.

We have seen that the mystics obtain an assurance of marvellous knowledge and abilities; a delightful impression of freedom and unlimited power; and, in the higher religions, an ethical purification and unification which, in their estimation, makes the universal Will their own Will. Much, but not all, of this is illusory. Speaking of Christian mysticism we shall say that the refreshment incident to the abandoning of the complications, the struggles, and the worries of life; the unification of the mind by purification (temporary though it may be) from egoistic tendencies and purposes; and the comfort and optimism of the belief in the sustaining presence of God are all vast and desirable realities.

Let it be recalled now that these results follow upon the practice of even those moderate forms of mystical worship which are common in the Christian churches. The first step in the production of the mystical state is Meditation, which is described as the focussing of attention upon some thought or object. Then comes Contemplation during which the discursive activity of the mind is further reduced. The mind is absorbed in some "simple affective thought." After that, if the mystical process continues, the characteristics of trance manifest themselves more clearly : the senses cease altogether to respond to external stimulation and the soul, conscious only of its closeness to God, seems entirely withdrawn within itself. Total unconsciousness may bring the experience to an end.

Now the early stages of this mystical journey, Meditation and Contemplation, constitute prayer when begging and intercessory prayer has given place to the higher form of it prevalent in Christianity.

Let it be recalled, further, that neither the production of the mental states characteristic of mystical worship, nor its essential effects necessitate a belief in the causal activity of a personal Agent, and that, when that causal conception is detached from the mystical method, its kinship to certain recent psychotherapeutic methods becomes obvious. It will be sufficient to mention here the therapeutic use made of suggestion during hypnosis and near-sleep states ; the related methods of various schools of mind-curors ; and, more recently still, the method of the psychoanalysts who aim at the re-establishment of mental wholeness, at the unification of consciousness.

At bottom the problem, in these cults and in these scientific or semi-scientific practices, is always to reorganize the mental life upon a more stable basis, to synthetize it and make it whole by removing excrescences, contradictions, suppressions, amnesias, and the like. And the method of cure, whatever its name, involves in every instance the placing of the subject in a state of relaxation, passivity, and mental simplification. His gaze is turned away from the unmanageable present, away from the changing surface of things, in the expectation that something deeper, truer, more lasting, will assert itself and assume a controlling and unifying rôle. And so psychotherapists and ethical teachers, even while rejecting the orthodox theology, may join with the mystic, John Woolman, when he writes : " The necessity of an inward stillness has appeared clearly to my mind, in true silence strength is renewed, the mind is weened from all things, save as they may be enjoyed in the divine Will."

We are thus led to regard the mystical method of soul-cure as an approximation to the present-day, more or less scientific, methods of psychotherapy. The effects of these related methods have a common two-fold source : (1) A moral and physical refreshment takes place, quite irrespective of any idea or purpose in the mind of the person. This is a direct consequence of the physiological change produced by the passage from the ordinary condition of consciousness to the trance-like state. We recall in this connexion Maupassant's striking description of the effects of a drunken bout : " A good bath of forgetfulness out of which one arises done up and yet renewed ; a great purge that scours, as with fire, body and soul." (2) The ideas and purposes dominant in the subject's mind exert an unusually powerful influence because all these related states constitute conditions of increased suggestibility.

Among the tasks of psychology is the determination of the mental condition which would make a person receptive in the highest degree to the influences, internal or external, to which it may be desirable to subject him. It is clear that to push the trance to complete unconsciousness is an error, for complete unconsciousness means entire unresponsiveness, instead of a condition of increased suggestibility.

*　　　　*　　　　*

The cry, raised on every hand, that Christianity has failed is answered by the counter-cry, " Christianity never yet has been tried ! " To this a sociologist makes the retort : " If a religion which has existed for two thousand years and has been held officially by the most powerful nations for fifteen hundred years has not been tried, it has failed."

. If the ideals of the Christian religion have conspicuously failed of realization, it is not only because they are *ideals ;* it is also because the causal conception embodied in Christian worship is largely inefficient to produce the desired results. Supplications to the Almighty Father for protection from physical and moral harm, thanks and praises to him for a share of prosperity and happiness, and the search, in prayer and in communion with the alleged personal Cause of all good things, for enlightenment and power, are methods possessing some degree of utility, but they are now known not to be the most effective methods available.

If more rapid progress is to be made towards the realization of the exalted aims of Christianity, its primitive conception of causation, and the methods of worship dependent upon it, will have to be replaced by a scientific understanding of causation and by methods in agreement with it. Spiritual improvement may then be expected to rival in rapidity the improvement in matters of health and longevity which have taken place as consequences of the discovery and of the application of medical knowledge.

*　　　　*　　　　*

It is not a replacement of the religious spirit by science which is indicated here, but the inclusion into religion of the relevant scientific knowledge. The hope of humanity lies in a collaboration of religious idealism with science—the former providing the ideal to be attained, and the latter, so far as it can, the physical and the psychological means and methods of achievement.

ANALYTICAL INDEX OF SUBJECTS

INDEX OF AUTHORS

Printed and bound by CPI Group (UK) Ltd, Croydon, CR0 4YY

01/11/2024

01782629-0011